ANNUAL EDITIONS

Nutrition 13/14

Twenty-Fifth Edition

EDITOR

Amy Strickland, MBA, MS, RD
University of North Carolina–Greensboro

Amy Strickland is an Academic Professional Assistant Professor and the Director of the Didactic Program in Dietetics in the Nutrition Department at the University of North Carolina at Greensboro.

Her current teaching responsibilities include a speaking and writing intensive Nutrition Education course, Nutrition Assessment, and Medical Nutrition Therapy. In past semesters she has taught multiple sections of Introductory Nutrition, Advanced Clinical Dietetics, Management Practices in Dietetics, and Food Safety/Sanitation as a certified ServSafe Instructor/Proctor with the National Restaurant Association.

Recent emphasis in her work at UNCG includes overseeing service learning projects in which UNCG students create and implement nutrition education programs for elementary-school-aged children, with special emphasis on educating children of low-income families.

Prior to working at UNCG, Amy worked six years as a clinical dietitian, one year as a consultant dietitian, and five years in a biomedical laboratory. She is a member of The American Dietetic Association, American Society for Nutrition, and American Society for Parenteral and Enteral Nutrition.

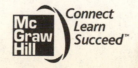
McGraw Hill

*Connect
Learn
Succeed*™

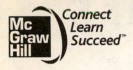

ANNUAL EDITIONS: NUTRITION, TWENTY-FIFTH EDITION

Published by McGraw-Hill, a business unit of The McGraw-Hill Companies, Inc., 1221 Avenue of
the Americas, New York, NY 10020. Copyright © 2014 by The McGraw-Hill Companies, Inc. All
rights reserved. Previous edition(s) © 2013, 2012, 2011, and 2010. Printed in the United States of
America. No part of this publication may be reproduced or distributed in any form or by any means,
or stored in a database or retrieval system, without the prior written consent of The McGraw-Hill
Companies, Inc., including, but not limited to, in any network or other electronic storage or transmission, or broadcast for distance learning.

Some ancillaries, including electronic and print components, may not be available to customers
outside the United States.

This book is printed on acid-free paper.

Annual Editions® is a registered trademark of The McGraw-Hill Companies, Inc.
Annual Editions is published by the **Contemporary Learning Series** group within the
McGraw-Hill Higher Education division.

1 2 3 4 5 6 7 8 9 0 QDB/QDB 1 0 9 8 7 6 5 4 3

MHID: 0-07-351563-9
ISBN: 978-0-07-351563-2
ISSN: 1055-6990 (print)
ISSN: 2158-4117 (online)

Developmental Editor: *David Welsh*
Content Licensing Coordinator: *DeAnna Dausener*
Marketing Director: *Adam Kloza*
Marketing Manager: *Nathan Edwards*
Senior Project Manager: *Melissa M. Leick*
Cover Designer: *Studio Montage, St. Louis, Missouri*
Buyer: *Nichole Birkenholz*
Media Project Manager: *Sridevi Palani*

Compositor: Laserwords Private Limited
Cover Image Credits: McGraw-Hill Companies [background]; Noah Clayton/Getty Images [inset]

Editors/Academic Advisory Board

Members of the Academic Advisory Board are instrumental in the final selection of articles for each edition of ANNUAL EDITIONS. Their review of articles for content, level, and appropriateness provides critical direction to the editors and staff. We think that you will find their careful consideration well reflected in this volume.

ANNUAL EDITIONS: Nutrition 13/14
25th Edition

EDITOR

Amy Strickland, MBA, MS, RD
University of North Carolina–Greensboro

ACADEMIC ADVISORY BOARD MEMBERS

Preface

In publishing ANNUAL EDITIONS we recognize the enormous role played by the magazines, newspapers, and journals of the public press in providing current, first-rate educational information in a broad spectrum of interest areas. Many of these articles are appropriate for students, researchers, and professionals seeking accurate, current material to help bridge the gap between principles and theories and the real world. These articles, however, become more useful for study when those of lasting value are carefully collected, organized, indexed, and reproduced in a low-cost format, which provides easy and permanent access when the material is needed. That is the role played by ANNUAL EDITIONS.

Many of the articles in Annual Editions: Nutrition 13/14 are based on the areas of concentration identified in the 2010 U.S. Dietary Guidelines. The Dietary Guidelines are published every five years by the U.S. federal government to address latest nutrition-related research findings and how they apply to the health of U.S. citizens. The 2010 Guidelines targeted obesity and other nutrition related chronic diseases, food insecurity, physical activity, and the food environment in the United States. The majority of the articles in this edition address the challenges to improving the health of our country and many of the articles suggest possible solutions.

Annual Editions: Nutrition 13/14 is composed of eight units that review current knowledge and controversies in the area of nutrition. The first unit describes current trends in the field of nutrition with emphasis on how consumer demand for healthy food is impacting the food industry and the role of federal, state, and local governments in improving the health of its citizens.

The second unit is centered on childhood nutrition in response to the increased national emphasis on childhood nutrition and the "Let's Move" campaign. Articles on the new guidelines for school meals and the importance of positive role models and family involvement in nutrition and health are the cornerstones of this unit.

Unit 3 includes seven articles on the function and food sources of nutrients. Vitamin D, sodium, potassium, and fats are all emphasized in the 2010 Dietary Guidelines as nutrients of concern for Americans and are represented in articles in this section.

Units 4 through 6 include topics that focus on the relationship between nutrition, obesity, and chronic diseases. Recent research findings on the role that nutrition plays in diabetes, heart disease, hypertension, and obesity are emphasized.

Unit 7 covers food safety and technology, including information on the safety of domestic and imported food and beverages. Several articles in this section will discuss the use and prevalence of genetically modified foods and other technologies that facilitate food production and preservation.

Unit 8 focuses on hunger, nutrition, and sustainability of our food supply. Articles on the growing prevalence of nitrogen added to our environment, agriculture practices in other countries, and sustainability efforts of the food industry make up this section.

Annual Editions: Nutrition is updated annually with the latest topics and controversies in the field as a way to keep students who study nutrition informed of the latest research findings, changes in policy, and trends in nutrition related topics. Keeping up with all of the nutrition research and policy changes is a challenging task, but thanks to books like the updated versions of Annual Editions, you can easily review the latest nutrition information taken from reputable sources.

Annual Editions: Nutrition 13/14 is to be used as a companion to a standard nutrition text so that it may update, expand, or emphasize certain topics that are covered in the text or present totally new topics not covered in a standard text. We hope that the reader will develop critical thinking and be empowered to ask questions and to seek answers from credible sources.

A Topic Guide assists students in finding other articles on a given subject within this edition, while a list of recommended Internet References guides them to the best sources of additional information on a topic.

There are two features in Annual Editions designed to assist students in their study and expand critical thinking. Located at the beginning of each unit, Learning Outcomes outline the key concepts that students should focus on as they are reading the material. Critical Thinking questions, located at the end of each article, allow students to test their understanding of the key concepts.

Your input is most valuable to improve this anthology, which we update yearly. We would appreciate your comments.

Amy Strickland
Editor

The Annual Editions Series

VOLUMES AVAILABLE

Adolescent Psychology
Aging
American Foreign Policy
American Government
Anthropology
Archaeology
Assessment and Evaluation
Business Ethics
Child Growth and Development
Comparative Politics
Criminal Justice
Developing World
Drugs, Society, and Behavior
Dying, Death, and Bereavement
Early Childhood Education
Economics
Educating Children with Exceptionalities
Education
Educational Psychology
Entrepreneurship
Environment
The Family
Gender
Geography
Global Issues
Health
Homeland Security

Human Development
Human Resources
Human Sexualities
International Business
Management
Marketing
Mass Media
Microbiology
Multicultural Education
Nursing
Nutrition
Physical Anthropology
Psychology
Race and Ethnic Relations
Social Problems
Sociology
State and Local Government
Sustainability
Technologies, Social Media, and Society
United States History, Volume 1
United States History, Volume 2
Urban Society
Violence and Terrorism
Western Civilization, Volume 1
World History, Volume 1
World History, Volume 2
World Politics

Contents

UNIT 1
Nutrition Trends

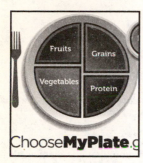

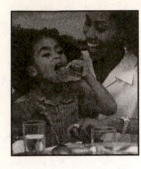

UNIT 2
Childhood Nutrition

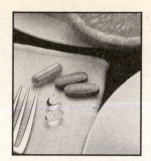

UNIT 3
Nutrients

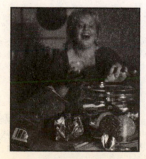

UNIT 4
Diet and Disease

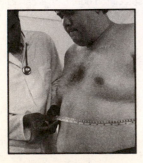

UNIT 5
Obesity and Weight Control

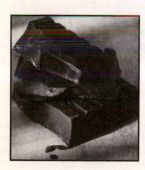

UNIT 6
Health Claims

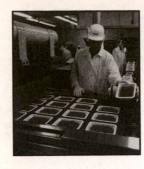

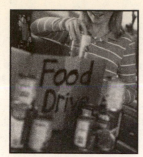

UNIT 8
Hunger, Nutrition, and Sustainability

Correlation Guide

The *Annual Editions* series provides students with convenient, inexpensive access to current, carefully selected articles from the public press. **Annual Editions: Nutrition 13/14** is an easy-to-use reader that presents articles on important topics such as *nutrition trends, obesity and weight control, sustainability,* and many more. For more information on *Annual Editions* and other *McGraw-Hill Contemporary Learning Series* titles, visit www.mhhe.com/cls.

This convenient guide matches the units in **Annual Editions: Nutrition 13/14** with the corresponding chapters in five of our best-selling McGraw-Hill Nutrition textbooks by Schiff, Wardlaw/Smith, and Byrd-Bredbenner et al.

Annual Editions: Nutrition 13/14	Nutrition for Healthy Living, 3/e by Schiff	Contemporary Nutrition: A Functional Approach, 3/e by Wardlaw/Smith	Contemporary Nutrition, 9/e by Wardlaw/Smith	Wardlaw's Perspectives in Nutrition, 9/e by Byrd-Bredbenner et al.	Perspectives in Nutrition: A Functional Approach, by Byrd-Bredbenner et al.
Unit 1: Nutrition Trends	**Chapter 1:** The Basics of Nutrition **Ch\apter 2:** Evaluating Nutrition Information **Chapter 3:** Planning Nutritious Diets	**Chapter 1:** What You Eat and Why **Chapter 2:** Guidelines for Designing a Healthy Diet	**Chapter 1:** What You Eat and Why **Chapter 2:** Guidelines for Designing a Healthy Diet	**Chapter 1:** The Science of Nutrition **Chapter 2:** Tools of a Healthy Diet **Chapter 3:** The Food Supply	**Chapter 1:** The Science of Nutrition **Chapter 2:** Tools of a Healthy Diet **Chapter 3:** The Food Supply
Unit 2: Childhood Nutrition		**Chapter 18:** Nutrition from Infancy through Adolescence	**Chapter 15:** Nutrition from Infancy through Adolescence	**Chapter 17:** Nutrition during the Growing Years	**Chapter 17:** Nutrition during the Growing Years
Unit 3: Nutrients	**Chapter 5:** Lipids **Chapter 9:** Nutrients Involved with Fluid and Electrolyte Balance **Chapter 10:** Nutrients that Function as Antioxidants **Chapter 11:** Nutrients Involved in Bone Health **Chapter 12:** Nutrients Involved with Energy Metabolism and Blood Health	**Chapter 4:** Carbohydrates **Chapter 5:** Lipids **Chapter 8:** Vitamins **Chapter 6:** Fats and Other Lipids	**Chapter 4:** Carbohydrates **Chapter 5:** Carbohydrates **Chapter 8:** Vitamins	**Chapter 5:** Carbohydrates **Chapter 6:** Lipids	**Chapter 5:** Carbohydrates **Chapter 6:** Lipids **Chapter 12:** Micronutrients: Vitamins and Minerals **Chapter 13:** Micronutrients in Energy and Amino Acid Metabolism
Unit 4: Diet and Disease	**Chapter 10:** Energy Balance and Weight Control	**Chapter 7:** Energy Balance and Weight Control **Chapter 13:** Nutrition for a Lifetime **Chapter 17:** Pregnancy and Breastfeeding **Chapter 18:** Nutrition from Infancy through Adolescence **Chapter 19:** Nutrition during Adulthood	**Chapter 7:** Energy Balance and Weight Maintenance **Chapter 15:** Nutrition from Infancy through Adolescence **Chapter 16:** Nutrition during Adulthood	**Chapter 2:** Tools of a Healthy Diet **Chapter 16:** Nutritional Aspects of Pregnancy and Breastfeeding **Chapter 17:** Nutrition during the Growing Years **Chapter 18:** Nutrition throughout Adulthood	**Chapter 2:** Tools of a Healthy Diet **Chapter 16:** Nutritional Aspects of Pregnancy and Breastfeeding **Chapter 17:** Nutrition during the Growing Years **Chapter 18:** Nutrition during the Adult Years
Unit 5: Obesity and Weight Control	**Chapter 10:** Energy Balance and Weight Control	**Chapter 7:** Energy Balance and Weight Maintenance	**Chapter 7:** Energy Balance and Weight Control	**Chapter 10:** Energy Balance, Weight Control, and Eating Disorders	**Chapter 10:** Energy Balance, Weight Control, and Eating Disorders

Correlation Guide

Unit 6: Health Claims	Chapter 8: Vitamins Chapter 9: Water and Minerals	Chapter 10: Nutrients that Function as Antioxidants Chapter 11: Nutrients Involved in Bone Health	Chapter 8: Vitamins Chapter 9: Water and Minerals	Chapter 12: Fat-Soluble Vitamins Chapter 13: Water-Soluble Vitamins Chapter 14: Water and Major Minerals Chapter 15: Trace Minerals	Chapter 12: Micronutrients: Vitamins and Minerals
Unit 7: Food Safety and Technology	Chapter 12: Food Safety Concerns	Chapter 16: Food Safety	Chapter 13: Safety of Food and Water	Chapter 3: The Food Supply	Chapter 3: The Food Supply
Unit 8: Hunger, Nutrition, and Sustainability	Chapter 13: Nutrition for a Lifetime	Chapter 15: Undernutrition throughout the World	Chapter 12: Undernutrition Throughout the World	Chapter 3: The Food Supply	Chapter 3: The Food Supply

Topic Guide

This topic guide suggests how the selections in this book relate to the subjects covered in your course. You may want to use the topics listed on these pages to search the Web more easily.

On the following pages a number of websites have been gathered specifically for this book. They are arranged to reflect the units of this Annual Editions reader. You can link to these sites by going to www.mhhe.com/cls

All the articles that relate to each topic are listed below the bold-faced term.

Internet References

The following Internet sites have been selected to support the articles found in this reader. These sites were available at the time of publication. However, because websites often change their structure and content, the information listed may no longer be available. We invite you to visit www.mhhe.com/cls for easy access to these sites.

Annual Editions: Nutrition 13/14

General Sources

Academy of Nutrition and Dietetics
www.eatright.org

This consumer link to nutrition and health includes resources, news, marketplace, search for a dietician, government information, and a gateway to related sites. The site includes a tip of the day and special features.

The Blonz Guide to Nutrition
www.blonz.com

The categories in this valuable site report news in the fields of nutrition, food science, foods, fitness, and health. There is also a selection of search engines and links.

CSPI: Center for Science in the Public Interest
www.cspinet.org

CSPI is a nonprofit education and advocacy organization that is committed to improving the safety and nutritional quality of our food supply. CSPI publishes the Nutrition Action Healthletter, which has monthly information about food.

Institute of Food Technologists
www.ift.org

This site of the Society for Food Science and Technology is full of important information and news about every aspect of the food products that come to market.

International Food Information Council Foundation (IFIC)
www.FoodInsight.org

IFIC's purpose is to be the link between science and communications by offering the latest scientific information on food safety, nutrition, and health in a form that is understandable and useful for opinion leaders and consumers to access.

My Plate
www.choosemyplate.gov

The USDA published My Plate to help simplify the message of eating a balanced diet. The site targets children, pregnant moms, and people who want to lose weight.

U.S. National Institutes of Health (NIH)
www.nih.gov

Consult this site for links to extensive health information and scientific resources. Comprised of 24 separate institutes, centers, and divisions, the NIH is one of eight health agencies of the Public Health Service, which, in turn, is part of the U.S. Department of Health and Human Services.

UNIT 1: Nutrition Trends

Food Science and Human Nutrition Extension
www.fshn.uiuc.edu

This extensive Illinois State University site links to latest news and reports, consumer publications, food safety information, and many other useful nutrition-related sites.

Healthy Hunger Free Kids Act of 2010
www.fns.usda.gov/cnd/governance/legislation/CNR_2010.htm

This piece of legislation, passed in December 2010, provides guidelines for breakfasts and lunches served in schools that receive federal funding as part of the breakfast and lunch program.

My Plate
www.choosemyplate.gov

The USDA published My Plate to help simplify the message of eating a balanced diet. The site targets children, pregnant moms, and people who want to lose weight.

American Society of Exercise Physiologists (ASEP)
www.asep.org

The goal of the ASEP is to promote health and physical fitness. This extensive site provides links to publications related to exercise and career opportunities in exercise physiology.

UNIT 2: Childhood Nutrition

Centers for Disease Control and Prevention— Obesity Trends
www.cdc.gov/obesity/data/trends.html

The CDC is the premier resource for statistics and latest research on diseases that impact U.S. citizens. This site is full of statistics on obesity among U.S. children and adults.

Centers for Disease Control and Prevention— Healthy Youth
www.cdc.gov/healthyyouth/obesity/facts.htm

The CDC is the premier resource for statistics and latest research on diseases that impact U.S. citizens. This site describes programs that are underway to help curtail the obesity epidemic.

U.S. Dept of Health and Human Services
http://aspe.hhs.gov/health/reports/child_obesity

This site describes the current research on how eating habits, lifestyle, socioeconomic status, parenteral influences, and marketing are impacting childhood obesity.

U.S. Dietary Guidelines
www.cnpp.usda.gov/DGAs2010-DGACReport.htm

A comprehensive view of the current state of nutrition and diet within the United States with recommendations for interventions, programs, and future research.

UNIT 3: Nutrients

Dietary Supplement Fact Sheet: Vitamin D
http://ods.od.nih.gov/factsheets/VitaminD-HealthProfessional

The Office of Dietary Supplements fact sheet on vitamin D provides comprehensive information on the vitamin.

Food and Nutrition Information Center
http://fnic.nal.usda.gov

Use this site to find dietary and nutrition information provided by various USDA agencies and to find links to food and nutrition resources on the Internet.

Internet References

NutritionalSupplements.com
www.nutritionalsupplements.com

This source provides unbiased information about nutritional supplements and prescription drugs, submitted by consumers with no vested interest in the products.

Office of Dietary Supplements: Health Information
http://ods.od.nih.gov/HealthInformation

The Office of Dietary Supplements, a division of the National Institute of Health is the leading source on nutritional and botanical supplements. This website provides comprehensive information on the supplement industry.

U.S. National Library of Medicine
www.nlm.nih.gov

This site permits you to search databases and electronic information sources such as MEDLINE, learn about research projects, and keep up on nutrition-related news.

UNIT 4: Diet and Disease

American Cancer Society
www.cancer.org

Open this site and its various links to learn the concerns and lifestyle advice of the American Cancer Society. It provides information on alternative therapies, tobacco, other Web resources, and more.

American Diabetes Association
www.diabetes.org

The American Diabetes Association is the primary resource for type 1, type 2, and gestational diabetes.

American Heart Association (AHA)
www.heart.org/HEARTORG

The AHA offers this site to provide the most comprehensive information on heart disease and stroke as well as late-breaking news. The site presents facts on warning signs, a reference guide, and explanations of diseases and treatments.

Medline Plus
www.nlm.nih.gov/medlineplus

This site provides health information from the National Library of Medicine and the National Institutes of Health.

National Eating Disorders Association
www.nationaleatingdisorders.org

This site offers information on the different types of eating disorders, programs, events, research, resources, insurance coverage, and a support line.

UNIT 5: Obesity and Weight Control

American Society of Exercise Physiologists (ASEP)
www.asep.org

The goal of the ASEP is to promote health and physical fitness. This extensive site provides links to publications related to exercise and career opportunities in exercise physiology.

Calorie Control Council
www.caloriecontrol.org

The Calorie Control Council's website offers information on cutting calories, achieving and maintaining healthy weight, and low-calorie, reduced-fat foods and beverages.

Overweight & Obesity
www.cdc.gov/obesity

The Centers for Disease Control and Prevention is a component of the U.S. Department of Health and Human Services. It monitors and tracks the general health of Americans, conducts research, and implements health prevention strategies.

Shape Up America!
www.shapeup.org

At the Shape Up America! website you will find the latest information about safe weight management, healthy eating, and physical fitness. Links include Support Center, Cyberkitchen, Media Center, Fitness Center, and BMI Center.

UNIT 6: Health Claims

Federal Trade Commission (FTC): Diet, Health & Fitness
www.ftc.gov/bcp/menus/consumer/health.shtm

This site of the FTC on the Web offers consumer education rules and acts that include a wide range of subjects, from buying exercise equipment to virtual health "treatments."

Food and Drug Administration (FDA)
www.fda.gov/default.htm

The FDA presents this site that addresses products they regulate, current news and hot topics, safety alerts, product approvals, reference data, and general information and directions.

National Council against Health Fraud (NCAHF)
www.ncahf.org

The NCAHF does business as the National Council for Reliable Health Information.

Office of Dietary Supplements: Health Information
http://ods.od.nih.gov/HealthInformation

The Office of Dietary Supplements, a division of the National Institute of Health, is the leading source on nutritional and botanical supplements. This website provides comprehensive information on the supplement industry.

QuackWatch
www.quackwatch.com

Quackwatch Inc., a nonprofit corporation, provides this guide to examine health fraud. Data for intelligent decision making on health topics are also presented.

UNIT 7: Food Safety/Technology

American Council on Science and Health (ACSH)
www.acsh.org

The ACSH addresses issues that are related to food safety here. In addition, issues on nutrition and fitness, alcohol, diseases, environmental health, medical care, lifestyle, and tobacco may be accessed on this site.

Centers for Disease Control and Prevention (CDC)
www.cdc.gov

The CDC offers this home page, from which you can obtain information about travelers' health, data related to disease control and prevention, and general nutritional and health information, publications, and more.

Internet References

FDA Center for Food Safety and Applied Nutrition
www.fda.gov/food/foodsafety/default.htm

It is possible to access everything from this website that you might want to know about food safety and what government agencies are doing to ensure it.

Food Safety Project (FSP)
www.extension.iastate.edu/foodsafety

This site from the Cooperative Extension Service at Iowa State University has a database designed to promote food safety education via the Internet.

Institute of Food Technologists
www.ift.org

This site of the Society for Food Science and Technology is full of important information and news about every aspect of the food products that come to market.

USDA Food Safety and Inspection Service (FSIS)
www.fsis.usda.gov

The FSIS, part of the U.S. Department of Agriculture, is the government agency "responsible for ensuring that the nation's commercial supply of meat, poultry, and egg products is safe, wholesome, and correctly labeled and packaged."

UNIT 8: World Hunger, Nutrition, and Sustainability

Food and Agriculture Organization of the United Nations (FAO)
www.fao.org/index_en.htm

The FAO is the premier site for information on food production, consumption, deprivation, malnutrition, poverty, and food trade of countries around the globe. The FAO hunger map is a tool that is commonly used to demonstrate the areas of the world that suffer from malnutrition and food insecurity.

International Food Information Council Foundation (IFIC)
www.FoodInsight.org

IFIC's purpose is to be the link between science and communications by offering the latest scientific information on food safety, nutrition, and health in a form that is understandable and useful for opinion leaders and consumers to access.

Population Reference Bureau
www.prb.org

A key source for global population information, this is a good place to pursue data on nutrition problems worldwide.

U.S. Sustainable Agriculture Research and Education Program, University of California–Davis
www.sarep.ucdavis.edu/concept.htm

This UC-Davis sponsored site describes the main concepts of sustainable agriculture principles and practices.

World Health Organization (WHO)
www.sarep.ucdavis.edu/sarep/about/def

This home page of the World Health Organization will provide you with links to a wealth of statistical and analytical information about health and nutrition around the world.

UNIT 1

Nutrition Trends

Unit Selections

Learning Outcomes

After reading this unit, you will be able to:

- Summarize the potential impact of the higher demand for "natural" products on the food industry.

- Describe the impact of animal welfare groups on the production of eggs in the United States.

- Describe how consumer's emotional attachment to food is influencing the food supply.

- Identify the programs and policies that are covered by the farm bill.

- Describe the implications of subsidizing the production of commodity crops at greater rates than fruits and vegetables.

- Defend the requirement that chain restaurants must post nutrition information on their menus.

- Identify the benefits of community gardens.

- Explain how governments can promote the consumption of fruits and vegetables and stimulate local economies.

- Describe how the Patient Protection and Affordable Care Act of 2010 will impact restaurants and vending companies with 20 or more locations.

- Explain the premise of tracking calories using physical activity equivalents.

- Evaluate the potential of using social media software within corporate wellness programs.

- Provide examples of how restaurants have eliminated trans fats from their menus.

- Explain how McDonald's in Europe has "cleaned up" its reputation.

Student Website

www.mhhe.com/cls

Internet References

Food Science and Human Nutrition Extension
    www.fshn.uiuc.edu
Healthy, Hunger-Free Kids Act of 2010
    www.fns.usda.gov/cnd/governance/legislation/CNR_2010.htm
My Plate
    www.choosemyplate.gov
American Society of Exercise Physiologists (ASEP)
    www.asep.org

The hottest trends in nutrition today revolve around reducing the incidence of obesity/chronic disease and improving the quality of food produced, marketed, and sold in the United States. Unit 1 addresses these current trends in nutrition with particular emphasis on the recent paradigm shift in the food industry and the role of government to provide a healthy food supply for its citizens.

Products that are grown naturally, ethically, and safely are at increasing demand in the United States and many other developed countries. The biggest restaurant chains, food producers, and grocery chains are changing the way they do business to address the consumer sentiment for healthy food and natural ingredients. Marketing plans are changing to portray more natural, local, and/or healthy foods that are, ideally, provided by family-run business models. The words "all natural," "cage free," "fair trade," and "naturally raised" are now a vital component of marketing campaigns of many food producers.

With the ease of sharing information via the Internet and social media sites, people have a venue for communicating their emotional ties to food. Food preferences are driven by emotion, and one of the strongest emotions that Americans currently have about their food is fear. Viral videos, books, and documentaries about food production in the United States are raising distrust of our industrialized food system. Whether it is concern about the use of pesticides, pink slime, growth hormones, preservatives, and antibiotics or the prevalence of *E. coli*, salmonella, or mad cow disease, Americans are vocalizing their sentiments about the U.S. food systems. U.S. consumers' emotional attachment to food is leading the food industry to change the way they produce and market food.

Increased attention to the ethical treatment of animals is changing the foods that are offered in popular restaurants and the nature of how some farmers raise their animals. Consumers want to feel better about how their food is raised. An example of these trends within the food industry can be seen in the changes that are occurring by fast food restaurants. McDonald's is taking strides to improve its image by offering healthier options in the United States and has changed its operations to more ethical and ecofriendly practices in Great Britain and Northern Ireland. McDonald's UK has made great strides to ensure no genetically modified foods are sold at its restaurants in Europe. Burger King promises to serve only cage-free pork and eggs by 2017.

Articles four through seven of this unit concentrate on the role of federal, state, and local governments to provide healthy foods and educate the public about proper nutrition. One of the most significant pieces of legislation that impacts the U.S. food production and supply is the Farm Bill. The Food, Conservation, and Energy Act of 2008 (i.e., "Farm Bill") is renewed every five years. The renewal often ignites conversation about the impact of the federal government's degree of financial backing for industrial growers of commodity crops in relation to the lesser support of fruit and vegetable production. The farm bill is a 1,770-page document that covers everything from nutrition

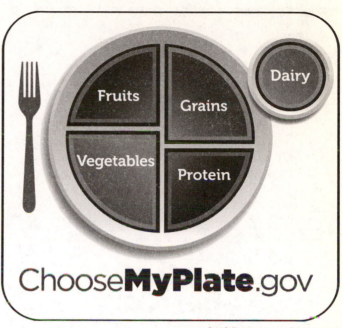

© US Department of Agriculture

assistance programs to land conservation. It determines agricultural subsidies and crop insurance policies in the United States. With the emphasis of increased vegetable and fruit intake in the latest MyPlate guidelines, many public health professionals are questioning our current agriculture policy. *Fresh Fruit; Hold the Insulin* is an editorial report that discusses the outcome of the Farm Bill on the U.S. food supply and, secondarily, its food intake.

Lawmakers of state governments are creating initiatives that support the USDA's latest nutrition education campaign, My Plate. Legislative support for improving access to locally grown fruits and vegetables, seafood, and dairy is becoming more prevalent at the state level. State governments are making attempts to have a positive impact on local economies through promotion of state agriculture. These efforts serve to improve not only the health of the states' people, but also their economies.

Federal health legislation now requires chain restaurants to post the calorie content of their menu items. Preliminary studies show that calorie posting positively influences food choices by consumers. Sara Bleich and colleagues investigated how consumer behavior is impacted by the way calorie information is presented. Bleich et al. tested three ways of presenting calorie information: a calorie count, percentage of daily intake, and physical activity equivalent. Information presented as physical activity equivalents had the most impact on purchasing behavior among low-income black adolescents in Baltimore, Maryland.

A recent trend in corporate wellness programs is the use of social media platforms to support employees adopting healthy lifestyle behaviors. Social media programs can provide a venue for participants to journal, create fitness challenges, and offer support to fellow participants. It provides social support and motivating factors such as accountability and friendly competition. The article by Michelle Rafter describes how one New Jersey hospital has made great progress to improve the health of its employees through a social-media-based corporate wellness program.

The eight articles in Unit 1 focus on a variety of trends seen in nutrition and health environments. The selection of articles includes topics that have been seen in popular media as well as trends observed within the profession of nutrition. These articles stretch across the topics commonly covered in general nutrition courses.

Have a Bite, It's Natural

Food giants are promising to use more natural, ethical ingredients, but will consumers pay?

CHRIS SORENSEN

With their soft, mashed potato insides and crispy exteriors stamped in the shape of a happy face, McCain Foods' frozen Smiles are marketed as a fun-to-eat children's snack. They're not supposed to explode. And yet, that's what happened inside the Canadian food giant's laboratory in Florenceville-Bristol, N.B., as researchers attempted to "reformulate" the Smile's long list of unpronounceable ingredients, part of a company-wide strategy to make its packaged foods more natural and wholesome.

Tony Locke, McCain's director of product development, says the trouble began while trying to ditch mono- and diglycerides, emulsifiers that help retain moisture in some packaged foods. Emboldened by previous success with frozen pizza pockets, Locke's team added a mixture of yeast, wheat gluten and flaxseed to the Smiles. "It was working very well in the lab," says Locke, referring to what was the 40th attempt to rejig the recipe. "But then when we went to scale it up, we actually had these little Smiles going down the line in the plant and coming out of the fryer and exploding. They would literally come out of the oil and burst."

And that, in the form of a combustible little potato snack, is the huge and complex challenge faced by food companies as consumers increasingly demand meals that are not only healthier, but more "natural" and therefore, it's reasoned, better for you. With the public spooked by everything from processed foods (too much salt, too many additives) to hormone-raised beef, food producers are suddenly bending over backwards to portray themselves as purveyors of local, fresh ingredients, and their suppliers as earthy, family-run outfits, as opposed to giant factory farms. The phrases "all-natural," "naturally raised" and "cage-free" are everywhere.

The latest big name to jump into the fray is Burger King. The fast-food giant recently promised to serve only "cage-free" pork and eggs at all of its 7,200 United States restaurants by 2017, marking the first time a big fast-food chain has made such a definitive pledge. McDonald's, meanwhile, has said it will work with its pork suppliers to phase out restrictive gestation crates used to house sows while they raise their piglets. And Tim Hortons is facing calls to go completely cage-free from the Humane Society of the United States, which holds a small number of shares and is proposing a shareholder vote at the company's annual meeting next week. The ethical treatment of animals is one argument driving the changes, but so too is the assertion that happier livestock translates into healthier food.

As for packaged foods, McCain is just one of several companies that's now focused on simple, easy-to-understand ingredients. Others include General Mills, with its Pillsbury Simply line of cookies, and Häagen-Dazs's Five ice cream (with just five ingredients).

But while the sudden shift in focus may seem like a welcome change, critics say it is as much about marketing as it is science. And it has left food producers faced with the prospect of spending billions to overhaul their operations, even though the new and improved approaches may, in reality, do little to improve the nutritional value of the food we eat. Everyone likes the idea of food that's "natural" and ethical, but, it must be asked, are they willing to pay the price?

FOR MANY BIG food companies, the pressure to change their ways intensified earlier this year. In February, Chipotle Mexican Grill (once owned by McDonald's) aired an animated ad during the Grammy Awards that became an Internet phenomenon, with some six million YouTube views. The spot depicted the evolution of factory farming over the years, starting with a farmer and his wife standing in a field with a pig and ending with hundreds of pigs being deposited by machines onto conveyor belts, where they were stuffed with pills, stamped into cubes and loaded into the back of trucks.

Then, in March, a long-simmering debate about "pink slime" (beef scraps ground into a slurry, treated with ammonia and used as hamburger filler) went from being a favourite whipping boy of celebrity chef Jamie Oliver to a mainstream public issue. By the end of the month, everyone from McDonald's to Safeway said they would no longer buy beef made with the stuff, while one of the product's major producers, Beef Products Inc., had to shut down several of its factories, and another ground beef processor, AFA Foods, filed for bankruptcy due to lack of demand.

It's against this backdrop that Burger King, under pressure from the humane society and shifting consumer sentiment,

ITIONS

...decision to promise to use only cage-free eggs and ...the United States within five years (there are no imme- ...plans to do the same in Canada). Other companies that ha..e offered similar promises include McDonald's, Wendy's, Subway, Costco and food giant Unilever, which makes Hell-man's mayonnaise. "We're going to continue to consume beef, pork, chicken, fish, but we want to feel better about the prac-tices," says Darren Tristano, the executive vice-president of Technomic, a food industry consulting firm in Chicago.

Driving the changes is the assertion that happier, healthier livestock translates into food that's better for you

The idea that getting rid of cages is more "natural" comes as news to many producers. Florian Possberg, 61, has been raising hogs in Humboldt, Sask., near Saskatoon, since 1975. Possberg started out raising sows in communal pens and then eventually switched to the more restrictive gestation crates in the 1980s. Research at the time suggested it was better for the animals and consumers, decreasing the risk of disease and injury. "Sows are pretty aggressive when they live in groups," says Possberg, a director of the Canadian Pork Council. He adds that roughly half of the 5,400 sows on his farms are housed in gestation crates, while the rest are in groups, estimating that it would cost more than $1 million to switch over the rest of the operation.

It's a similar story with egg farmers, who, several decades ago, moved to caged systems because it was viewed as cleaner and helped prevent the birds from attacking and eating each other. But animal welfare groups claim the use of small "battery" cages that each house several laying hens are too cramped, preventing the birds from engaging in natural behav-iours such as scratching, nesting or flapping their wings. With pressure mounting south of the border, the United Egg Produc-ers reached a deal last year with the United States humane soci-ety to promote the use of so-called "enriched" cages, which are bigger and offer extras like perches and nesting areas. The two groups are also calling for Congress to pass laws requiring new standards in a bid to avoid a costly patchwork of state regu-lations, and also to ensure individual operators who make the switch aren't put at a "competitive disadvantage." Translation: if everyone has to absorb the same costs, they can more easily be passed on to consumers via higher prices.

In Canada, both pork and egg producers are looking to the National Farm Animal Care Council for guidance. The seven-year-old group devises codes of practice for the industry with input from producers, scientists, government and animal wel-fare groups. It's in the process of updating several of its codes, including those for hogs and poultry, although results aren't expected for a few years. "It takes a long time," says Jackie Wepruk, the council's general manager, of the typically Cana-dian consensus-oriented approach. "But if you look south of the border, you'll see the divisive way animal welfare is being tackled there. Most decisions are being made in a knee-jerk, reactionary sort of way."

But Peter Clarke, chairman of the Egg Farmers of Canada, says the industry may have to move more quickly depending on what happens in the United States "The major food purchas-ers won't accept significantly different practices on one side of the border or the other," he says, adding the cost of such an industry-wide switch would be significant.

Whether it's instant noodles or the oft-mocked Twinkie, most products that come in a bag or a box have histori-cally been marketed based on their convenience, not prov-enance, and come loaded with artificial colours, flavours and other additives—all designed to maintain taste while boosting shelf life.

At McCain, the decision to reformulate its entire lineup of products (more than 80 since 2010) to include only "real" or natural ingredients represented the biggest-ever undertaking for the company's research and development team, accord-ing to Locke. The move was based on extensive customer research that suggested consumers were growing wary of additives that were synthetic-sounding. Nor was the chal-lenge strictly limited to McCain's own operations. "We might buy a seasoning mix from a primary supplier, but of course they're getting all of the components to assemble the mix from another group of suppliers," Locke says. "So it was a complicated effort."

All of the tinkering has translated into big business for another sector of the food industry: flavour companies. Though many consumers don't realize it, many ingredients now viewed as undesirable—salt, sugar and other additives—do a lot of heavy lifting when it comes to taste. Once they're taken out, new flavours must be added to maintain a product's appeal. And not just any flavouring solution will do. Bob Eilerman, the head of science and technology at Switzerland's Givaudan, one of the biggest flavour and fragrance companies in the world, estimates that more than 50 percent of Givaudan's customers now want "natural" flavourings, as opposed to artificial ones, even though there's not much difference (other than cost). "Natural has good connotations behind it," says Eilerman. "But at the end of the day, it's all about chemicals. Whether it's a strawberry flavour that came from crushed strawberries or from one of our laboratories, the chemical composition that we're trying to create is very similar."

It raises the question of whether the current fixation on nat-ural and ethical is ultimately worth the price. McCain seems to think so. Calla Farn, a company spokesperson, says sales of some reformulated McCain products have enjoyed gains of up to 10 percent. As for the cost, Farn admits that the new-and-improved products are more expensive to make, but says the company "worked hard to identify savings in other areas to ensure our products remained cost-neutral."

Not all companies may be so lucky. In the case of cage-free eggs, Tristano estimates that the cost per egg will go up by 25 cents to 40 cents per dozen, which threatens to squeeze the margins on a simple breakfast sandwich. That's because fast-food operators typically have a much tougher time passing on rising commodity prices than do grocery stores because of intense competition. "It's about three cents an egg on a product that sells for $2 or $3, so it doesn't seem like a lot," he says.

4

"But when you can only increase prices by about two per cent and you're getting hit by a per cent and a half just to have cage-free, that's a big deal."

Ultimately, a bigger risk to the industry may come from the public's new heightened expectations from food companies. As they change the way food is made, there is every likelihood consumers will turn their attention to some other unappetizing aspect of the mass-production process. "Once you move forward, there's no turning back," warns Tristano. "And let's be honest: if we really cared that much, we'd all be vegetarians."

Critical Thinking

1. Summarize the potential impact of the higher demand for "natural" products on the food industry.

2. Describe the impact of animal welfare groups on the production of eggs in the United States.

3. Explain why restrictive gestation cages for pigs and cages for hens were adopted during the 1980s.

4. Critique the statement, "Happier livestock translates into healthier food."

Behind the Brand: McDonald's

In the first of a major new series following on from the ground-breaking "Behind the Label," Peter Salisbury takes a look at one of the biggest brands in the world—McDonald's—and asks: Has the burger giant done enough to clean up its act?

PETER SALISBURY

Chances are that you have had a McDonald's meal in the past or if not, you certainly know a lot of people who have. It's the biggest fast food chain in the world, with 32,000 outlets in 117 countries. The clown-fronted burger outfit employs a staggering 1.7 million people, and in the first three months of 2011 alone it made $1.2 billion in profits on the back of revenues of $6.1 billion. The company has come in for huge amounts of criticism over the past 20 years, for the impact it has on the diets of people worldwide, its labour practices and the impact its business has had on the environment. From *Fast Food Nation* to *Supersize Me* by the way of the McLibel trials of the 1990s, plenty has been written and broadcast to tarnish the golden arches' shine.

Declining sales in the early 2000s, which saw franchises being shut for the first time in the company's history, caused a major rethink of the way McDonald's operates, and its recent rhetoric has been that of a firm with a newly discovered zeal for ethical end eco-friendly practices, garnering praise from champions as unlikely as Greenpeace and the Carbon Trust. But is this just marketing hype or has McDonald's had a genuine change of heart?

The answer is yes and no. First of all, because of the way the company is run, it's hard to generalise. Around 80 per cent of McDonald's outlets are run by franchisees who have to meet standards set by the company, but who can—and do—go above and beyond them. Further, McDonald's branches are run by country and regional offices, each of which is subject to domestic standards. The production of much of the raw products which go into McDonald's meals, from burger patties to sauces, is subcontracted to different suppliers, making it impossible to assess the company in terms of a single golden standard. Its sole global supplier (for soft drinks) is Coca-Cola.

The UK branch of the company has certainly made great strides since the 1990s, when it became embroiled in the 1997 McLibel court case, in which McDonald's Corporation and McDonald's Restaurants Limited sued Helen Steel and Dave Morris, a former gardener and a postman, for libel after they published a series of leaflets denouncing the company.

Exploitation

The judge overseeing the case decided that, although the pair could not prove some of their accusations—that McDonald's destroyed rainforests, caused starvation in the third world or disease and cancer in developed countries—it could be agreed that the company exploited children, falsely advertised their food as nutritious, indirectly sponsored cruelty to animals and paid their workers low wages: a major blow to the brand in an age of increasing consumer-consciousness.

Since then, the UK branch has committed to a number of initiatives to improve its image, running an aggressive marketing campaign at the same time to portray itself as an ethical employer which is both farmer and eco-friendly. It has also moved to become more transparent, putting ingredients lists for all of its products on its website and setting up another website, Make Up Your Own Mind, inviting customers to voice concerns and publishing accounts of critics' visits to its production sites.

All of this should be taken with a grain of salt however. It's not surprising that a multibillion-dollar corporation, which has been hurt in the past by concerns over its practices, will do its utmost to sell itself as a reformed character. And it's suspicious that any web search of the company brings up a hit list of sites almost exclusively maintained by the company.

Yet research conducted by the *Ecologist* shows that in many areas the company has improved its record of ethical and environmental awareness over the last decade. The company's burgers, for example, are now 100 per cent beef, and contain no preservatives or added flavors whatsoever. All of McDonald's UK's burgers are provided by Germany's Esca Food Solutions, which claims to maintain rigorous standards at its abattoirs and production plants, and which works closely with 16,000 independent farmers in the UK and Ireland to maintain high standards.

Since the early 2000s, McDonald's UK has maintained that none of its beef, bacon or chicken is fed genetically modified grain. Farmers working for McDonald's have independently confirmed to the *Ecologist* and Esca that they have a 'decent' working relationship with the company.

In 2007, Esca won the UK Food Manufacturing Excellence Awards for its burgers, and in 2010 McDonald's announced that it was launching a three-year study into reducing the carbon emissions caused by the cattle used in its burgers (cattle account for four per cent of the UK's emissions). Meanwhile, all of the fish used in Filet-O-Fish and Fish Finger meals in Europe are sourced from sustainable fisheries certified by the Marine Stewardship Council. Fries are largely sourced from McCain's, the world's biggest potato supplier, and McDonald's claims that the vast majority are produced in the UK, again by independent farmers. The fries are prepared in-store and are cooked in vegetable oil containing no hydrogenated fats. At the beginning of the potato-growing season, dextrose—a form of glucose—is added as a sweetener, and salt is added after cooking (the company claims to have reduced the amount of salt used by 23 per cent since 2008).

The bread for McDonald's buns and muffins is sourced from a single unnamed supplier based in Heywood, Manchester, and Banbury, Oxfordshire. McDonald's would not comment on where it sources the grain for the bakeries but says once more that it does not buy genetically modified crops. Meanwhile, the company has been working with its suppliers and franchise-holders to make sure that they are as energy efficient as possible. In 2010, the Carbon Trust awarded McDonald's its Carbon Trust Standard for reducing its overall carbon emissions by 4.5 per cent between 2007 and 2009. The company is currently experimenting with a series of energy initiatives based around turning its waste, from packaging—which is 80 per cent recycled—to vegetable oil into energy.

Certification

Since 2007, the company—which is one of the world's biggest coffee retailers—has committed to selling only Rainforest Alliance certified coffee. Although the certification body has certainly been responsible for improving conditions and practices in many farming operations worldwide, it has been the subject of controversy—most recently after an undercover investigation by the *Ecologist* revealed allegations of sexual harassment and poor conditions for some workers at its certified Kericho tea plantation in Kenya which supplies the PG Tips brand.

Certification issues aside, McDonald's has undoubtedly become considerably better at taking criticism. In 2006, Greenpeace activists stormed McDonald's restaurants across the world dressed in chicken suits in protest at the destruction of the Amazon rainforest, which they attributed to greedy soy producers—who in turn were selling their produce to chicken farms, of whom McDonald's was a major customer. They subsequently praised the fast food chain for leading a unified response among soy buyers, pressuring producers to adopt a 'zero destruction' approach to growing their crops. Despite praise from Greenpeace, the Carbon Trust and personalities such as Jamie Oliver who have praised the company for its ethical stance on meat and buying its produce locally, the firm is by no means perfect.

One of the biggest incongruencies in its newly discovered zeal for ethical practices comes from its seemingly differing approaches to the conditions chickens live in depending on whether they produce eggs or are used as meat in Chicken McNuggets and similar meals. The firm proudly trumpets that its UK branch only buys eggs from Lion-certified free-range producers, a laudable effort from a huge buyer of eggs, and that the meat in each nugget is 100 per cent chicken breast (the final product is around 65:35 meat and batter).

Factory Farming

Yet by the same token, the company buys most of its chicken from two suppliers, Sun Valley in the UK and Moy Park in Northern Ireland, who are in turn owned by the controversial American firm, Cargill, and Brazil's Marfrig. Sun Valley has been accused of using intensive chicken farming methods to produce their meat, which campaigners say can typically involve birds being cooped up in giant warehouses for much of their natural lives with barely any space to move. Sun Valley was embroiled in a scandal in 2008 when the activist group Compassion in World Farming secretly filmed poor conditions at its supplier Uphampton Farm near Leominster.

Furthermore, although McDonald's is happy to advertise the provenance of its beef, dairy products and eggs, it is more circumspect about chicken meat. This may be because up to 90 per cent of the meat it uses in the UK is sourced from Cargill and Marfrag facilities in Thailand and Brazil, where regulations in the farming sector are perhaps less stringent than in the UK.

Meanwhile, the fact remains that despite attempts in recent years to cultivate a more healthy image, McDonald's primary sales come from fast food in a time when there is increasing recognition that obesity has reached epidemic proportions in the UK and the US. Although the European, and in particular the UK, arm of the company have become increasingly ethically aware, the same cannot be said for the US arm, which uses livestock farmed using intensive methods and fed in some cases on GM crops. And by buying McDonald's in the UK, you are still buying from the same clown.

Critical Thinking

1. Identify a US city that has a population equal to the number of people employed by McDonald's worldwide.
2. Explain why McDonald's made the decision to "clean up" its reputation. When did this begin?
3. Justify the following statement: "It's impossible to assess the operations of McDonald's in terms of a single golden standard."
4. Explain why McDonald's restaurants in Europe do not sell foods containing genetically modified (GM) ingredients, whereas in the United States, McDonald's produces foods with GM ingredients.

Go On: Eat Your Heart Out

BRUCE HOROVITZ

There are few things parents are more passionate about than the food and drink that their kids consume. So it's no accident that Honest Tea, the organic tea maker recently swallowed-up by Coca-Cola, is revamping its wildly successful Honest Kids beverage line into one that this fall will be sweetened with fruit juice instead of cane sugar. A white blaze on the front of the pouch will proclaim: Sweetened *only* with fruit juice.

"They're nutritionally the same," concedes Seth Goldman, cofounder of Honest Tea. "But parents don't want to see added sugar. They can get very emotional about this."

What Americans eat and drink has become such an emotional roller coaster for so many of us that it's utterly changing the way the nation's biggest restaurant chains, foodmakers and grocery chains do business. Food used to feed our bodies. Now it also needs to feed our brains. Our egos. Our nostalgic memories. And maybe even our social-media appetites.

"While we have always had an emotional relationship with food, what's different is we talk about it more, and the discussion is much louder," says Harry Balzer, food guru at researcher NPD Group. "Food is fashion. You wear your diet like you wear your clothes."

Talking about food has become so fashionable that we may be doing more of it than ever. Social-media chatter about food—which is where we do much of it—is up more than 13% over the past year, says Nielsen Media Incite, which tracks buzz across social networks, blogs, forums and consumer review sites. That's millions of additional social morsels just on food. The hunger for food news seems insatiable. Food Network, which had 50,000 viewers per night in the mid-'90s, now averages more than 1.1 million.

Foodmakers are listening in. They know that one of the strongest emotions that many American consumers feel toward the food they eat is fear. One week the fear is over pink slime. Then, it's about chemicals in milk. Or mad cow disease. Or too many calories stuffed into a large, sugary drink. Or even some worker's fingertip getting chopped into an Arby's roast beef sandwich.

"Every week, something raises distrust for our industrialized food system," says Gary Hirshberg, co-founder of Stonyfield Farms. "There's a real-time awareness that our food may be making us sick."

The emotional hits or misses that people feel toward the food they eat can determine everything from what Whole Foods stocks to the thickness of Stonyfield's next yogurt to the look, taste and smell of a new appetizer that Applebee's will add to its menu this fall.

Our emotional attachment to food is leading foodmakers to:

Respond to consumer concerns. Consumer research revealed to Honest Tea executives something they didn't expect: The most important word in the company's name isn't "tea." It's "honest," Goldman says. That's honest as in: We can trust what this brand stands for.

In other words, consumers just want to know what's actually in a product, and they want to know that it's beneficial to eat or drink. So, the Honest brand is looking into a better-for-you carbonated soft-drink line by next year. And it's even looking into Honest-branded foods, he says.

Consumers want to be able to look the brand straight in the eye without the brand blinking, Goldman says. They want to trust it. But that trust is always on the line. Consumers complained, for example, about a new bottle last year that was 22% lighter and which was specifically designed to create less waste. What made consumers balk was that the design change—to use less plastic—made it look like the bottle had less product. "They thought we were selling them air," says Goldman. So the bottle was quickly redesigned again to make it clear that there were no shenanigans.

Folks also want to trust the Honest brand to keep them healthy. "Fifteen years ago, people were choosing organic to save the world," Goldman says. Now, he says, they're choosing it "to save themselves—and that's a much more powerful driver."

Concoct nostalgic food. When football season begins this fall, it won't be an accident if you find this appetizer on the menu at your local Applebee's: brew pub pretzel and beer cheese dip.

"The trick for us was giving customers the sense that they were at the stadium, but in a way that would be unique," says Melissa Hunt, who has been a senior chef at Applebee's for six years. After all, she asks, what's more emotional than fall, football and gathering with friends?

So, instead of a traditional salt pretzel, Applebee's opted to rethink how to make a culinary connection between the bond at a ballpark and taste expectations at an Applebee's. That meant less salt and more pepper and herbs on the pretzel. It meant a pretzel that was crispy on the outside but soft on the inside. And, of course, what to add to the cheese dip to give it the cosmic flavor and smell of sitting in stadium seats: beer, of course.

Sell better-for-you stuff. At Panera Bread, the internal name used for its food-development team is the "lust" team, because "food is such a sensual experience," says co-founder Ron Shaich.

Shaich said Panera's basic goal is to prod consumers to "fall in love" with the restaurant: "That's what I wake up first thing in the morning thinking. If you love this place, that's all that matters. Everything else will take care of itself."

So he works on the emotional cues that hit consumers at their core: no artificial stuff, antibiotic-free meats, fully posted calorie information and intangibles, he says, such as serving food on china plates instead of paper.

The chain recently starting selling a Fuji Apple Roasted Turkey Salad with turkey meat that doesn't taste like it's from the deli. Rather, he says, it looks, feels, smells and tastes like it's from one of the most memorable spots of all: the Thanksgiving table.

"This is real turkey," says Shaich. It's cut 1/3-inch thick. It's also a hit, he says, with early sales surpassing expectations.

Cater to "mouth feel." Some 29 years ago, Gary Hirshberg started with seven cows and an idea: to make organic yogurt for the masses. His company, Stonyfield Farms, is now the nation's fourth-largest yogurt maker.

Much of his free time is spent combing yogurt aisles of stores throughout Europe, searching for the next big thing in the U.S. thicker, cheesier yogurts. Europeans, who he says are more emotional about their food than Americans, want a "thicker, creamier mouth feel" when they eat yogurt. Americans eventually will, too, which helps explain why Greek yogurt sales have grown so quickly in the United States And that's the next generation of yogurt he's searching for: thicker and cheesier than Greek.

Get more local. Whole Foods executives know there are few things folks are more passionate about than where their food comes from.

Next year it will open a store in Brooklyn, N.Y., with something none of its stores have: a 10,000-square-foot rooftop garden. "You can't get more locally grown than that," says David Lannon, executive vice president of operations.

Most recently, it took that consumer passion for all-things-local to a new store in Kailua, Hawaii. The store has a fish bar that serves locally caught, sustainably sourced fish chopped with items such as onions and soy sauce to create an "emotional connection" to what locals ate as kids, Lannon says. The store targets locals, not tourists, with three porches where folks can sit, eat and socialize. "It brings folks full circle to their memories of growing up in Hawaii."

There's also a Whole Foods in Petaluma, Calif., where eggs are sold—when available—from a local farmer whose 200 chickens are never kept inside or in cages. Never mind that the eggs cost twice as much as conventional eggs. "Customers call the store and ask if that egg delivery arrived," Lannon says. "Some decide to come based only on that."

Serve "comfort" at 30,000 feet. Then, there's British Airways. It recently realized that its first-class passengers don't want fancy-dancy desserts. Last fall, it started serving what passengers told them they wanted most: comfort food. Its Crumb Crumble cobbler was such a smash, when caterers tried to replace it on the menu with a different dessert, passengers went ballistic, says Lynn McClelland, head of catering. It's all about emotions—even the most primitive, childhood emotions, she says. When stuck high above the ground for hours in a plane, she says, "Passengers tell us what they want most is what their moms used to feed them when they were 12."

Critical Thinking

1. Describe how consumers' emotional attachment to food is influencing the U.S. food supply.

2. Explain how social media is impacting the U.S. perspective of food.

3. Interpret the following statement: "One of the strongest emotions that American consumers feel toward food is fear."

Fresh Fruit, Hold the Insulin

While health officials wage a costly war on obesity and diabetes, taxpayers are subsidizing foods that make us fatter. It's time to rewrite the farm bill.

Some years ago two nutrition experts went grocery shopping. For a dollar, Adam Drewnowski and S. E. Specter could purchase 1,200 calories of potato chips or cookies or just 250 calories worth of carrots. It was merely one example of how an unhealthy diet is cheaper than a healthy one. This price difference did not spring into existence by force of any natural laws but largely because of antiquated agricultural policies. Public money is working at cross-purposes: backing an overabundance of unhealthful calories that are flooding our supermarkets and restaurants, while also battling obesity and the myriad illnesses that go with it. It is time to align our farm policies with our health policies.

In past years farm subsidies have been a third rail of American politics—never to be touched. But their price tag, both direct and indirect, has now brought them back into the debate and created an imperative for change. Conditions such as heart disease, diabetes and arthritis are strongly correlated with excess poundage and run up medical bills of nearly $150 billion every year. The government has poured billions of dollars into dietary campaigns, from the U.S., Department of Agriculture's new MyPlate recommendation (half of daily food consumption should be fruits and vegetables) to programs aimed at providing more produce in schools and in military cafeterias.

Agricultural subsidies undercut those efforts by skewing the market in favor of unhealthful calories. Much of the food we have to choose from—and how much it costs—is determined by the 1,770-page, almost $300-billion Food, Conservation, and Energy Act of 2008 (commonly known as the "farm bill"). This piece of legislation, up for renewal this year, covers everything from nutrition assistance programs to land conservation efforts. It also determines how much money gets paid out to agricultural operations in subsidies and crop insurance programs. Federal support for agriculture, begun in earnest during the Great Depression, was originally intended as a temporary lifeline to farmers, paying them extra when crop prices were low. Nearly eight decades later the benefits flow primarily to large commodity producers of corn and soy, which are as profitable as ever.

The current bill gives some $4.9 billion a year in automatic payments to growers of such commodity crops, thus driving down prices for corn, corn-based products and corn-fed meats. Cows that are raised on corn, rather than grass, make meat that is higher in calories and contains more omega-6 fatty acids and fewer omega-3 fatty acids—a dangerous ratio that has been linked to heart disease.

Cheap corn has also become a staple in highly processed foods, from sweetened breakfast cereals to soft drinks, that have been linked to an increase in the rate of type 2 diabetes, a condition that currently affects more than one in 12 American adults. Between 1985 and 2010 the price of beverages sweetened with high-fructose corn syrup dropped 24 percent, and by 2006 American children consumed an extra 130 calories a day from these beverages. Over the same period the price of fresh fruits and vegetables rose 39 percent. For families on a budget, the price difference can be decisive in their food choices.

But fruits and vegetables do not have to be more expensive than a corn-laden chicken nugget or corn syrup-sweetened drink. One reason they are costly is that the current farm bill categorizes them as "specialty crops" that do not receive the same direct payments or crop insurance that commodity crops do.

With the government tightening its belt, some of those old subsidies finally look ready to fall. Many lawmakers across the political spectrum, including President Barack Obama and the leaders of the U.S., Senate Committee on Agriculture, Nutrition and Forestry, have recommended cutting direct commodity payments, which would save money and help us stay healthier.

There is no dearth of policy options. Research groups such as the Robert Wood Johnson Foundation in Princeton, N.J., recommend leveling the playing field by extending subsidies and insurance programs more widely to fruit and vegetable producers. The government can also use its own purchasing power, through school lunch programs and institutional buying decisions, to fill people's plates with healthy choices. The imperative, however, is clear: any new farm bill should at the very least remove the current perverse incentives for people to eat unhealthily.

Critical Thinking

1. Define the farm bill. Identify the programs and policies that are covered by this bill.

2. Identify the implications of fruits and vegetables being categorized as "specialty crops" in the farm bill.

3. Contrast the price trends of sweetened beverages and fruits/vegetables from 1985–2010.

4. Identify the original intention of agricultural subsidies. When did the subsidies begin?

The New Healthy

Lawmakers are cooking up ways to encourage better eating and cultivate local economies.

AMY WINTERFELD

As Americans leap into the New Year, many will resolve to eat healthier to make up for holiday indulgences. New guidelines for what eating healthy means, released last year by the U.S. Department of Agriculture, include a new "MyPlate" icon: a dinner plate that divides fruits, vegetables, grains, protein and dairy into appropriate portions on a colorful place setting.

With more than 33 percent of American adults overweight or obese—resulting in medical costs of about $147 billion a year, according to 2009 study in Health Affairs—and 17 percent of children and adolescents also above a healthy weight, eating more nutritiously is paramount.

"We need to make sure we have the most nutritious food that we can," says Texas Representative Carol Alvarado. "A child who receives a healthy meal will be a better student, a healthier adult and less likely to have heart disease and diabetes."

Healthy eating is an issue many lawmakers have already tackled. Some support comes from those who want to encourage healthy choices by bringing more fruit and vegetables to their communities. Others see a silver lining in the salad plate: a lift to local economies by promoting state agriculture products.

Fill Half Your Plate With Produce

The new dietary guidelines recommend a plate half full of fruits and vegetables. Yet 32 states scored at or below the national average, in a 2011 report by the Centers for Disease Control and Prevention. The report looked at the availability of supermarkets, produce stands and farmers' markets that typically sell healthy foods such as fresh produce, whole grains and low-fat dairy products.

"My district is underserved by grocery stores and has more convenience stores that don't provide fruits and vegetables," says Alvarado. "I support community gardens—it teaches children about where food comes from and how it grows and also teaches them to take pride in their community."

State legislatures in Illinois, Louisiana, New York and Pennsylvania have supported public-private partnerships to bring healthy food sellers into urban, suburban and rural communities currently starved of produce. Not only can this help local diets, it also may give a boost to local economies. Grants, loans and tax credits are offered to grocery operators to build new full-service stores or improve existing facilities by adding refrigerated storage for fresh produce, for example. In Pennsylvania, over a five-year span, 5,000 jobs were created or retained as a result. New federal funding is available to states for these efforts.

California legislators in 2011 enacted a tax credit for farmers who donate fruits and vegetables to food banks. In 2010, Mississippi lawmakers exempted food grown or processed in Mississippi and sold at farmers' markets from the sales tax. Laws in California, Illinois, Nebraska and Washington support electronic card readers at farmers' markets to encourage public benefit recipients to use their cards to buy fresh produce.

Lawmakers have also looked at promoting healthier habits for school children while supporting local economies by purchasing local food for schools. In 2011, Michigan legislators created a school purchasing preference for food grown or produced by Michigan businesses. New Jersey lawmakers enacted a "Jersey Fresh" program that allows schools to adopt price preferences for local agricultural and farm products, improve kitchen facilities to incorporate more fresh, locally grown produce, and add information about the value of eating fresh, locally grown produce to school curricula.

"Educating our children about our state's diverse and delicious agricultural fare and the nutritious value of local and safe 'Jersey Fresh' produce will help them cultivate healthier food choices and make them aware of the importance of supporting local farmers," says New Jersey Assemblyman John McKeon.

A Rutgers University report found that $1.1 million spent in New Jersey in 2000 to promote local fare had an economic impact of $63.2 million. It also generated an increase in state and local tax revenue by $2.2 million for the year. In 2011–2012 Oregon legislators created grants to reimburse districts for buying local food products and for conducting certain food-based educational activities.

Last year, Missouri Representative Casey Guernsey sponsored legislation that established a Farm-to-Table Advisory Board to "link schools and state institutions with local and regional farms for the purchase of locally grown agricultural products; increase market opportunities for locally grown agricultural products; and assist schools and other entities to teach children and the public about nutrition, food choices, obesity, and health; and the value of having an accessible supply of locally grown food."

In Colorado and Massachusetts, lawmakers established food policy advisory councils in 2010. Massachusetts directed its council to increase local food production and state use of local products. Colorado's council is charged with fostering a healthy food supply while enhancing agricultural and natural resources, encouraging economic growth, promoting "Colorado Proud" products and improving community health.

In Texas, a "Go Texan" agricultural marketing and promotion effort by Senator Craig Estes supports programs for rural economic development, marketing and promotion of agricultural and other products grown, processed, or produced in the state. Vermont also enacted legislation in 2011 to encourage economic development by marketing state foods and products.

In 2011, legislators in at least six other states—Georgia, New Mexico, New York, South Carolina, Virginia and Washington—proposed legislation to encourage local food purchasing or "buying from the backyard" by state agencies or schools. Five of those bills carried over into 2012.

Bring on the Amber Waves

Grains cover another quarter of the USDA-recommended plate. The new dietary guidelines advise "make at least half your grains whole grains." An Oregon law enacted in 2011 puts whole grain flours on an equal footing with enriched flour. Previously, only enriched flour met health requirements for manufacturers of bread, rolls or buns.

Guidelines for healthy school foods and snacks in North Carolina and Rhode Island call for increasing whole grain and grain products. Texas has just created a grain producers indemnity fund to protect farmers from economic hardship.

Pack in the Protein

Most Americans eat enough protein, but the new guidelines encourage leaner and more varied selections of protein-rich foods. Meat, poultry, fish, beans, eggs, peanut butter and nuts or seeds all provide protein. Legislators focused on fish last year in at least two states.

Rhode Island's fishing community will benefit from a newly created Seafood Marketing Collaborative to support local fishermen and small businesses. It will be promoting the health and vitality of the state's seafood populations, identifying regulatory restrictions that inhibit local seafood businesses, and increasing consumer demand for local seafood through marketing.

Even in land-locked Nebraska, legislators appropriated funds to enhance fisheries by improving hatcheries and buying and developing fishing facilities that improve access for fishermen.

Washington appropriated $3.47 million for improving recreational fisheries. Legislators also directed state agencies to look for partnerships that will help keep fish hatcheries operating with less reliance on state money. In 2009, another New England state, Vermont, established a milk and meat pilot program to encourage purchasing local milk and meat for school meals and to provide technical assistance to schools to help them provide the most local fruits and vegetables possible.

In Arkansas and Indiana, lawmakers established liability protection for agritourism, which encourages education, entertainment or recreation on farms and ranches.

Get in the Moo-ed

MyPlate places a cool blue glass of milk next to the plate as a reminder that the dietary guidelines recommend switching to fat-free or low-fat milk. Dairy products add protein, as well as calcium, vitamins D, B12 and A, phosphorus, and potassium.

Licensed child-care facilities in California must now provide water and serve only low-fat or nonfat milk to children older than 2. Minnesota appropriated $500,000 for each of the next two years to the state's six Second Harvest food banks to purchase milk from Minnesota processors.

Massachusetts legislators, in 2010, directed the state's public health department to use scientific guidelines to set standards for school snacks and beverages that encourage greater consumption of water, low- and nonfat milk, fresh fruits and vegetables, and reduction of fat and sugar in snacks. Beverage standards set by Louisiana legislators in 2009 require high schools to serve low-fat milk or skim milk.

In New York, a Calcium Purchasing Preference Initiative is pending that would require foods and beverages that contain a higher level of calcium to be purchased for government buildings so long as they are same quality, and equal or lower in price.

Critical Thinking

1. Assess how local economies can benefit from the MyPlate guidelines.
2. Discuss the benefits of community gardens.
3. Identify five examples of how local, state, and federal government can promote the consumption of fruits and vegetables and stimulate local economies.

AMY WINTERFELD tracks nutrition issues for NCSL.

Calorie Posting in Chain Restaurants

SARAH H. WRIGHT

Nutrition labeling on packaged food has been mandatory in the United States since the early 1990s, and printing tiny lists on cans and bags has long been accepted practice. Yet, in spite of this improvement in providing information, the share of Americans who are obese has continued to rise, increasing from 15.9 percent in 1995 to 26.6 percent in 2008.

The fraction of calories consumed in restaurants also has risen in recent years. In 2008, New York City extended nutrition labeling to chain restaurants, requiring them to post clearly the number of calories in every one of their foods and beverages. In March 2010, new federal health care legislation mandated calorie posting for chain restaurants nationwide beginning in 2011. Will these point-of-purchase postings have any public health effect? Could menus with "350 calories" printed beside "eight grain roll" drive a consumer to buy a banana (100 calories) instead?

In **Calorie Posting in Chain Restaurants** (NBER Working Paper No. 15648), study authors **Bryan Bollinger, Phillip Leslie,** and **Alan Sorensen** ask whether mandatory calorie posting influences consumers' purchase decisions. They use detailed data from Starbucks stores in New York City, where calories are posted; from Starbucks in Boston and Philadelphia, where calories are not posted; and from Starbucks stores throughout the nation. The researchers find that mandatory calorie posting influenced consumer behavior at Starbucks in New York City, causing average calories per transaction to drop by 6 percent (from 247 to 232 calories). They also find that these effects are long lasting: after the posting began, the calorie reduction persisted for at least 10 months (the duration of the sample period). There is also evidence of persistent learning effects: commuters who lowered their calories per transaction on weekdays in New York City also lowered them in transactions at Starbucks outside the city, where calories were not posted.

Mandatory calorie posting influenced consumer behavior at Starbucks in New York City, causing average calories per transaction to drop by 6 percent.

The researchers also find that almost all of the calorie-reduction effects in Starbucks are related to food—not beverage—purchases.

Following calorie posting, average food calories per transaction fell by 14 percent. The effect is larger for high-calorie consumers: individuals who averaged more than 250 calories per transaction reacted to calorie posting by decreasing calories per transaction by 26 percent—dramatically more than the 6 percent average reduction for all consumers.

Beverage consumption was largely unaffected by calorie posting. Consumers tended to underestimate the calories contained in Starbucks' food and bakery items, but they overestimated the calories contained in Starbucks beverages. According to the researchers, consumers who discovered by calorie posting that an Iced Cafe Latte contains just 130 calories were pleasantly surprised—continued buying.

Noting that calorie reductions on the order of 6 percent at chain restaurants would yield only modest decreases in body weight, the researchers suggest that the direct effect of calorie posting on U.S. obesity may be small. The most meaningful effect of the calorie posting law may be its long-run impact on menu choices, as restaurants will have an economic incentive to offer low-calorie options. The new policy may also benefit public health as consumers grow accustomed to counting calories and choose or demand healthier foods.

The study also explores how calorie posting affected corporate profits. The authors find that it did not cause any significant change in Starbucks' overall revenue. At Starbucks stores located within 100 meters of a Dunkin Donuts store, revenue actually increased by 3 percent—suggesting that calorie posting may have caused some consumers to substitute away from Dunkin Donuts toward Starbucks.

Critical Thinking

1. What year will mandatory calorie posting be enforced for chain restaurants?
2. Describe how calorie posting affected consumer behavior of Starbucks customers.
3. Predict the long-term impact on restaurant's menu offerings considering the likely increased demand for lower calorie items.
4. Defend the requirement that chain restaurants must post nutrition information on their menus. In your response, consider the perspective of a restaurant owner, a politician, and a nutritionist.

Cause + Effect

Nutrition labels might be informative, but they're not worth the package space if consumers don't understand them. One Johns Hopkins researcher explains how public policy experts could use marketers' help—and messaging prowess—to alter unhealthy consumer behaviors and develop a solution to America's obesity epidemic.

ELISABETH A. SULLIVAN

The link between marketing and public policy stands in stark relief against America's struggle with obesity. For years, critics have questioned the potency of marketing messages aimed at younger audiences that promote sugary cereals, high-fat and high-calorie foods or otherwise less-than-optimal consumables. At the same time, advocates have championed marketers' ability to help promote healthier consumption behaviors and encourage consumers to balance their caloric intake with more active lifestyles. Marketers wield considerable power over what consumers choose to consume—and public policy experts such as Sara Bleich want to harness that power to help alleviate the obesity problem in the United States and beyond.

Bleich, an assistant professor at Johns Hopkins' Bloomberg School of Public Health, is working to help check obesity and related diseases by researching, as her bio says, "the intersection between public policy and obesity prevention/control," including "novel environmental strategies to reduce caloric intake." Marketing, she says, plays a central role both in her research and in possible remedies to the country's obesity problem.

Late last year, Bleich and co-authors Bradley Herring, Desmond Flagg and Tiffany Gary-Webb released the results of a study that examined the effect of store signage on teens' purchase of sugary beverages. The study involved 1,600 beverage purchases made by 12- to 18-year-olds in four corner stores in Baltimore. The article, called "Reduction in Purchases of Sugar-Sweetened Beverages Among Low-Income, Black Adolescents After Exposure to Caloric Information," was published in the *American Journal of Public Health* and garnered considerable media attention, partly because it deals with the hot-button issue of obesity but mostly because it presents a noteworthy finding: that consumers' purchase decisions might be influenced by products' nutritional information that replaces the traditional calorie number with what Bleich calls the "physical activity equivalent."

Marketing News caught up with Bleich to discuss how her consumer behavior research was carried out and what the findings might mean for food and beverage marketers.

Q: Why did you decide to study the power of messaging regarding sugary, high-calorie drinks, in particular?

A: We know that people generally don't have a good understanding of the amount of calories that are in the food that they eat, and Americans typically have low numeracy skills and poor skills when it comes to calorie literacy. Basically, they don't have a good sense of what's in the foods that they eat in terms of calories and they're not good at doing mental math.

Since health reform is going to require that if you're a chain outlet with more than 20 stores, starting in the middle of this year, you're going to have to post calorie information, we thought, Well, maybe the current standard, which is calorie counts, won't be the most effective way to get people information. What we wanted to do was test three different ways of giving them information, the first being absolute calorie counts and then two others, which are much easier for people to understand without doing any mental math, and look at the effect on sugar-sweetened beverage purchases.

And we specifically focused on sugar-sweetened beverage purchases [because] when it comes to thinking about dealing with the obesity problem, there's a close link between sugar-sweetened beverage consumption and obesity. It also, in terms of a category, is very easy to isolate beverages and try to get people to consume less of them, whereas obviously food is something where it's a little bit harder. But if you can get someone to not buy soda and maybe buy water, you can actually pull a lot of empty calories out of their diet pretty easily.

Nutrition Tips in the Chip Aisle

In an attempt to participate in consumers' nutritional education with an industry-led initiative, several grocery store chains now feature third-party-provided nutritional ratings systems on their shelves to help guide consumers toward healthier choices within product categories. One such system, developed by Braintree, Mass.-based NuVal, takes into account more than 30 nutritional elements such as protein, calcium and vitamins, as well as sugar, sodium and cholesterol, and uses a point system to signify that higher-rated products are the healthier choices within the given category. The NuVal System currently is offered in stores such as Meijer, Kroger and Pick 'n Save, among others.

Menus Are About to Get a Whole Lot Lengthier

Nutrition-related federal legislation introduced in March 2010 is about to take effect, requiring restaurant chains—and vending machine companies—to make calorie counts and nutritional information readily available. As part of the Patient Protection and Affordable Care Act of 2010, restaurants with 20 or more locations must list calorie information for their standard menu items on all menus—including drive-through menus. Restaurants also must have other nutritional information available for consumers who request it, including a listing of the product's total calories, fat, saturated fat, cholesterol, sodium, total carbohydrates, sugars, fiber and protein.

Q: How did you decide on the messaging to test?

A: We knew we wanted to do absolute calories, which is the current standard, and then two different types of relative information, so we just sat down and brainstormed and figured out, Let's do a percentage of daily intake, which is another way that we often see calories represented. And then the third was the physical activity equivalent, which is just novel and we thought that it would be more meaningful to people than both absolute calories and the percent daily value.

In terms of how we picked jogging as opposed to yoga or dancing or basketball, or a million other things that we could choose from, there's research that suggests that negative messaging is a little bit more powerful than positive messaging, so we purposefully did not pick something like dancing or basketball, which may have been attractive to our target population, which was black adolescents between the ages of 12 to 18. We chose jogging, which may be perceived as a little bit less desirable.

We calculated, for the average 110-pound adolescent, how many minutes of jogging they'd have to do to burn off a 250-calorie bottle of soda and that was about 50 minutes. And that [physical activity equivalent] sign was the most effective at reducing sugar-sweetened beverage purchasing.

[Editor's note: The study found that the signs listing the "absolute calorie" and "percentage of daily intake" information reduced the likelihood of sugar-sweetened beverage purchases by 40 percent compared with the baseline of no signage, while the "physical activity equivalent" sign reduced the likelihood of such purchases by 50 percent.]

Q: You tested this in corner stores in Baltimore. How was it logistically set up? You had the signage in there, and then did you have field researchers watching kids come in and gauging their reactions when they saw the signs? Did you have video set up or were you interviewing them?

A: I've been asked this question so many times and it's a good question. What we did is, basically, you walk into a store and you're a customer, and there are these walls of beverage cases. On the beverage cases is an 8 ½-by-11-inch sign. There's one type of sign, but there could be multiple signs if there are multiple beverage cases. But basically, it's at eye level, it's 8 ½ by 11 and it has a message on it, and it's one of three messages, which are randomized across the stores and you're only going to see one message at a time.

So you walk into the store, you go to open up the beverage case and the sign is right in front of you, and you make your selection. We had a research assistant sitting in the store in sort of an out-of-the-way place with a full, clear view of the counter and, for a random sample of adolescents who were purchasing beverages, he would record the beverage that they purchased. We purposefully did not intervene and say: 'Are you, a.) black, b.) between the ages of 12 and 18, and, c.) what did you purchase?' because we knew that the minute we started asking questions, it would mitigate the effect of information on purchasing, so we simply observed. And in the instance where an adolescent was buying two different beverages, we simply recorded the one that hit the counter first, but that was a very rare occurrence. That research assistant was consistent across all the stores and he would just observe the purchases and record them, and then we'd analyze the data later.

The other thing I should add is that to ensure that we'd get our target population, the stores had to be in zip codes that had at least 70 percent black population and they had to be located within walking distance—so less than five city blocks—of middle and high schools because that was the target age group.

Q: What was the timeline for the study?

A: It was about six months. It started in May and ended in October. It was a total of four stores and we started data collection at two of the stores first, had about a month or so of overlap time and then concluded with the second two stores. The primary reason for that was because of possible issues of seasonality because it could be that people drink differently in the summer than they do when it's a little bit colder outside, so we adjusted for all of that in the models but purposefully staggered the data collection periods.

Q: And the results were quantitative, mainly? You were really just gauging what sold after people encountered the signage?

A: Exactly. Our denominator was all purchases and we were looking at the percentage of sugar-sweetened beverage purchases.

Q: Was the researcher taking note of whether the customer looked at the signs?

A: We qualitatively talked about this. Weekly, we'd check in and he'd tell me about the signs. . . . [The research assistant] certainly said that adolescents noticed the signs, but again, we purposefully didn't stop them and say, 'Did you notice the sign and did it affect your purchasing behavior?' We simply observed the purchase.

But we have been funded to do this study again and in that, we will both be doing focus groups on the front end to ask adolescents—this time including Hispanic adolescents, too—'What sorts of things are most effective? Is it a physical activity equivalent? Is it the number of teaspoons of sugar in a can of soda?' Then on the back end, we'll do exit interviews among a sample of adolescents and ask them, 'Did you see the signs and how did it affect your behavior?'

Q: Are you also going to test whether this kind of signage or messaging would work on a label versus on a sign?

A: I think, logistically, that would be very hard because that would require a partnership with Coca-Cola or some other bottling company and I would imagine that they would be somewhat hesitant to allow us to do that. I mean, if they would, I would love to, but I think that would be somewhat tough. But it's something that would be interesting to try.

Another thing that we will look at in the follow-up study is we've [already] observed: Signs are posted and what's the immediate effect on purchasing behaviors when it comes to sugary beverages? But there could be some post-intervention effects, such that the signs come down and for three to six to nine months out, people are still being affected by what they saw previously, and we'll also test that post-intervention effect in the follow-up study.

Q: If we're going to extrapolate on these findings and guess at what kind of lasting consumer behavioral changes might take place, what do you think such signage would do? Do you think that this will increase consumers' food literacy and nutritional literacy so that they might reconsider imbibing so many sugary beverages a day? What are you hoping that this kind of educational tool will result in?

A: My sense is that this sort of information is not necessarily educating the consumer, but really it's making information more interpretable. Right now, anything that you buy that's packaged has calories on it—cookies have 200 calories, a bag of chips has 300 calories—but if you don't have a good sense of, a.) how many calories you should have in a

given day and, b.) what the tradeoff is in terms of how much exercise you have to do to burn that off, I don't think people realize how much they're consuming.

What I hope this type of information will do is it will cause people to pause and say: 'I'm going to have to run for an hour and a half to burn off a bag of chips? Maybe I'll just forego the bag of chips. Maybe I'll get something that's lower-calorie instead.' By increasing the transparency around the, sort of, tradeoff between consumption and expenditure, I think it would make it easier for people to make more educated decisions about their consumption.

Q: How about from a marketplace perspective, though? Are you hoping, ultimately, that marketers will start to change their labels to be exercise-related rather than calorie-focused, or are you hoping that this will inspire more of a public service announcement approach across the industry in which this kind of educational messaging will be pumped out?

A: I think both would be wonderful. A challenge that we have in private industry is that the way that nutrition information is reported varies quite a bit by product line and by the type of item that it is. The way you see things on a can of Coke may be different than you see things on a box of sugary cereal. . . . One thing that would need to happen that's going to be really important is that assuming that we were able to provide calorie information in the form of a physical activity equivalent, it would have to be something that's standardized across the different products because if you see minutes of running in one place, minutes of yoga somewhere else and minutes of basketball in a third place, my guess is that it may lose its meaning with consumers. But if it's the same message consistently, I think that could actually have an effect.

We have to figure out, what kind of physical activity is most meaningful when it comes to changing behavior? My guess, from the literature and from this study, is that it's probably something that's more on the negative side because if you pick something that people enjoy doing, they're going to say, 'Oh, well, I'll go dancing for an hour and burn off that piece of pizza.' But if they have to run or do sit-ups or push-ups, it's not really as desirable. I guess that's the first thing.

The second is that there's obviously logistical concerns. If you're putting on a can of soda '150 or 250 calories,' that takes up a certain amount of space. If you then want to try to say, 'This is the equivalent of 50 minutes of jogging,' that'd take up a lot more space, so I think you have to figure out the best way to present this information. And if you standardized it across all of the different product lines, I think that would allow you to condense it even more because people would be used to seeing that information presented in a certain way. But I would say that, in the case of chain restaurants, the information has to be posted by the middle of this year per federal legislation, so from a public health perspective, how can we maximize something that, from a legislative perspective, is going to happen? I think that what this study tells me is that simply using calorie counts is probably not the most effective way to alter behavior.

Q: Based on studies like yours that show that exercise-related messaging could be effective, do you think that the federal government is going to step in and mandate that that sort of language be used on labels or would it be an industry-led initiative?

A: I would be surprised if there were legislation largely because I think, the industry could make the argument, which is compelling, that the information is already there and it's already required to be there. You turn this package over and it says how many calories per serving are in something. There's been a lot of industry-led initiatives when it comes to anti-obesity, anti-calorie things over the past four or five years and I think a lot of that seems to be an effort to, sort of, make sure that the heavy hand of government doesn't come down or to stay ahead of it.

Sure, I think we could see different companies thinking about ways to put information on product labeling by pulling stuff out of the bag that's supposedly useful to consumers. I would say that if you are PepsiCo, for example, maybe you could think about looking at your product line and saying: 'A bag of Fritos would be 50 minutes of running, but a bag of 'x' would be 20 minutes of running. Why don't you instead choose a bag of 'x'?' By using the substitution effect, it would be cost-neutral in the sense that you're not losing consumers; you're just driving them to a different product line.

I think the key with any of these types of studies where you're trying to change consumer behavior is that from a public health perspective, we're excited when people change what they do, but from a private industry perspective, it's got to be cost-neutral because if it's the case that I put these signs up in stores and people choose not to buy anything, then the stores aren't going to want to participate. What we found is that sugar-sweetened beverage purchases went

down, but then water purchases went up. We don't know, exactly, whether or not it was perfectly cost-neutral, but what the results suggest is that if you're thirsty, you're going to buy something, but that information will sway what that something will be.

Q: What role, ideally, would marketers play in this effort to reduce consumers' caloric intake? As you're talking about here, it's a profit question and changes might impact bottom lines if Coke, for example, all of a sudden does have to put this messaging on its cans to dissuade a consumer from buying the product. That's obviously not appealing to Coke's interests, yet marketers certainly have a role to play in fostering good public health.

A: I'm one of those people who think that private industry is not the devil and that there's lots of things that public health [organizations] could do to partner with industry and think about, what are some ways that we can marry the interest in maximizing health on the public health side and the fiduciary responsibility that private industry has to maximize profits for their shareholders? How can you marry those two objectives and find things that actually work? . . .

What should happen is that these sorts of messages should be tested in a larger audience using focus groups and other sorts of mechanisms to figure out, what is the most effective way to influence people and influence different types of people? We focused on a small swath of the population, black adolescents. My sense is that this is a group who's at very high obesity risk and may or may not have strong concerns when it comes to calories and exercise and that sort of thing. If you took a swath of the population, say, middle-income white women for whom those concerns are very strong, and you gave them this sort of information, I think the effect would be much, much larger.

So I think the role that marketing could possibly play is thinking about how you take these sorts of interventions and do them on a grander scale, and then spin them in a way that's really effective. I have no background in marketing, so who knows if someone could come in that has a lot of expertise and make these signs a million times more effective by just changing a few words, or changing the colors or changing the images and that sort of thing? . . .

People are not stupid, but messages have to be simple and easily understandable in a very short amount of time when you're about to make a purchase. Where research needs to go and what marketing can possibly do is to think about how you take this complicated information, when you're combining items on a menu or having combo meals, and give it to people in easily interpretable formats. Just telling them these broad calorie numbers is not very meaningful to the average person.

Q: Is the marketer's job done when the communication has been effectively made? Corporations can change their messaging, their labeling and packaging methods, and then can they stop there? Or should they be investing in other public service or public policy initiatives to try to get people to be healthier?

+ Food Label Literacy

59 percent of respondents to a global study conducted by Nielsen have trouble understanding nutrition labels. In the U.S., while the food label literacy rates compare favorably with that global average, more than four in 10 consumers (42 percent) still report having trouble understanding the nutritional information on packaging.

Globally, 33 percent of respondents trust calorie counts to be "always accurate" and 58 percent say that they're "sometimes accurate."

When it comes to more ambiguous nutritional claims such as "fresh," "all-natural" and "heart-healthy," approximately 80 percent of consumers doubt their veracity.

The Nielsen Global Survey of Food Labeling Trends was conducted in March and April, and August and September of 2011, and polled more than 25,000 respondents in 56 countries.

A: Is it the case that you stop once you get information to consumers and you allow them to run with it? From a marketing perspective, if you have a good message, you've done your job by putting it out there. I think the bigger question is, what are you putting out there?

"Its not going to fix the problem of obesity, but more transparency about what we're eating and helping people make better decisions at the point of purchase can be effective, so I think marketing has a huge role to play."

I do think that more effort should be made to think about how you change the messages to create healthier environments. Obviously, marketing can't change the fact that there are lots of convenience stores or lots of fast-food restaurants, but marketing can change how different product lines are marketed and to whom they're targeted. Again, I strongly believe that if you are one of these big multinationals like Coca-Cola or Pepsi, you have a very diverse product line, so simply encouraging people toward the healthier side will, hopefully, not hurt your bottom line. It will just diversify what people are actually purchasing. . . . I think the key is using marketing to actually change demand—we know it's possible, that you can actually induce demand—and try to help people and steer them in the right direction when it comes to healthier eating. . . .

What's going to have to happen is to do the good public health research, we have to figure out what the most effective messaging is and that's going to come directly from marketing. That's an area where I have no expertise, so we're going to have to collaborate in terms of figuring out the most convincing way to tell people. The punch line that I try to get across is the reason that we are getting bigger as a country and across all developed countries is not because, on average, we're exercising too little. It's because we're simply eating too much. So how do you pull some calories out of the diet? I think that these messages can move us in that direction. It's not going to fix the problem of obesity, but more transparency about what we're eating and helping people make better decisions at the point of purchase can be effective, so I think marketing has a huge role to play.

Critical Thinking

1. Describe how the Patient Protection and Affordable Care Act of 2010 will impact restaurants and vending companies with 20 or more locations.

2. Explain the premise of tracking calories using physical activity equivalents.

Can Social Media Produce Wellness Results?

MICHELLE V. RAFTER

For years, *Chilton Hospital* tried to get employees to take better care of themselves.

The northwest New Jersey hospital's human resources staff launched diabetes and other disease management initiatives to improve employee well-being and reduce health care costs. But the resulting behavior changes were minor, and the programs only covered a small number of employees.

That changed, though, when Chilton switched gears to a wellness program that asked employees to get social and competitive.

In March 2011, Chilton entered a countywide fitness challenge where employees vied in teams of six against other local businesses to see who could eat the healthiest, walk the most or drop the most weight. During the 100-day challenge, competitors logged onto a private, Facebook-like social network to share results and cheer each other on. To get employees to participate, the 256-bed hospital offered $150 to each member of the winning team and $500 to the employee who shed the most pounds. All told, 56 teams signed up, about 37 percent of the staff. In the end, though, it wasn't the money that drew the workers in. It was the online camaraderie, and the challenge. "People wanted to be on the winning team," says Julie McGovern, Chilton's vice president of administration and HR.

Experiences like Chilton's are playing out across the country as companies rebuild their employee wellness programs on Internet-based social networks that are equal parts health journal, fitness challenge and online support group.

Companies hope the programs will curb escalating costs for health care benefits. In 2008, the first year American Financial Group, or AFG, ran a social media-based walking program through vendor *WalkingSpree,* the insurance company saved $9.27 in employee health care costs for every $1 spent on the program. The insurance company's health care premiums stayed flat that year because employees were healthier, according to a testimonial from AFG, which continues to use the program.

Aside from cutting costs, online-based wellness applications can help retain talent. The programs generally make employees feel better about themselves, and by extension, with the place they work, so they'll stick around longer.

"Employers are starting to recognize that incorporating elements of social media into a wellness program can boost participation and engagement and help create that buzz and culture around health and wellness that traditional engagement" methods aren't generating, says Kristie Howard, a vice president at *Longfellow Benefits,* a Boston-based benefits consultant.

Social wellness games represent a confluence of some of today's most significant online and workplace trends. One of the biggest is "gamification," or adding gamelike features to software and other business processes to make them more fun and engaging. Technology analyst Gartner Group predicts that by 2014, *70 percent* of the 2,000 largest companies in the world will use at least one "gamified" enterprise software application.

With more companies using internal social networks such as Yammer and Socialtext to improve workforce collaboration, *replace email* or streamline other aspects of work, it's easing the way for workplaces to adopt Internet-based platforms for wellness games and challenges. When wellness tech vendor *ShapeUp Inc.* polled 351 U.S. corporate wellness executives this spring, 56 percent said that they were using some type of online competition or challenge, and another 40 percent were considering it. "It's a natural migration for wellness programs," says Shawn LaVana, ShapeUp's marketing vice president.

Like other tech innovations that started out as consumer products before migrating to the world of work, many social wellness services had their roots in the personal health care apps that appeared after the iPhone and other smartphones became commonplace. Software as a Service-based internal networks such as ShapeUp let employees chart their progress toward losing weight or getting fit, or to record their standings in team or group challenges. Others such as Walkingspree work with pedometers or other devices that employees wear while working out, and then plug into a PC to download data to an online fitness journal.

As more employees bring smartphones to work, it has become easier for employers to offer wellness games and other social media-based content that can be accessed from a mobile device or laptop or desktop computers. But apps don't have to be that sophisticated. Employees can use ShapeUp, for example, to receive fitness-related text messages on a standard cellphone, a selling point for companies with large contingents of blue-collar workers who don't or can't use a smartphone on the job.

Enough companies are interested that industry organizations, such as the Society for Human Resource Management, are holding sessions on social media-based wellness programs at various 2012 annual conferences.

Although some companies stick to Facebook and Twitter or corporate blogs for wellness tips and to promote challenges, more employers are paying monthly or yearly subscription fees to outside vendors to run online programs for them.

To run its social wellness program, Chilton chose *Keas,* a 4-year-old online game platform co-founded by the former head of the now shuttered Google Health. The platform lets employees create profiles, share updates to a Facebook-like news feed, take online health quizzes and keep tabs on their teams and challenges. Wellness program managers use the platform to generate reports on participation, physical activity and other statistics.

During the hospital's first 100-day challenge, 336 employees used the platform to track losing an aggregate 1,230 pounds, eating 8,918 additional servings of fruit and vegetables and putting in 1,274 extra days of exercise, according to McGovern, the facility's administration and HR vice president. "It wasn't just exercise and eating better," she says. "People made a commitment to stop smoking, take stress management classes and control ongoing diseases."

The hospital's already committed to hosting two more challenges this year. But it will take time for the program to affect the hospital's bottom line. To gauge that impact, Chilton is doing free biometric screenings—height, weight, blood pressure, cholesterol and body mass index—once every six months for employees who participate in the challenges. "Because if people can keep the weight off, it will ultimately be a positive thing," for them and the company, McGovern says.

Elsewhere, reception of the new generation wellness programs has been strong. In ShapeUp's survey, 75 percent of companies offering some type of online fitness challenge said it had improved employees' perception of their corporate wellness program, and 71 percent said employees were using more wellness resources because of the programs. "It's getting people to take ownership of their health," says Fran Melmed, an employee wellness communications consultant who conducted the survey for ShapeUp.

For some companies, social wellness programs are already paying off. Sprint Nextel Corp. *estimates it saved approximately $1.1 million* through a companywide fitness challenge launched in 2011 as employees' healthier lifestyles led to fewer medical claims. In the company's first 12-week Sprint Get Fit Challenge, run by ShapeUp and benefits provider OptumHealth, about 16,000 employees in teams of up to 11 lost a collective 41,000 pounds, took more than 4.8 billion steps and logged nearly 22 million exercise minutes, according to the company.

Other employers and social wellness vendors are still calculating the return on investment such products can have. Traditional wellness programs such as Weight Watchers have a head start because of their longevity, Melmed says, but new vendors are taking steps to quantify how well their programs work. ShapeUp and Healthways Inc.'s *MeYou Health,* for example, are doing studies to compile hard data, she says.

A weight-loss study that ShapeUp conducted in 2009 is one of the first analyses of online-based employee-wellness programs to be published in a peer-reviewed medical or scientific journal. The results are based on data from 3,330 overweight or obese people in 987 teams that completed a 12-week online challenge. The results, published online in March by *Obesity,* a research journal, support the theory that online programs that let people work out with teammates can help workers lose weight, according to the report.

Despite the advantages social wellness programs offer, some employees worry about their personal information being compromised, says Howard of Longfellow Benefits who helped start the *Worksite Wellness Council of Massachusetts* last year. Howard isn't aware of any breaches, "but due to the potential for issues with HIPAA privacy,

social media is an area employers and wellness vendors should approach cautiously," she says. Also to avoid privacy issues, social wellness product vendors are being careful to use their platforms to share health and wellness information but not dispense personalized health care advice, Howard says.

Melmed agrees. "Employers should look to insurers and other third parties to help them expand their programs with sensors or devices," she says. "That way the employer gets a better sense of movement, activity or engagement but doesn't get into how many steps Suzy or Jack took today. It makes for an easier, cleaner message to the employee as well."

It may be easy to get employees excited about an eight- or 10-week weight-loss challenge or a one-time companywide biometric screening. But for long-term success, social media-based programs need to be part of a larger commitment, wellness experts say.

In addition to online challenges, a wellness program has to foster ongoing discussion of healthy lifestyles, whether through a digital network, blog, e-newsletter or old-fashioned print materials, says Jennifer Benz, founder of a San Francisco-based employee wellness communications consultancy. Companies also need to offer a healthy work environment, one with fitness facilities, nutritious options in the cafeteria and a culture that doesn't prize overtime at the expense of its employees' well-being, says Benz, who partnered with wellness application vendor Limeade on a wellness app platform called *Limeade GreenLine.* "You have to address all those structure things that get in the way of people achieving their optimal health," she says.

Chilton Hospital has taken that advice to heart. Since that first 100-day challenge a year ago, the hospital put a walking path around campus and organized walking groups and a hiking club. McGovern scaled back the prizes she's offering for signups and winners because workers no longer need as much persuading.

McGovern says she believes that the combination of the online wellness challenge, biometric screenings and running a separate disease management program will eventually help the hospital cut health care costs. The social media wellness campaign is a major part of that, especially because so many of the facility's employees who don't sit at a desk all day can use it. And they are—everyone from nurses to the cleaning crew and cafeteria staff. "They're finding ways to use it on their breaks, or on their smartphones at home," she says. "To have so many people participating, it shows you how much they want to do it."

Critical Thinking

1. Evaluate the potential of using social media software to encourage weight loss and the adoption of healthy lifestyles.

2. Define gamification. Explain how gamification can be used in corporate wellness programs.

3. Summarize the wellness program developed by Chilton Hospital in New Jersey.

MICHELLE V. RAFTER is a Workforce Management contributing editor.

UNIT 2
Childhood Nutrition

Unit Selections

Learning Outcomes

After reading this unit, you will be able to:

- Explain the state of nutrition, dietary intake, eating behavior, and physical activity among U.S. children.

- Summarize the condition of the "food environment" in the United States. Explain why many health professionals refer to our food environment as toxic to the health of U.S. children.

- Identify the nutrients that are commonly consumed in inadequate amounts in the diet of U.S. children.

- Describe how families and teachers can improve food behavior of kids during lunch or snack time.

- Develop recommendations of how families can effectively impact the nutrition and health of their children.

- Summarize how the federal school lunch program has changed since it was formed in 1946.

- Evaluate the nutrition standards set by the Healthy, Hunger-Free Kids Act for meals served in the National School and Breakfast programs. Critique the breakfast and lunch standards.

- Describe the effects of the federal law passed in 2004 regarding vending in schools.

- Describe reasons children are at greater risk of harm from exposure to agricultural chemicals.

- Critique the association between pesticide exposure and neurobehavioral conditions in children.

Student Website
www.mhhe.com/cls

Internet References

Centers for Disease Control and Prevention—Obesity Trends
www.cdc.gov/obesity/data/trends.html
Centers for Disease Control and Prevention—Healthy Youth
www.cdc.gov/healthyyouth/obesity
Food Science and Human Nutrition Extension
www.fshn.uiuc.edu
U.S. Dept. of Health and Human Services
http://aspe.hhs.gov/health/reports/child_obesity
U.S. Dietary Guidelines
www.cnpp.usda.gov/DGAs2010-DGACReport.htm

According to the Centers for Disease Control, childhood obesity has more than tripled in the past 30 years. In the United States 20 percent of 6- to 11-year-olds and 18 percent of 12 19-year-olds are considered obese and 30 percent of U.S. children are considered overweight. Because of this, childhood obesity has gained much needed attention in the media and in health and political arenas.

The Let's Move initiative prompted a task force on childhood obesity prevention. This task force derived 70 recommendations for government, healthcare, communities, schools, and families to take action against childhood obesity in the United States. A goal of reducing the childhood obesity rate from 17 percent to 5 percent by 2030 was set by the task force.

Recent data from the National Health and Nutrition Examination Survey (NHANES) indicates that typical diet eaten by children is below recommendations for vitamins and minerals and above recommendations for added sugar and saturated fat. Foods that are commonly marketed to children are often high in calories with low nutrient density. Excess calories contribute to children being overweight and diets of low nutrient density may impact learning and behavior, resistance to viruses and disease, and dental caries.

Data from 2008 NHANES indicates that 90 percent of children over eight years old do not eat the recommended servings of vegetables and 75 percent consume less than recommended amounts of fruit. Over 50 percent of boys aged 9–18 years and 90 percent of girls do not consume the recommended amount of dairy. The outcome of this results in diets low in calcium, potassium, fiber, and vitamin's A, C, D, and E among many other micronutrients.

Major changes in the diet of U.S. children were first noticed in the 1977 NHANES data. Shifts in beverage consumption from milk to sugar sweetened drinks, higher daily consumption of calories, snacking on "junk food," and more food eaten outside of the home were all documented by NHANES over 35 years ago.

Overweight and obese children often mature into unhealthy adults who are plagued by obesity-related chronic diseases such as heart disease, diabetes, gallbladder disease, osteoarthritis, and some cancers. Obesity related chronic diseases burden our current healthcare system and government-supported healthcare reimbursement programs with exorbitant costs, which is adding to the national debt and bankrupting our country.

The most cost-efficient and effective method of action to curtail childhood obesity is in prevention of the condition. A great deal of funding and resources are devoted in an attempt to curtail the childhood obesity epidemic in the United States. Efforts are being focused on the environmental factors, improving the quality of foods available to kids, and increasing physical activity. This unit concentrates on environmental factors such as the impact of parents and teachers as role models for proper nutrition and the quality of foods served in schools.

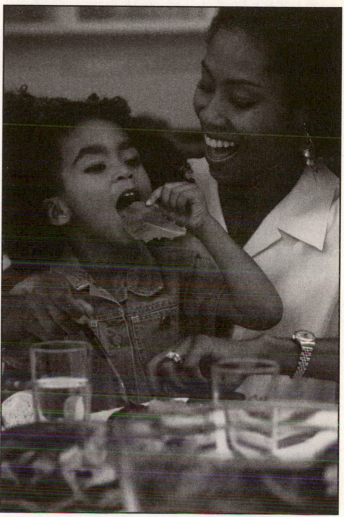

© Rolf Bruderer/Blend Images LLC

The recent passage of the Healthy, Hunger-Free Kids Act has prompted the USDA to modify the standards for the National School Lunch and Breakfast programs. The new standards for schools that participate in the federal program that supports free and reduced price breakfasts and lunches are addressed in the article written by Nirvi Shah, "Ultimate Food Fight Erupts as Feds Recook School Lunch Rules." Schools who participate in the National School Lunch and Breakfast program are now required to put the new guidelines in place in their schools.

When the school food policies were tightened, thousands of vending companies fled the school vending market, leaving room for new concepts in healthy vending options. Nick Lieber focuses on some of the changes seen in the school vending market in the article, "Junk Food-Free Vending Machines Go to School."

Another hot topic in childhood nutrition is the effect of agricultural chemicals from fruits and vegetables on the health of young children. Recent research is supportive of a possible connection between chemicals in foods and attention, cognition, behavior, and sensory issues in children, particularly ADHD.

The articles in Unit 2 were compiled to demonstrate different views of nutrition that impact the health of children, particularly childhood obesity. Many of the articles provide solutions to the problem; however, solving the obesity epidemic in the United States is a challenging task. The problem is multifactorial and took decades to occur. The solutions, which will essentially be a change in our entire societal culture, will also have to be multifactorial and will take years to see marked results. The articles in this unit can be used as supplemental information for topics on childhood nutrition and the obesity epidemic.

The State of Family Nutrition and Physical Activity

Are We Making Progress?

AMERICAN DIETETIC ASSOCIATION AND AMERICAN DIETETIC ASSOCIATION FOUNDATION

Executive Summary

Ten years ago, the U.S. Surgeon General released a landmark report: "The Call to Action to Decrease and Prevent Overweight and Obesity." The Surgeon General warned that, if overweight and obesity were not controlled, the number of obesity-related deaths would soon surpass the number of tobacco-related deaths.[1] This news caught the nation's attention and led to many public and private efforts targeting two of the root causes of overweight and obesity: poor nutrition and lack of physical activity.

The Surgeon General's report, and many subsequent government and science-based institutions' reports, called for changes in five key areas: communities and families, schools, healthcare, worksites and media. As these reports have concluded, poor nutrition and inactivity stem from many factors deeply rooted in our culture, factors that have become part of the societal norm. Changes will not necessarily come quickly and will require ongoing, vigilant attention from public and private sectors.[2]

In a major step to drive changes further, First Lady Michelle Obama launched the Let's Move! initiative, and the White House convened a Task Force on Childhood Obesity Prevention. In May 2010, the task force released 70 recommendations for childhood obesity prevention and announced the goal of reducing the childhood obesity rate from the current 17 percent to 5 percent by 2030.[3] The recommendations for government, healthcare, communities, schools and families help to focus resources, and the Let's Move! campaign brings the vital momentum required to keep prevention efforts moving forward.

Over the past decade, the American Dietetic Association (ADA) and its Foundation (ADAF) committed resources toward efforts to treat, reduce and prevent childhood over weight and obesity. This commitment is further strengthened now with the launch of *Kids Eat Right,* a platform designed to ensure that sound nutrition recommendations are part of childhood obesity prevention. A member-driven public education campaign, *Kids Eat Right* mobilizes ADA's 71,000 members to support families, schools and communities in their pursuit of quality nutrition for all children—especially for our most at-risk populations.

With all of this exciting momentum, we must also give care and consideration to actions taken and messages sent regarding food and nutrition. It is critical that nutrition policies and practices take a total diet approach that supports all the foods required for optimal growth and development. An inadequate amount of food or lack of nutrient-dense foods may negatively affect children's health today and disease prevention for the future.[4] Without daily consumption of foods providing the necessary nutrients, children are at risk for iron-deficiency anemia, poor academic performance, development of psychosocial difficulties and an increased likelihood of developing chronic diseases such as heart disease, diabetes and osteoporosis during adulthood.[5]

Nutrition policies and practices need a total diet approach supporting eating patterns that provide nutrients required for normal growth and development.

Kids Eat Right **is designed to ensure that sound nutrition recommendations are part of childhood obesity prevention. This initiative mobilizes the American Dietetic Association's 71,000 members to support families, schools and communities in their pursuit of quality nutrition for all children— especially for our most at-risk populations.**

Review of recent food consumption data from the National Health and Nutrition Examination Survey (NHANES) indicates that there are gaps between children's recommended and actual intake of key nutrients, gaps that sadly are the same as ten years ago, despite increasing efforts to close them.[6,7,8] Along with low intake of vitamins and minerals, these data show higher-than-recommended consumption of sugar and saturated fat. The consumption of sweetened beverages, desserts and snack foods adds calories without necessary nutrients and may also displace the eating of nutrient-dense foods, resulting in a negative effect on the quality of kids' diets and their nutritional status.[9,10] Failure to address these nutritional gaps puts the nation at risk of raising a generation of children who suffer negative consequences to their social and physical well-being regardless of their weight.

We must assess, re-calibrate and redouble our efforts to address children's total nutrient needs while promoting healthy weights. *Kids Eat Right* recognizes the powerful role that registered dietitians can play in this effort. With a unique blend of skills and knowledge, dietitians can balance the concurrent needs of normal growth and development along with prevention of chronic illnesses.

This report outlines the premise behind *Kids Eat Right* and highlights the eating and activity habits of families and subsequent nutritional gaps or deficiencies in kids' eating patterns. A newly released survey conducted by the ADAF—the *Family Nutrition and Physical Activity Survey* of children and their parents—reveals that families have made changes since the initial survey in 2003 and are ready to make more changes. The child-parent pairs were asked the same questions to determine if parents were aware of behaviors and if they connected with children's views. Obviously, being aware of eating and activity habits is the starting point; without that, change cannot occur. The survey provides insight into eating and activity behaviors and can help to explain why kids' diets are inadequate in key nutrients. Kids are not always eating three meals a day and eat many times throughout the day. This is reflected in the NHANES data that documents kids' snack foods are often high in calories without necessary nutrients; this may lead to unhealthy weights in kids.[11,12] Importantly, the survey indicates that there are many opportunities for positive change. By building on children's and parents' desire to eat healthy and be active—and by identifying drivers of positive habits— solutions to the chronic problems associated with under-nourishment, inactive lifestyles and unhealthy weights can be more successful.

The time is now. With communities across America focused on the issue, with the Let's Move! initiative in place and with children and their parents showing a new stage of readiness for change, this is the time to help *Kids Eat Right*.

Are We Making Progress?

The December 2001 Surgeon General's report made headlines: it found that 13 percent of 6- to 11-year-old children and 14 percent of 12- to 19-year-olds were obese (at that time, the terminology was overweight).[1] Since then, information about obesity and two of the primary causes—poor nutrition and inactivity—has been regularly in the news. Although researchers say the rapid rise in obesity is leveling off, nearly a decade later 17 percent of 2- to 19-year-olds are obese, with the highest prevalence among Mexican American boys (27 percent) and African American girls (29 percent).[13,14]

Since 1980 when the first Dietary Guidelines for Americans were released, there have not been the types of improvements in the diets of Americans as hoped for by health professionals working as advisors on the Guidelines.[15] The aim of the Guidelines is to provide advice about how good dietary habits can promote health and decrease risk for major chronic disease.[16] The messages have been generally consistent: Americans have been called upon to maintain a healthy weight, to limit sugar, sodium and saturated fat and to eat plenty of fruits, vegetables, whole grains and low-fat and fat-free dairy foods. Unfortunately, the majority of children do not meet the recommended servings from the five food groups, and adults consume below recommended intake on four or more nutrients.[17]

In light of these trends, this *Kids Eat Right* report examines the state of family nutrition and physical activity using data from the National Health and Nutrition Examination Survey (NHANES 2005–2006, 2007–2008),[17,18] statistics from the Centers for Disease Control and Prevention 2009 Youth Risk Behavior Surveillance Survey[19] and new findings from the American Dietetic Association Foundation's (ADAF) *Family Nutrition and Physical Activity Survey*. Conducted initially in 2003 and again in 2010, the ADAF survey assesses children's attitudes and behaviors related to nutrition and physical activity and parents' understanding

Family Nutrition and Physical Activity Survey Methodology

The American Dietetic Association Foundation Family Nutrition and Physical Activity Survey was developed to gain a better understanding of factors related to healthy weights. The survey explored children's attitudes and behaviors regarding nutrition, eating habits and physical activity, as well as parents' awareness of their children's attitudes and behaviors.

The survey was first fielded in January 2003 to 615 pairs of children and parents representative of the U.S. population. In 2010, the survey instrument was amended to include new content domains based on results from an environmental scan, literature review on factors related to childhood obesity and prevention as well as information and insights gained from focus groups conducted in spring 2009 with parents (low-income white, Hispanic, African American, men and women) and their children of middle-school age (boys and girls).[20] Changes to the survey instrument included adding questions about potential drivers of healthful behaviors and the role of registered dietitians. Nearly two-thirds of the original questions were repeated in the 2010 survey.

Knowledge Networks, a custom survey research company, administered the 2003 and 2010 surveys. Beginning in 1999, Knowledge Networks recruited and established the first online research panel through probability-based sampling. Panel members were randomly recruited through random-digit dialing and address-based sampling methods and were representative of the entire U.S. population. To cover both online and offline populations, households were provided with access to the Internet and hardware if needed.

The most recent survey was administered online in February 2010 to three population samples of youth aged 8 to 17 and their parents. The population samples included 754 pairs of children and parents who are representative of the U.S. population, 230 Hispanic pairs and 209 African American pairs. The participants were randomly selected from Knowledge Networks' panel, and the survey was offered in English or Spanish.

A sample of 420 white child-adult pairs taken from the 754 pairs in the U.S. population sample was used to assess differences between white, Hispanic and African American child-adult pairs. For analysis by race and income, income brackets were matched to the USDA's nutrient data. "Low" income includes household incomes below $25,000, "medium" income includes household incomes between $25,000 and $74,999, and "high" income includes household incomes of $75,000 or more.

of and connectedness to their children's behaviors. (See sidebar for more information on the ADAF survey.)

What Kids Are Not Eating

At the same time that many children are overweight or obese, many children have diets that are deficient in one or more nutrients, leaving them in a state of under-nutrition, or malnourishment.[21] Data from the National Health and Nutrition Examination Survey (NHANES) from 2007–2008 indicate that 90 percent of children over 8 years of age do not consume recommended servings of vegetables and that 75 percent consume less than recommended amounts for fruits. For milk and milk products, more than 50 percent of boys aged 9 to 18 years and over 90 percent of girls do not consume recommended amounts.[21] The grain group now distinguishes between refined and whole grain foods, and while all kids exceed recommended servings for refined grains, 95 percent do not consume the recommended amount of whole grains. Lastly, consumption of meat, poultry, fish, eggs, soy products, nuts and seeds is low for 75 percent of girls aged 9 to 18 years, while other kids meet or exceed recommended servings.[21]

At the same time that many children are overweight or obese, many children have diets that are deficient in one or more nutrients, leaving them in a state of under-nutrition, or malnourishment.

The 2010 Advisory Committee to the Dietary Guidelines for Americans is concerned about the food kids do *not* eat. Because kids do not consume recommended amounts of core food groups, their diets are low in Vitamin D, calcium, potassium and dietary fiber.[21] Eighty percent of girls and 75 percent of boys ages 4 to 18 have inadequate intake of calcium, and nearly half of all kids' diets are deficient in Vitamin D. The low intake of vegetables, whole grains and fruits is evident in the inadequate consumption of dietary fiber and potassium by 95 percent of all kids.[21] This is not a new problem. Over the past decade, children's eating patterns have been markedly low in vitamins A, C, D and E.[22,23,24]

Poor eating habits not only contribute to unhealthy weights, but negative effects from poor nutrition may also include learning and behavior problems, lowered immunity or resistance to colds and flu and dental caries.[4,5] These nutrition-related problems can affect children's academic achievement due to missed days of school, poor classroom behavior and diminished ability to concentrate and problem solve.[25,26,27] Chronic under-nutrition and/or not eating breakfast before going to school (or work) can have a negative effect on problem solving and other cognitive tasks.[28,29] A review of studies linking nutrition and learning found that even a well-nourished child who misses breakfast could have diminished problem-solving capacity to a degree that lowers test scores.[30]

The State of Childhood Overweight and Obesity

According to the National Health and Nutrition Examination Survey (NHANES), prevalence of overweight and obesity has doubled among 2- to 11-year-olds and tripled among 12- to 19-year-old adolescents.

Among children surveyed in NHANES 2003–2006, 16 percent of 2- to 19-year-old children and teens were obese, with body mass index (BMI) levels at or above the age and gender-specific 95th percentile, and almost one-third were over-weight or obese, with BMI levels at or above the 85th percentile.

Based on 2007–2008 NHANES data, obesity is more prevalent among Hispanic males aged 6 to 19 years (27 percent) than among non-Hispanic white (18 percent) and non-Hispanic African American (19 percent) males in that same age group. For females, obesity is more prevalent among non-Hispanic African American females (26 percent) than among non-Hispanic white females (16 percent). No significant differences in prevalence of overweight by race and ethnicity were observed among either males or females aged 6 to 19 years.[31]

Weight Status	Percentile Range
Underweight	Less than the 5th percentile
Healthy weight	5th percentile to less than the 85th percentile

Weight Status	Percentile Range
Overweight	85th percentile to less than the 95th percentile
Obese	*Equal to or greater than the 95th percentile*

Definition of Overweight and Obesity

For children and adolescents (aged 2 to 19 years), the BMI value is plotted on the CDC's growth charts to determine the corresponding BMI-for-age percentile.

- Overweight is defined as a BMI at or above the 85th percentile and lower than the 95th percentile.
- Obesity is defined as a BMI at or above the 95th percentile for children of the same age and sex.

These definitions are based on the 2000 CDC Growth Charts for the United States and expert committee. A child's weight status is determined based on an age- and sex-specific percentile for BMI rather than by the BMI categories used for adults. Classification of overweight and obesity for children and adolescents are age- and sex-specific because children's body composition varies between boys and girls and by age.

For more information, see Prevalence of Obesity Among Children and Adolescents: United States, Trends 1963–1965 Through 2007–2008 *by Cynthia Ogden, Ph.D., and Margaret Carroll, M.S.P.H., Division of Health and Nutrition Examination Surveys (www.cdc.gov/mmwr/preview/mmwrhtmlmm5940a7.htm).*

What Kids Are Eating

Most children and teens eat enough calories, and some eat more calories than needed for their activity level, which could lead to unhealthy weight gain. The majority of kids, whether at a healthy weight or not, are not eating the right foods—those foods that provide "quality calories." The NHANES survey of 1977–1978 and 2001–2002 identified, major changes in food and drink choices during this period of time; these changes coincided with increases in weight in all age-sex categories. Children shifted from drinking milk to high-sugar drinks and ate more foods that were higher in calories yet lower in nutrients.[9] More kids now eat food from outside the home, and daily snacking has increased, with calories in the snacks increasing as well. As noted above, consumption of the food groups kids need more of did not increase over this period.[21,23,24]

Foods that provide the most calories in children's diets are also high in solid fats and/or added sugar. In fact, about one-third of total calories consumed by 2- to 18-year-old U.S. children and adolescents come from the intake of solid fats and added sugars that are commonly viewed as nutrient-poor calories. Grain-based desserts, such as cakes, cookies, donuts, pies, cobblers and granola bars, are the largest source of calories for adults and kids, without contributing any important nutrients.[9,10,21]

The shift toward consumption of sweetened beverages, desserts and snack foods is a major contributor to daily calorie intake without contributing valuable nutrients.[10,21,32] Substituting nutrient-dense foods, such as vegetables, fruits, low-fat and nonfat dairy and non-dessert whole grain foods, would benefit calorie balance and diet quality.

The chart on page 32 lists foods that represent the largest source of calories from sugar in kids' diets. The results vary slightly by race/ethnicity and income levels but are generally consistent among all groups of kids.[32] Dominating the list are soda/energy/sports drinks, which contribute nearly one-third of the calories in children's diets.[21,32]

Foods that provide the most calories from saturated fat include the grain-based desserts (11 percent calories from solid fat), regular cheese (8 percent), sausage, franks, ribs and bacon (together 7 percent), pizza (6 percent), French fries (6 percent) and dairy-based desserts (5 percent). Kids ages 14 to 18 get more solid fat calories from French fries and beef.[9,10,21] The Advisory Committee recommends that no more than 5 percent to 15 percent of total

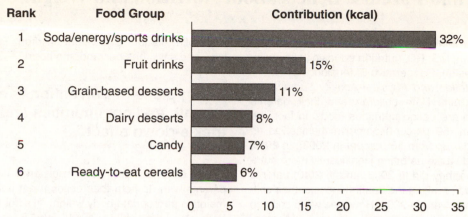

Percent Contribution of Foods to Calories from Added Sugar in Kids' Diets

Rank	Food Group	Contribution (kcal)
1	Soda/energy/sports drinks	32%
2	Fruit drinks	15%
3	Grain-based desserts	11%
4	Dairy desserts	8%
5	Candy	7%
6	Ready-to-eat cereals	6%

Source: Mean Intake of Added Sugar & Percentage Contribution (kcal) of Various Foods Among US Children & Adolescents, by Race/Ethnicity & Family Income, NHANES 2005-06. National Cancer Institute. See http://riskfactor.cancer.gov/diet/foodsources/added_sugars/table4a.html. Accessed Oct. 11, 2010.

calories come from solid fats and added sugar to allow for more nutrient-dense foods and maintain caloric balance.

To both meet recommended nutrients and limit added sugar and solid fat, major changes to eating patterns will be required. Changing the foods kids eat requires attention to taste-appeal. Because taste drives eating habits, modifying favorite foods to improve kids' total diet is a key prevention strategy, especially when those preferred foods are also a good source of nutrition. For example, popular "kids foods" like pizza and whole milk provide Vitamin D, calcium and potassium, although because kids eat these at higher frequency, they are also a source of saturated fat. Reduced-fat and fat-free alternatives to whole milk are available, and many school lunch programs now serve pizzas made with whole grain crusts and lower fat cheese. On the other hand, some of the sources of saturated fat, like grain-based desserts, do not provide beneficial nutrients. Focusing on increasing the foods and drinks that supply missing nutrients could displace foods that provide a high amount of "nutrient-poor calories".[33]

The chronic nature of low nutrient consumption combined with higher intake of sugar and solid fats is cause for alarm. Poor nutrition from the over-consumption of foods high in calories and low in required nutrients can result in weight gain along with low nutrient intake. However, it is important to note that, whatever a child's weight, it is likely that the child is not consuming the recommended servings from all required food groups.[21,31]

Physical Activity Stagnates

Nutrition and physical activity are addressed simultaneously for healthy weights and overall health. As with nutrition, time kids spend being physically active and their fitness levels are important determinants of health;

higher fitness levels are also correlated with better moods, behaviors, concentration and learning.

The 2009 Youth Risk Behavior Surveillance Study (YRBSS) found that the percentage of high school students who had been physically active for a total of at least 60 minutes per day on seven days has not significantly changed in the past half decade.[19] In the 2005 YRBSS, only 18 percent of high school students were active at least 60 minutes on all seven days, and in 2009, 18 percent of students reported seven days of activity.[19] Additionally, the percentage of students who do not participate in 60 minutes of physical activity on any day decreased from 25 percent in 2005 to 23 percent in 2009, although this too was not statistically significant.[19]

Inactivity is just as important to monitor as activity. YRBSS data show a significant increase in the percentage of students using computers three or more hours a day for non-school work such as video games: 22 percent fit this description in 2003 while the figure increased to 25 percent in 2009.[19] Concurrent with this increase in computer time has been a significant decrease in the percentage of students who watch three or more hours per day of television, from 43 percent in the 1999 YRBSS to 33 percent in the 2009 YRBSS.[19] It may be that sedentary activities are traded one for another and that it is harder for youth to switch to being physically active on most, if not all, days of the week.

Similarly, the ADAF *Family Nutrition and Physical Activity Survey* finds mixed results to questions about physical activity. For example, between 2003 and 2010, there was a significant increase in the percentage of kids being physically active with their parents three or more days a week (from 16 percent in 2003 up to 31 percent in 2010). However, during the same time period, there also was a significant increase (from 57 percent in 2003 to 64

Children's and Parents' Beliefs about Nutrition and Weight

"In general, people think they eat better than they do." So says Gayle Coleman, MS, RD, nutrition educator, University of Wisconsin-Extension, Cooperative Extension.

The *Family Nutrition and Physical Activity Survey* confirms Coleman's claim. Both children and their parents report that children are eating nutritious foods. In fact, the majority of children (59 percent) perceive themselves as eating healthy foods (up from 46 percent in 2003). In 2010, kids rank their food intake as being significantly more nutritious (p <.001) than they did in 2003, and in 2010, parents are more aligned with ranking the healthfulness of their children's diets than they were in 2003. However, while children report that they are eating nutritious foods, studies demonstrate that children's diets have serious nutrient shortfalls.

Children also have misperceptions of their body size. Significantly more children in 2010 report being at the "right weight" than in 2003, with 22 percent of the surveyed children reporting that they are overweight, down from 32 percent in 2003. Registered Dietitians interviewed explained that many over-weight adults underreport their weight; this is happening with some kids too. The national data do not agree that kids are slimming down quite like kids tell us: over the 2003-2010 period, weight was still increasing, though in some categories it was starting to stabilize.[13, 14, 31]

These disconnects may reflect a shift in what is perceived as "normal" food intake and body weight. Because high-calorie, low-nutrient foods are more available than high-nutrient options, poor food choices have become the standard. At the same time, society in general has become desensitized to over-weight. Lucille Beseler, MS, RD, LD/N, CDE, president and founder of the Family Nutrition Center of South Florida, points out that television commercials now more often feature overweight children. Seeing overweight kids, she says, has become "the norm."

"A big piece of prevention is educating parents and communities and having the trickle-down effect."

Yet despite these gaps, registered dietitians find that parents want to help their children eat healthier foods and maintain appropriate body weight. "It's not that parents don't understand their child is overweight," Beseler says. "They're busy and overwhelmed without a lot of time or a lot of resources." Coleman agrees. People have a "general sense of what's healthy and what they should do," she says, but they may need help putting that information into action.

"Many, if not the majority of, parents want to know what they can do to improve their families' diets," says Beseler. This desire for greater nutrition literacy gives registered dietitians a real opportunity to help parents understand the most healthful food choices and recognize healthy weights.

"A big piece of prevention is educating parents and communities and having the trickle-down effect," Beseler remarked about her experiences working with families for over 20 years.

Parents are the behavior leaders at home, and as the Let's Move! initiative also calls for, we must empower parents to be the best role models possible. Registered dietitians can help to improve parents' self-efficacy by teaching skills and information essential for putting a balanced meal on the table. We need to help parents see the immediate benefits of eating and serving healthier options consistently.

---

percent in 2010) in the number of kids and parents spending time watching TV, viewing a movie or playing a video game together three or more days a week.

In 2010, the percentage of kids who played on a sports team or participated in group physical activity decreased a few percentage points, although not significantly (from 63 percent in 2003 to 60 percent in 2010). Also in 2010, there was an increase in the number of kids preferring outdoor activities to sedentary indoor activities (21 percent preferring out door activities in 2010 compared to 15 percent in 2003), although it was also not statistically significant. The *Family Nutrition and Physical Activity Survey* also finds that the percentage of children having 60 minutes of physical activity seven days a week was similar to the national YRBSS findings. The survey further finds that parents' knowledge of their kids' activity level is consistent with their children's self-report, with no differences by race: 17 percent white, 17 percent Hispanic and 16 percent African American kids report getting 60 minutes of activity daily.

Between 2003 and 2010, there was a significant increase in the percentage of kids being physically active with their parents, according to the *Family Nutrition and Physical Activity Survey* results.

Ready for Change

The *Family Nutrition and Physical Activity Survey* results provide a new level of confidence that changes are occurring and will continue to occur. Perhaps the most compelling survey finding is that children and their parents are at a different place in awareness and that they are even trying new behaviors, more so than they were in 2003.

When the *Family Nutrition and Physical Activity Survey* was first conducted in 2003, a primary aim was to understand the child-parent connection as it related to activity and eating attitudes and behaviors. The big news in 2003 was the disconnect that existed between parents and their children.

This year's survey results show a marked improvement in the parents' connection to eating and activity patterns for their kids. Child-parent pairs are much more aligned, showing an awareness that was not there in 2003. Changes in kids' behaviors cannot take place without parents being aware and making nutrition and activity important priorities for the family. There was statistically significant agreement in the child-parent pairs in 2010 on nearly every question. This alignment signals a shift in children's and parents' connectedness on these topics. This higher awareness relates to a new stage of "readiness" to make healthy changes.[36]

The "Stages of Change Model" is a framework that can help visualize the process or sequence of behavior states or stages that occur between not knowing there is a problem to a changed behavior that has now become a habit. This framework can help explain changes in population samples too. Until there is an awareness of a behavior—precontemplation—there is not a move forward.[36,37] Precontemplation moves to contemplation once there is an awareness of the problem.

The Family Factor

For youth to experience lasting changes in nutrition and physical activity, the entire family system needs to change.[38] Generational habits and behaviors can prevent change from happening, so it's important to have buy-in from the family system.[40] As such, slow and gradual changes usually are more effective. It is also important to identify which family behaviors can help meet the goals of healthy weights and quality nutrition.[38,39,40] Research over the past decade has identified child-parent interactions that can promote healthy or unhealthy weights.[38,39,40,41] Eating family meals at home has positive benefits, while eating away from home can have a negative effect on the quality of kids' diets.[42,43,44,45] Other positive effects on healthy eating habits are seen with regular daily routines and with children and parents spending time together.[46,47]

"Both parents and children are aware that there is a problem and that they need to be eating healthier and they're willing to think about eating healthier. I think this is a major step. In my experience over the decades in treating overweight children and their families, a lot of times the hardest thing is to move a person from a stage of inaction to a stage of contemplation, to saying 'Gee, maybe I want to do something.' I think that this is the opportunity for dietitians to help patients."

Nancy Copperman, MS, RD, CDN,
Director of Public Health Initiatives, North Shore Long Island Jewish Health System

"It seems like parents are more aware of what the kids are doing. And I think that's good. That's the first little mini-step into trying to do something differently."

Aida Miles, MMSc, RD, CSP, LD, CNSD,
Director of the Coordinated MPH Program,
Division of Epidemiology and Community Health,
University of Minnesota School of Public Health

More family meals

Many benefits are found in sharing meals as a family.[42,43,44,45] Studies of teens who regularly have meals with their families find that these teens are at lower risk of using drugs and that they experience better connectedness at home, enjoy improved mental health and exhibit better eating patterns, including higher consumption of fruits and vegetables.[46,47,48,49] Data indicate that when kids eat meals with their parents/families, without watching television, this meal time is an important opportunity for bonding and teaching good nutrition and eating behaviors.[42,44,49,50,51] The *Family Nutrition and Physical Activity Survey* finds a significant increase in family meals, with 73 percent of families eating at home daily in 2010 up from 52 percent of families in 2003. A closer look at 2010 data reveals significant racial/ethnic differences in the percentage of children eating with their parents at home daily. African American children (61 percent) eat dinner with their parents daily, significantly less often than white (72 percent) and Hispanic children (72 percent).

While the percentage of families eating dinner at home has increased since 2003, the percentage of children reporting that they eat out with their parents has remained constant and much less than the percentage eating at home. Children's and parents' responses to these questions are significantly correlated across all racial groups, indicating a high level of parental awareness and validation of children's responses in 2010.

Increase in regular routines

Another family factor correlated with healthy behaviors is the existence of family routines. Routines—or regular daily activities—are important in organizing daily life and reflect family characteristics.[41,46,47] Family routines, including regular family meals and regular bedtimes, are positively linked to multiple positive child outcomes, including academic achievement, self-esteem and both behavioral and psychosocial adjustment. Families that are organized and have predictable routines produce children with more positive outcomes.[46,47,52]

Changes Between 2003 and 2010: Percent of Children Reporting Behaviors

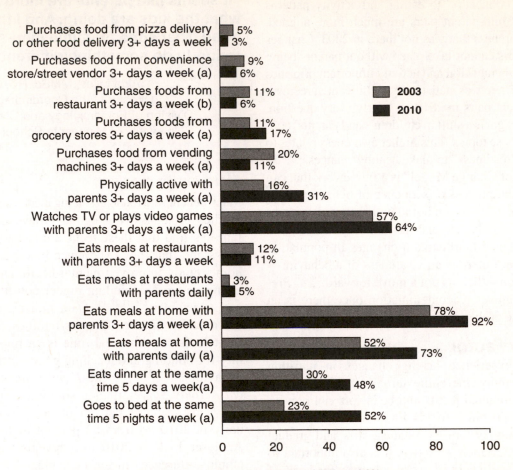

Purchases food from pizza delivery or other food delivery 3+ days a week: 2003 5%, 2010 3%
Purchases food from convenience store/street vendor 3+ days a week (a): 2003 9%, 2010 6%
Purchases foods from restaurant 3+ days a week (b): 2003 11%, 2010 6%
Purchases foods from grocery stores 3+ days a week (a): 2003 11%, 2010 17%
Purchases food from vending machines 3+ days a week (a): 2003 20%, 2010 11%
Physically active with parents 3+ days a week (a): 2003 16%, 2010 31%
Watches TV or plays video games with parents 3+ days a week (a): 2003 57%, 2010 64%
Eats meals at restaurants with parents 3+ days a week: 2003 12%, 2010 11%
Eats meals at restaurants with parents daily: 2003 3%, 2010 5%
Eats meals at home with parents 3+ days a week (a): 2003 78%, 2010 92%
Eats meals at home with parents daily (a): 2003 52%, 2010 73%
Eats dinner at the same time 5 days a week (a): 2003 30%, 2010 48%
Goes to bed at the same time 5 nights a week (a): 2003 23%, 2010 52%

a: Behaviors are different with statistical significance between 2003 and 2010, $p < 0.001$.
b: Behaviors are different with statistical significance between 2003 and 2010, $p < 0.05$.
Source: ADAF Family Nutrition and Physical Activity Survey, *2003 and 2010*

Percent of Kids Reporting Eating with Parents

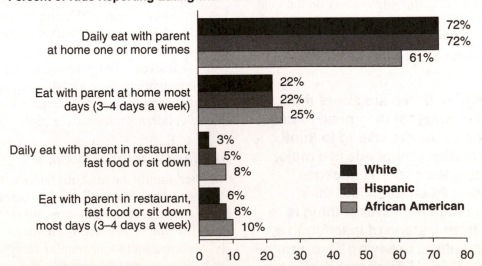

Daily eat with parent at home one or more times: White 72%, Hispanic 72%, African American 61%
Eat with parent at home most days (3–4 days a week): White 22%, Hispanic 22%, African American 25%
Daily eat with parent in restaurant, fast food or sit down: White 3%, Hispanic 5%, African American 8%
Eat with parent in restaurant, fast food or sit down most days (3–4 days a week): White 6%, Hispanic 8%, African American 10%

There are differences among races in the frequency of children and parents eating meals at home, with African Americans having meals together significantly less often than Hispanic and white parent-child pairs, $p < 0.05$.

Source: ADAF Family Nutrition and Physical Activity Survey, *2010*

Another family factor correlated with healthy behaviors is the existence of family routines. Routines—or regular daily activities—are important in organizing daily life and reflect family characteristics.

Many more children report eating dinner at or about the same time five nights a week in the 2010 *Family Nutrition and Physical Activity Survey* (48 percent) than they did in 2003 (30 percent). The 2010 survey also shows a significant increase in the percentage of children going to bed about the same time five nights a week; over 50 percent of kids in 2010 report regular bedtimes on all school nights compared to only 23 percent of children in 2003.

There are, however, racial differences observed in 2010 survey results. Significantly more white children report regular meal times five nights a week (52 percent) than do African American children (40 percent); the difference is not significant between white and Hispanic children at 48 percent. The 2010 survey also finds significantly more white children (55 percent) than Hispanic (46 percent) and African American (45 percent) children reporting regular bed time five days a week. But overall, daily routines are up—a step in the right direction for healthy eating habits and proper nutrition.[42,46,47]

More time together

Time parents spend with children is an important factor affecting children's health and nutrition for a variety of reasons.[51,52,53] Parents model behaviors, good or bad, and children in both the 2003 and 2010 surveys name their mothers as their number one role model and their fathers as number two. What parents eat, whether they value being physically active and whether they spend time with their children engaged in healthy behaviors—all are examples of positive, powerful role modeling that can shape children's eating and activity behaviors.[43] The quality of the time parents and children spend together is critical. As parents are stretched for time, they can convey all-important lessons by preparing meals with their children, shopping for foods and cleaning up after the meal.[46,47,52,53]

The good news is that, according to the *Family Nutrition and Physical Activity Survey* results, parents are spending time with their children. Children and parents enjoy activities together—such as eating and watching movies or TV—on a daily basis. The increase in parents spending time being physically active three or more days a week is sizable, moving from 16 percent in 2003 to 31 percent in 2010. However, as noted above, more children

and their parents are watching TV and playing video games together three or more days a week, a significant increase in this behavior from 2003 (57 percent of children and parents) to 2010 (64 percent).

Race and income have an effect on where children purchase foods, and the general decrease in poor purchase habits from 2003 to 2010 was not uniform across race and income levels.

Where and When Kids Eat

Despite the positive trends, there is still room for improvement. From skipping meals and frequent snacking to buying food and drinks from a variety of places, troubling patterns stand in the way of children consuming adequate nutrients. By understanding behaviors related to kids' eating and activity, decision makers, health professionals and families are better equipped to make changes that have an impact on the lives of children.

A recent U.S. Department of Agriculture (USDA) report concluded that foods eaten from fast food outlets, restaurants and other commercial sources negatively affect the quality of kids' diets.[45] The study shows that away-from-home eating increases caloric consumption and decreases dietary quality in kids aged 6 to 18.[45] Food consumption data from 2007–2008 show on average that one-third of children's calorie intake is away-from-home food; in 1977, it was less than one-fourth of calorie intake in children.[45,54,56] This is an area where educational efforts are necessary to help improve children's choices of away-from-home foods and beverages.[54]

The 2010 ADAF *Family Nutrition and Physical Activity Survey* indicates that parents and children are infrequently eating meals at restaurants. Survey results show that only 9 percent to 18 percent of children and parents eat away-from-home foods three or more days a week. A significant difference between 2003 and 2010 is the decrease in the percentage of kids buying food or drink from school vending machines and snack bars, convenience stores and restaurants. It is worth noting that the survey found a statistically significant increase in the percentage of kids buying from grocery stores three or more days per week, from 11 percent in 2003 to 17 percent in 2010. Purchase data are not available, making it unclear if an improvement in nutrition follows this trend. However, this is a sign that kids have access to nutrient-dense foods, and this could mean new opportunities for healthier snacking.

Race and income have an effect on where children purchase foods and the general decrease in poor purchase habits from 2003 to 2010 was not uniform across race and income levels. Significantly more African American children from low-income homes (less than $25,000 a year) report buying foods from vending and snack bars at school, convenience stores and restaurants. Low-income African American children buy food three or more days a week from pizza or other food delivery (22 percent), significantly more often than Hispanic children at all income levels (5–7 percent) and white children in medium- (1 percent) and high-income (2 percent) households.

Kids eat day and night

Meals aside, most kids report eating several times throughout the day. The majority of kids eat snacks after school at least some of the time (81 percent white, 88 percent Hispanic and 87 percent African American). Kids eat while watching TV, doing homework, playing computer games and talking on the phone; however, some kids do so more than others. African American children report snacking more often—while watching TV (significantly more than white children), while doing homework, while playing computer games, while talking on the phone (significantly more than white and Hispanic) and before bedtime (significantly more than Hispanic children).

Recently published data on kids' snacking patterns find that the overall quality of the diet, or nutrient density, lowers as snacking increases.[11,12,32] Foods eaten as snacks provide more sugar and saturated fat and fewer vitamins and minerals.[9,10,11,12] Since the late 1970s, the percentage of 12- to 19-year-olds who snack increased from 61 percent to 83 percent, the number of snacks increased from 1.0 to 1.7 snacks per day, and daily calories from snacks increased from 300 to 526.[12,57]

Three Square Meals a Day—Not Always

The meal kids skip most frequently is breakfast, probably the worst meal to miss given the connection between breakfast and learning and given that after a night's sleep immediate

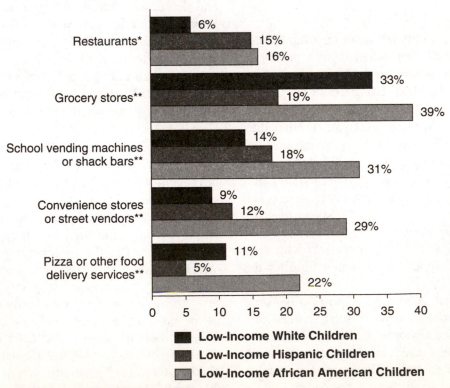

Percent of Low-Income Kids Purchasing Snacks and Meals
Kids purchase foods three or more days a week from the following places ...

- **Low-Income White Children**
- **Low-Income Hispanic Children**
- **Low-Income African American Children**

*Statistically significant differences by race, p < 0.05

* * Statistically significant differences by race, p < 0.001

Source: ADAF Family Nutrition and Physical Activity Survey, *2010*

Percent of Kids Eating All, Most or Some of the Time …

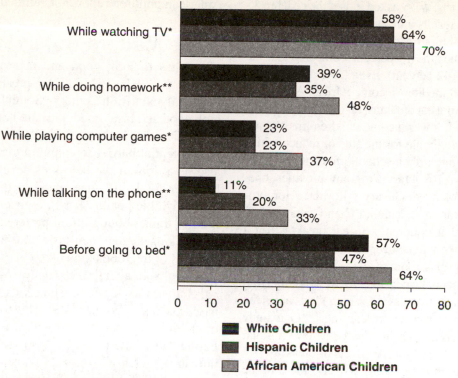

* Statistically significant differences by race, p < 0.05
" Statistically significant differences by race, p < 0.001
Source: ADAF Family Nutrition and Physical Activity Survey, 2010

"The *[Family Nutrition and Physical Activity]* study tells us that for children to eat healthier foods, they have to look and taste good. Schools have financial, time and other resource-related limitations. We need new approaches, such as partnerships with local restaurants, farmers, food producers and local dietetic associations, especially to address cultural preferences and nutritional issues of the children attending schools in those communities."

"For example, restaurateurs, chefs and registered dietitians in the community could help schools make culturally relevant tasty meals that also meet dietary guidelines for the children. Help in the area of food and nutrition has to be continuous if it is going to make a positive difference in the children's nutritional status and their acceptance of school foods."

Judith Rodriguez, PhD, RD, FADA, LDN, President, American Dietetic Association

"A lot of people only look at macronutrients when thinking about nutrient standards and stop there. They feel that if we meet our macronutrient goals, then the food is okay. I think the public needs to look at guidelines that are based on meeting micronutrient standards as well."

"In order to meet micronutrient and macronutrient standards, schools would then be supported in offering more fruits, vegetables and low-fat dairy products that are high in folic acid, Vitamin C, Vitamin A, calcium and fiber. One way of meeting this goal is to fund schools so that they can incorporate more whole foods into their menus."

Nancy Copperman, MS, RD, CDN, Director of Public Health Initiatives, North Shore Long Island Jewish Health System energy stores in the body are running low. The *Family Nutrition and Physical Activity Survey* asked kids if they eat breakfast all of the time and results indicate that many children do not do so. Significantly more African American children do not eat breakfast all of the time (59 percent) compared to white and Hispanic children (42 percent). Even higher numbers of low-income whites and medium-income African Americans (both at 67 percent) do not eat breakfast all of the time. It is of particular concern when lower income children miss breakfast, as many would be eligible for the free or reduced price School Breakfast Program if their school offered it.

The USDA School Breakfast Program provides one-fourth of the Recommended Dietary Allowance for protein, calcium, iron, Vitamin A, Vitamin C and calories.[58,59] Studies have shown that children who eat breakfast on a regular basis are less likely to be overweight.[58] Schools that provide breakfast in the classroom to all students have shown decreases in tardiness and suspensions as well as improved student behavior and attentiveness.[28] Which foods are eaten for breakfast also has an impact on learning.[60] One study showed that eating foods high in fiber and low in sugar helped students sustain the cognitive effects of breakfast.[61]

Children also have an opportunity to participate in the National School Lunch Program, which is available at most schools. While school lunch often gets a "bad rap," it offers the most nutritious foods available at school. The *Family Nutrition and Physical Activity Survey* results reveal that 44 percent of white children, 35 percent of Hispanic children and 25 percent of African American children do not eat from the school lunch line on most days. Kids report not eating school lunch because they "do not like what is served or how it tastes" (50 percent white, 59 percent Hispanic and 63 percent African American) or because "their parents want them to bring lunch from home" (56 percent white, 45 percent Hispanic and 37 percent African American). Of those not eating the school lunch, most bring their lunch from home (88 percent white, 70 percent Hispanic and 60 percent African American).

One of the few areas in which parents are disconnected from what their kids are doing is that of alternative lunch sources. For kids who do not eat from the school lunch line each day, African American children more than white or Hispanic children buy food from vending machines (27 percent) or from stores or restaurants close to school (29 percent). And of those African American children who do not eat lunch from the school lunch line, more than a third—34 percent—do not eat lunch at all.

Dinner is a meal many parents and kids say is their healthiest because it is eaten at home. Despite the high numbers reporting regular meal times and eating at home with parents, a good percentage of kids report they do not eat dinner all of the time: 22 percent of white children, 38 percent of Hispanic children and 34 percent of African American children report not eating dinner every night.

Taste Matters

"Food has to look good and taste good," says Lucille Beseler, MS, RD, LD/N, CDE, president and founder of the Family Nutrition Center of South Florida. "If it doesn't look good and taste good, kids are not going to eat it."

In other words, kids eat for taste. But while taste can be a potential barrier to eating nutrient-rich foods, it can also be a draw if we help kids develop a taste for these healthier foods. To meet kids' taste expectations while also providing healthy foods, registered dietitians say we need to think about cultural preferences, work gradually to help kids change their taste buds and prepare healthier versions of the foods kids like.

Again and again, the *Family Nutrition and Physical Activity Survey* found that kids eat—or don't eat—based on taste. When asked why they ate, the majority of children selected hunger and taste over other reasons. Eating "all of the time" because "food tastes good" significantly increased, from 23 percent in 2003 to 31 percent in 2010. Likewise, a majority of kids who don't eat from the school lunch line said they do not do so because they don't like how the school meal tastes. And an overwhelming majority of kids (89 percent white, 90 percent Hispanic and 94 percent African American) reported that they'd eat healthier foods if those foods tasted better.

However, trying to decipher what kids mean by "taste" can be challenging.

One key factor in taste is cultural preference, says Nancy Copperman, MS, RD, CDN, director of Public Health Initiatives at North Shore Long Island Jewish Health System. Kids are used to certain flavors that are associated with particular cultural foods. As we prepare school meals, she asks, "are we really bringing in the cultural foods that these particular ethnicities enjoy as taste?"

Just as they are accustomed to certain cultural flavors, kids also become accustomed to certain tastes from processed foods. "As we help kids shift to healthier foods with lower sugar and salt content," says Gayle Coleman, MS, RD, nutrition educator, University of Wisconsin-Extension, Cooperative Extension, "we need to realize that taste for many foods is acquired. Healthier foods, like vegetables, may not meet kids' taste needs initially, but they can learn to like them." Thus, change needs to be gradual.

When asked why they ate, the majority of children selected hunger and taste over other reasons.

Judith Rodriguez, PhD, RD, FADA, LDN, President, American Dietetic Association, notes that taste has always been an important factor. "It may be because of an increased availability of sweet and saltier foods that choice for those foods is impacted," she says. "If a child has a greater access to foods that are high in sugar, fat and sodium and also has preference for it, he or she is likely to select it. Over time, if other foods do not have that sweet and salty taste, they will not taste as good as what is now preferred. It is an interesting research question: does the taste take on greater significance because there is more choice? Also, how does the exposure to a variety of flavors and tastes impact choices and preferences? The data seem to indicate that it does, so early education and modeling are important."

Finally, it's important to give kids great-tasting, healthier versions of their favorite foods, argues Elizabeth M. Ward, MS, RD, nutrition consultant, mother of three and author of several books about feeding children. For example, Ward says, "Pizza is the number one food on kids' plates, and that's a good thing because pizza supplies several nutrients, such as protein, calcium and magnesium. However, there are ways to reduce the calories, total fat and saturated fat in pizza that preserve the important nutrients while better promoting good health."

As we work with cultural food preferences and help kids get used to new tastes and create healthier versions of kids' favorite foods, we need to remember that change won't come overnight, Copperman says. "It's kind of retraining the taste buds."

Perspectives from the Field

Registered dietitians from around the country were interviewed about their reactions to the *Family Nutrition and Physical Activity Survey*. These leading professionals reflected on the survey and shared their observations of the current nutrition environment.

People have general knowledge, but they need skills, techniques, tips they can use within their lifestyle. They need to know how to make changes that work with the way they live. The survey data on why children eat were striking relative to hunger and taste. Taste is always a primary factor, and it may seem more important because of greater access to tasty foods. The increase in hunger needs to be looked at because hunger is a physiological response, where taste or appetite is a sociological phenomenon because something looks, appealing.

Judith Rodriguez, PhD, RD, FADA, LDN, President, American Dietetic Association

We need strategies that are flexible enough to accommodate different types of families and culture.

Gaye Coleman, MS, RD, University of Wisconsin-Extension, Cooperative Extension

There seems to be a need and a readiness. Both parents and children have a new level of awareness that there is a problem and a willingness or desire to make changes. This is the opportune time for registered dietitians to help families.

Nancy Copperman, MS, RD, CDN, Director of Public Health Initiatives, North Shore Long Island Jewish Health System

A big piece of prevention is educating families and communities. All health professionals have to be saying the same thing when addressing healthy eating and healthy weights for children. It is imperative to find a way for registered dietitians to share their expertise while educating other professionals. This could be a vital role for dietitians—training other health professionals. Getting more dietitians into the community does require us to be innovative, creative educators. As part of my business, I have had great response to registered dietitians being part of sports events, health fairs and festivals. There are tremendous opportunities to reach parents where they are, even in health fairs in retail outlets.

Lucille Beseler, MS, RD, LD/N, CDE, President and Founder of the Family Nutrition Center of South Florida

Staying positive about healthy eating means focusing on what kids should include in their diets on a daily basis, rather than what to avoid. Taking that approach typically displaces high-calorie foods that offer little in the way of nutrients that kids need to grow and develop to their fullest potential. The data say that soda is the number one contributor of sugar in children's diets, yet flavored milks, which are often the nutritional scapegoat, don't even make the list of the top five sources. Any type of milk provides vital nutrients, including calcium, potassium and vitamin D, three nutrients that experts say kids do not get enough of. We want kids to drink milk, and their preference for flavored milk should be taken into consideration at home and at school.

Elizabeth M. Ward, MS, RD, Nutrition Consultant and Author

"The data say that soda is the number one contributor of sugar in children's diets, yet flavored milks, which are often the nutritional scapegoat, don't even make the list of the top five sources."

Elizabeth M. Ward, MS, RD,
Nutrition Consultant and Author

"Staying positive about healthy eating means focusing on what kids should include in their diets on a daily basis, rather than what to avoid."

Elizabeth M. Ward, MS, RD,
Nutrition Consultant and Author

We're looking at prevention and we're looking at what's going to make a difference 20 years from now, but we still have the now. Policy and environmental change efforts may be a bit longer term. We need short-term strategies that help parents or schools immediately too. Students are working with local grocery chains and chefs to collaborate in developing nutritious meals that match the weekly food sales; cooking demonstrations are given by the chef, and the student dietetic professionals walk people through the menu for that week.

Aida Miles, MMSc, RD, CSP, LD, CNSD, Director
of the Coordinated MPH Program, Division of
Epidemiology and Community Health, University
of Minnesota School of Public Health

Moving Forward: Opportunity Areas

The *Family Nutrition and Physical Activity Survey* finds several key "opportunity areas"—family habits and children's behaviors. Parents' increased connectedness with their children on wellness as well as parents' improved understanding and awareness of their children's behaviors signal a shift in "readiness" to change eating and physical activity habits. Additionally, the majority of children responded positively to approaches that would help them eat healthier.

Parents also responded positively toward seeing a registered dietitian to get help with making better food choices and preparing healthier meals for their children. These drivers to positive change should be at the forefront of efforts to educate, support and work with children and their parents to improve kids' healthy eating and activity habits.

Opportunity #1: Parent Power

The majority of children identified their parents as their number one role model, with mothers as the first choice and fathers as the second choice. If parents display healthful eating and activity habits themselves, children are likely to emulate those behaviors. Indeed, children say that it would help them eat healthier foods if their parents ate these foods at home, with significantly more Hispanic and African American children reporting that this would help them.

Parents have many opportunities to set a good example when it comes to healthy habits. According to the *Family Nutrition and Physical Activity Survey* results from 2010, parents spend time with their children in numerous ways and thus have many opportunities to have an impact on children's health behaviors, especially when they eat together. Despite the prevalent belief that children and parents do not eat at home any more, the 2010 survey shows that more than 80 percent of white, Hispanic and African American children and parents say they eat meals at home together at least three days a week. Families that eat at home daily comprise the largest segment of this group, with 72 percent of white and Hispanic children and 61 percent of African American children reporting eating at home with family at least once a day. Not only does eating together as a family lead to lower rates of overweight and obesity as well as higher quality, more nutrient-dense diets;[42] mealtimes are also an excellent time to demonstrate healthy eating choices. Even the away-from-home eating could be improved with education, especially the times, although infrequent, that parents and kids are eating out together.[40,43,45]

Kids name their parents as the number one role model. More than 70 percent of kids said that, if parents ate healthy at home, this would help them do the same.

Kids Who Say Their Number One Role Model Is . . .	White	Hispanic	African American
Their Mother	18 percent	23 percent	30 percent
Their Father	17 percent	18 percent	16 percent

Nearly all parents base purchases on nutrition, fat and calorie content. Parents report that health attributes are important determinants to foods brought home.

The *Family Nutrition and Physical Activity Survey* finds that, in the majority of households, mothers have primary responsibility for meals. Moreover, in their role as primary food preparer, mothers buy food for the family's meals and snacks. As the number one role model and primary meal provider, mothers have a great responsibility to model

Percent of Parents Finding Health Attributes as "Very Important" When Buying Food

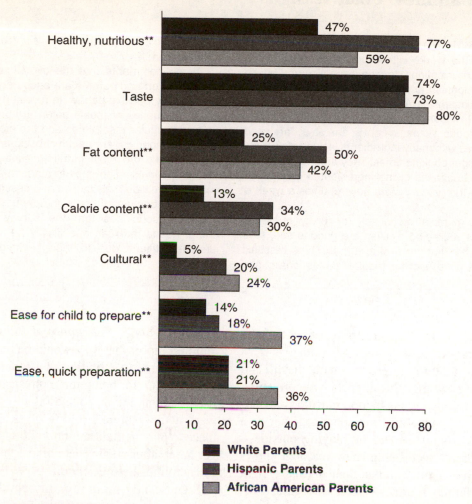

** Statistically significant differences by race, p < 0.001

Source: ADAF Family Nutrition and Physical Activity Survey, *2010*

healthy behaviors. Thus, working with mothers through nutrition and health education efforts should pay dividends in teaching healthy dietary habits to young people.

Parents play an especially important role as they make decisions about which foods to purchase—both for the nutrient quality of food that is available in the home and for the example they set as they select foods. Although not statistically different than others, more African American parents selected taste as a very important reason for buying foods. Parents have other "very important" reasons for purchasing foods, reasons that differ significantly by race (see chart on this page). For example, a significantly higher percentage of African American parents reported ease of preparation for their child and ease in general more than for white or Hispanic. Even more important to parents, however, are the health attributes of the foods they purchase, with significantly more Hispanic parents ranking the nutritious aspects of a food as a "very important" determinant. Similarly, fat and calorie

content is significantly less important to white parents than to Hispanic or African American parents—yet when combining responses for "somewhat important" and "very important," nearly all parents use nutrition, fat and calorie content to determine which foods are purchased.

Overall, parents have a powerful opportunity to model healthy behaviors for their children. Whether they're shopping for nutritious groceries or playing with their kids outside, parents set the tone for their families. Thus, parent education can be a key factor in improving children's healthy eating and activity habits.

Opportunity #2: The Rhythm of Family Routines

As noted throughout this report, children exhibit a range of healthy behaviors when their families observe regular routines.[46,47] When kids eat meals at home, when they eat with their parents regularly, when they spend time with their parents and when they go to bed at about

Hispanic Families: Positive Signs

Maria C. Alamo, MPH, RD, is president and founder of Salud Consulting Inc. She works with clients to develop culturally relevant communications, translate nutrition and health information into Spanish and develop recipes for nutritious meals for Hispanic families. Alamo explains that the primary characteristics of Hispanic meals are flavor, color and presentation of the foods. Hispanic cooks, she says, "are used to lengthier recipes with many ingredients including a variety of spices and longer cooking times. They are not afraid of a long recipe. The freshness of the ingredient is very important, so going to the grocery store several times a week is not unusual."

The Hispanic parents' responses to survey questions about talking to a registered dietitian are good to see, says Alamo, although not that much of a surprise. "The Hispanic culture has a lot of respect for medical professionals," she says, "so it is easy to see why they want to meet with a registered dietitian."

Alamo comments that the overall responses by Hispanic children and parents are encouraging. She points to several very positive behaviors revealed in the survey: the higher frequency of meals eaten at home, the pattern of eating at regular meal times and the practice of eating as a family. Hispanics "are health conscious and want to learn how to make the most nutritious meals for their family," Alamo observes. "The gaps in nutrition and foods that are missing from kids' diets can be addressed with the Hispanic community because there is an openness and readiness."

Alamo concludes that the survey findings indicate unmet needs that can specifically be addressed by registered dietitians due to their background in food and nutrition.

the same time each night, they are more likely to have healthier behaviors, including eating behaviors.[38,42,47]

Sharing meals as a family improves mental health and leads to better eating patterns; this important bonding time can be a great opportunity to teach good nutrition and eating behaviors.[40,42,43,44] Quality time spent together as a family—whether cooking a meal or playing outside—can enhance children's well-being; new research shows it may be protective against higher than normal weight gain.[45,53,55] And family routines—such as regular bedtimes—can lead to stronger academic achievement and higher self-esteem.[46,47,52]

The *Family Nutrition and Physical Activity Survey* results indicate there are differences in the percentage of families that practice these behaviors by race and income. Regular schedules may be more difficult for lower- and middle-income parents; some may have several jobs, varying work schedules and longer transportation times to and from work.[51,52] Families could benefit from learning cooking techniques and skills for parents and older children.[51,55] Overall, the trend for all races is quite promising, though significantly fewer Hispanic and African American families have the same regularity of routines as white families. These regular rhythms can provide a strong foundation as we seek to improve children's healthy eating and activity habits.

Opportunity #3: Kids' Desire to Move More

We know that the majority of children don't get the recommended 60 minutes of physical activity each day—but kids tell us they would move more if they had more opportunities to do so.[19]

In the *Family Nutrition and Physical Activity Survey* children report that they would be more physically active if there were fun activities after school. Other motivations they mention for being more physically active are: if their friends wanted to do something physically active, if there were activity breaks during class, if there were a safe place to play in their neighborhood, if there were a way to get home after staying late after school and if there were fun activities before school.

Significantly more minority children than white children express an interest in opportunities to be physically active before, during and after school. Other motivators include transportation home from afterschool activities and safe places to play; these motivators are significantly less important to whites than to Hispanic and African American children. These findings show that children want to be more physically active, and they need encouragement and support to do so.

Opportunity #4: Quality Nutrition, Wherever Kids Eat

The *Family Nutrition and Physical Activity Survey* results from 2010 indicate a decrease in kids purchasing foods at restaurants, vending and other commercial locations from 2003 survey results. However, a large majority of kids are purchasing foods away from home at least some of the time each week. Children say that they would eat healthier foods at school and other locations if the foods tasted better. Additionally, results show it would help kids eat healthier if healthy food and drinks cost less money, if their parents ate healthy foods at home and if there were less "junk food" in stores on the way to and from school.

Percent of Children Who Would Be More Active If ...

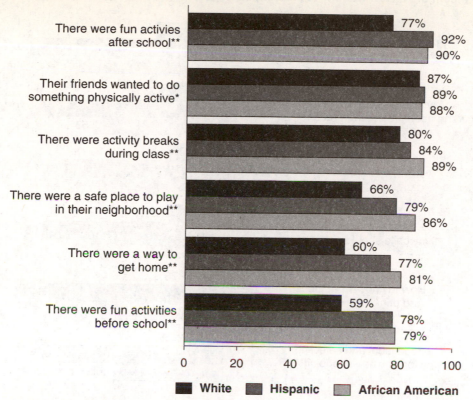

There were fun activies after school**
- White: 77%
- Hispanic: 92%
- African American: 90%

Their friends wanted to do something physically active*
- White: 87%
- Hispanic: 89%
- African American: 88%

There were activity breaks during class**
- White: 80%
- Hispanic: 84%
- African American: 89%

There were a safe place to play in their neighborhood**
- White: 66%
- Hispanic: 79%
- African American: 86%

There were a way to get home**
- White: 60%
- Hispanic: 77%
- African American: 81%

There were fun activities before school**
- White: 59%
- Hispanic: 78%
- African American: 79%

■ White ■ Hispanic ■ African American

*Statistically significant differences by race, p < 0.05

**Statistically significant differences by race, p < 0.001

Source: ADAF Family Nutrition and Physical Activity Survey, 2010

Percent of Children Who Would Eat Healthier If . . .

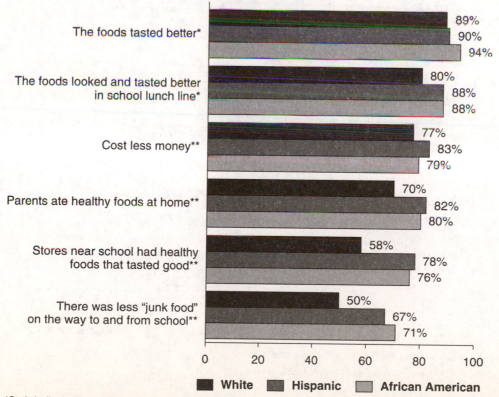

The foods tasted better*
- White: 89%
- Hispanic: 90%
- African American: 94%

The foods looked and tasted better in school lunch line*
- White: 80%
- Hispanic: 88%
- African American: 88%

Cost less money**
- White: 77%
- Hispanic: 83%
- African American: 70%

Parents ate healthy foods at home**
- White: 70%
- Hispanic: 82%
- African American: 80%

Stores near school had healthy foods that tasted good**
- White: 58%
- Hispanic: 78%
- African American: 76%

There was less "junk food" on the way to and from school**
- White: 50%
- Hispanic: 67%
- African American: 71%

■ White ■ Hispanic ■ African American

*Statistically significant differences by race, p < 0.05

** Statistically significant differences by race, p < 0.001

Source: ADAF Family Nutrition and Physical Activity Survey, 2010

Percent of Parents Wanting to Meet with a Registered Dietitian to Discuss . . .

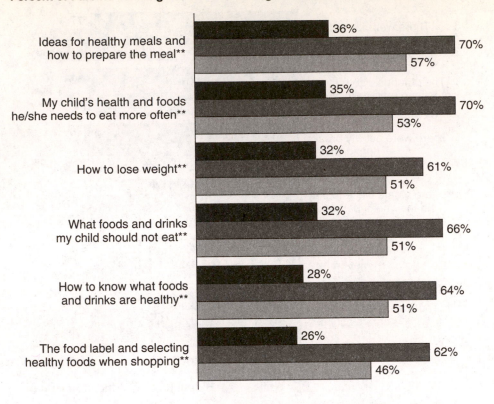

Ideas for healthy meals and how to prepare the meal**
- 36%
- 70%
- 57%

My child's health and foods he/she needs to eat more often**
- 35%
- 70%
- 53%

How to lose weight**
- 32%
- 61%
- 51%

What foods and drinks my child should not eat**
- 32%
- 66%
- 51%

How to know what foods and drinks are healthy**
- 28%
- 64%
- 51%

The food label and selecting healthy foods when shopping**
- 26%
- 62%
- 46%

Percent of Children Wanting to Meet with a Registered Dietitian to Discuss . . .

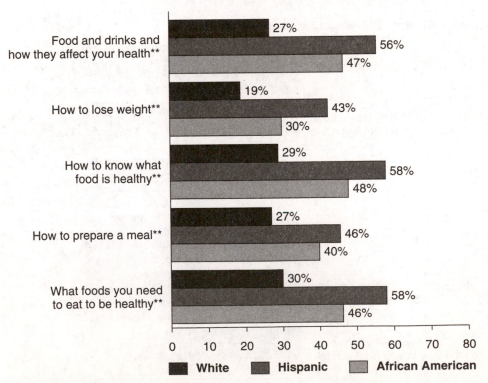

Food and drinks and how they affect your health**
- 27%
- 56%
- 47%

How to lose weight**
- 19%
- 43%
- 30%

How to know what food is healthy**
- 29%
- 58%
- 48%

How to prepare a meal**
- 27%
- 46%
- 40%

What foods you need to eat to be healthy**
- 30%
- 58%
- 46%

0 10 20 30 40 50 60 70 80

■ **White**   ■ **Hispanic**   □ **African American**

** Statistically significant differences by race, $p < 0.001$

Source: ADAF Family Nutrition and Physical Activity Survey, *2010*

Because kids do eat at school and do purchase foods away from home, we need to ensure that these foods are both healthy and kid-appealing.[45,57] Kids want foods that taste good—and public/private partnerships can take steps to enhance the flavor of the foods kids need to consume more of. Working together, community restaurants, registered dietitians and chefs can help schools improve the flavor and presentation of the foods they offer through their meal programs. Local funding could be made available so that schools could purchase fresh ingredients, use more scratch cooking and reduce dependence on processed foods. Local stores and restaurants—especially those near schools—can be encouraged to carry healthier foods that kids will eat.

Along with where the food is prepared, when kids eat is also an important consideration. Survey findings indicate that kids snack throughout the day. Current snacking patterns are problematic because of the food choices; however, snacking can be an opportunity to increase kids' consumption of the foods they need to eat more of—the nutrient-dense options.

If we focus on providing access to the nutrient-dense foods kids need to eat, making them look and taste great, these foods may displace high-sugar, high-calorie, low-nutrient foods.[33] This "displacement theory" may work in reverse too, unfortunately, as high-calorie, low-nutrient foods may displace nutrient-dense foods. In short, eating snacks does not have to mean eating high-calorie, low-nutrient foods.[33] Instead, kids can be encouraged to snack on foods that are good for them.

Poised for Healthy Change

It has been nearly a decade since the release of the Surgeon General's pivotal report on the obesity epidemic. Now is the time to ask: Are we making progress? This question must look beyond weight to nutrition and physical activity patterns in children. We also must ask: Are we addressing this comprehensively?

On one level, it would seem that we're making few, if any, strides. Looking at the current landscape, epidemic numbers of kids are overweight or obese, and the majority of kids' diets are deficient in one or more nutrients needed for growth and development.[4,6,21] The gap between children's recommended and actual intake of key nutrients remains alarmingly wide, regardless of weight status. Along with low intake of vital nutrients, data show that kids continue to consume a large percentage of calories from foods with sugar and saturated fat.[9,10]

The gap between children's recommended and actual intake of key nutrients remains alarmingly wide, regardless of weight status.

Additionally, the *Family Nutrition and Physical Activity Survey* shows kids' eating behaviors are inconsistent. Kids are grazing on foods throughout the day; frequent snacking throughout the day and evening is the norm, and there are less consistent patterns for meals for some kids, especially when race and income are factors. Recent food consumption data from NHANES found that increased snacking leads to lower quality of children's diet based on snack food choices high in calories and low in nutrients.[11,12] Snacking still occurs during school, with food purchased from school snack bars and vending machines. There are more kids who could benefit from school meal programs, so there are opportunities to increase participation. To do this, more attention on the taste and kid-appealing qualities of the foods is necessary, especially considering cultural differences in flavor and presentation of foods.

At the same time that kids' eating behaviors are less than optimal, activity levels are not adequate either.[19] In fact, the vast majority of youth are not achieving the national recommendation of 60 minutes of physical activity daily. This was the finding from the *Family Nutrition and Physical Activity Survey* and from the YRBSS 2009 results.[19]

Despite these real trouble spots, the *Family Nutrition and Physical Activity Survey* also reveals that on a deeper level the news about children's eating and activity behaviors may be more promising than first appears. Representing a crucial move forward, the survey findings suggest that a significant percentage of children and their parents are making or are ready to make changes in eating and activity patterns. How did we get to this new readiness for change, and how can we make the most out of this occurrence and not miss an opportunity?

The nation's attention to obesity and its causes has steadily increased over the last ten years, resulting in new policies, practices, food products and healthcare priorities. Although slight with respect to the magnitude of the problem, it seems that the national attention and subsequent changes have translated into more children and parents making changes in nutrition and physical activity on multiple levels. For example, compared to the 2003 report, children are engaging in healthier behaviors, such as maintaining more regular schedules and purchasing meals and snacks from vending machines and convenience stores less frequently. Children also say they want to eat healthier and be physically active. Both children and their parents indicate their trust in registered dietitians as credible sources as well as their desire to see them for guidance on what to eat and drink for health and wellness. All of this suggests that parents and children are ready to be supported as they work toward healthier behaviors.

Kids Eat Right

Kids Eat Right is the American Dietetic Association and Foundation platform of childhood obesity prevention initiatives. As part of **Kids Eat Right,** registered dietitians are mobilizing to support First Lady Michelle Obama's Let's Move! campaign and are working to ensure that childhood obesity prevention efforts are taking a quality nutrition approach.

Kids Eat Right recognizes that registered dietitians can provide evidence-based nutrition guidance supporting quality nutrition and healthy weights. Registered dietitians are uniquely qualified—through years of education and training—to advocate, educate and demonstrate the importance of meeting the total nutrient needs of all youth.

The public outreach effort brings more registered dietitians into community and school settings with tools and resources for shaping positive, lifelong habits of good nutrition and physical activity in youth. As part of this effort, registered dietitians are providing families with the tips they need to "Shop Cook Eat" to support quality nutrition and healthy weights in children.

The public education component shines a light on the deficiencies in nutrients that have become a common occurrence in children's diets along with unhealthy weights. Research shows that, while childhood obesity is at epidemic proportions, even higher numbers of youth are not eating the recommended number of servings from all food groups and therefore are missing nutrients vital to normal growth and development. ADA members are fighting these trends by working with families, parents, children, schools, community settings and media.

are uniquely qualified to apply the science of food and nutrition to increase health and to prevent and treat disease.

The *Family Nutrition and Physical Activity Survey* makes clear that children and their parents are poised for healthy change. It's time to build on this readiness for change, to seize this positive momentum. Together, we can tackle the twin problems of obesity and undernourishment—and help *Kids Eat Right*.

Special thanks to the following:

VANGUARD NETWORK
Kathryn A. Brown, EdD, RD, LD
Constance Brown-Riggs, MSEd, RD, CDE, CDN
Ruth Ann Carpenter, MS, RD
Gayle Coleman, MS, RD, CD
Jessica Donze-Black, RD, MPH
Robin Hamre, RD, MPH, LD
Kim Stitzel, MS, RD
Dorcas Ukpe, MS, RD, LD
Elizabeth M. Ward, MS, RD

RD COMMUNICATOR NETWORK
Maria C. Alamo, MPH, RD, LD
Stacey A. Antine, MS, RD
Susan T. Borra, RD
David Grotto, RD, LDN
Janet Helm, MS, RD
Cathy Kapica, PhD, RD, LD, CFCS, FACN
Shelley Maniscalco, MPH, RD
Susan D. Moores, MS, RD
Mary Mullen, MS, RD, LDN
Carolyn O'Neil, MS, RD
Jodie Shield, M.Ed, RD, LD
Liz Weiss, MS, RD

CONTRIBUTORS
Lucille Beseler, MS, RD, LD/N, CDE
Leslie Bonci, MPH, RD, CSSD, LDN
Nancy Copperman, MS, RD, CDN
Sheri Doucette, RD, LDN
Tab Forgac, MS, RD
Debra French, RD, CD
Niki Gernhofer, MS, RD
Lorry Luscri, MPH, RD, LDN
Aida Miles, MMSc, RD, CSP LD, CNSD
Theresa Nicklas, DrPH
Jean Ragalie, RD
Judith Rodriguez, PhD, RD, FADA, LDN
Bonnie Spear, PhD, RD

DIETETIC PRACTICE GROUPS
Food and Culinary Professionals
Sanna Delmonico, MS, RD
Amy Myrdal Miller, MS, RD

Hunger and Environmental Nutrition
Christopher Wharton, PhD, RD

Bottom line, the 2010 survey indicates new areas for intervention and support from registered dietitians. It also points to a shift in children's and parents' readiness for change that must be taken advantage of by efforts currently underway.

We must focus renewed attention on the total diet, ensuring that nutrient requirements are met as part of obesity prevention and health promotion efforts. The chronic poor eating habits have become intertwined with the problems of undernourishment and overweight. Kids' diets need to be shaped around eating the nutrient-dense food first. This approach can help to ensure kids consume the more than 50 nutrients necessary for proper growth, development and good health while simultaneously addressing obesity and undernourishment.[17,62] We need to encourage them not only to avoid unhealthy foods but also to eat plenty of nutrient-rich foods: fruits, vegetables, whole grains and low-fat and fat-free dairy foods, meat and beans.

As we work together to educate parents, support schools, reach out to children and take a "total diet" approach, we must call upon the expertise of registered dietitians, who

Pediatric Nutrition
Beverly W. Henry, PhD, RD
Susan Konek, MA, RD
Melissa Pflugh, MS, RD

Public Health/Community Nutrition
Carol J. Boushey, PhD, MPH, RD
Christina E. Ferroli, PhD, RD
Laura A. Nelson, MPH, RD, FADA
Gloria Stables, PhD, MS, RD

School Nutrition Services
Dayle Hayes, MS, RD
Mary Kay Meyer, PhD, RD
Constance Mueller, MS, RD, SNS

Sports, Cardiovascular and Wellness Nutrition
Liz Hobbs, MS, RD, LDN
Carol Lapin, MS, CSSD, RD, LD

Weight Management
Michele Doucette, PhD
Pat Harper, MS, RD
Anne Mathews, PhD, RD
Christine Weithman, MBA, RD, LDN

MEMBER INTEREST GROUPS
Latinos and Hispanics in Dietetics and Nutrition
Aurora Buffington, MS, RD
Julie Plasencia, MS, RD

AFFILIATE GROUPS
Colorado
Athena Evans, MS, RD, LD, CDE
District of Columbia
Sara Beckwith, RD
Florida
Eunshil Shim-McKenna, RD
Illinois
Anna Shlachter, MS, RD, LDN
Iowa
Jill Lange, MPH, RD, LD
Monica Lursen, RD
Molly Pelzer, RD
Lois Stillman, MPH, RDLD
New York
Susan Branning, MBA, RD, CNSD, CDN
North Carolina
Patricia J. Becker, MS, RD, CNSC
Ohio
Suzanne Cryst, RD
Tamara Randall, RD
Puerto Rico
Elba Gonzalez, RD
Tennessee
Tracy Noerper, RD
Deborah L. Slawson, PhD, RD, LDN
Texas
Karen Beathard, MS, RD, LD
Carol Bradley, MA, RD, LD

References

1. US Department of Health and Human Services, Public Health Service, Office of the Surgeon General. The Surgeon General's call to action to prevent and decrease overweight and obesity. www.surgeongeneral.gov/topics/obesity/. Published 2001. Accessed August 31, 2010.

2. Koplan JP, Liverman CT, Kraak VI, eds. *Preventing Childhood Obesity:* Health in the Balance. Washington, DC: The National Academies Press; 2005.

3. White House Task Force on Childhood Obesity Report to President. Solving the problem of childhood obesity within a generation, www.letsmove.gov/obesitytaskforce.php. Published May 2010. Accessed September 15, 2010.

4. American Dietetic Association. Position of the American Dietetic Association: Nutrition guidance for healthy children ages 2–11. J Am Diet Assoc. 2008;108:1038–1047.

5. American Dietetic Association. Position of the American Dietetic Association: Child and adolescent nutrition assistance programs. J Am Diet Assoc. 2010;110:791–799.

6. US Department of Agriculture. What we eat in America, NHANES 2007–2008: Nutrient intakes from food: Mean amounts consumed per individual, by gender and age. Agricultural Research Service Web site, www.ars.usda.gov/ba/bhnrc/fsrg. Published 2010. Accessed October 15, 2010.

7. US Department of Agriculture. Dietary Guidelines for Americans, 1980 to 2000. Center for Nutrition Policy and Promotion Web site. www.cnpp.usda.gov/DGAsPreviousGuidelines.htm. Published May 30, 2000. Accessed October 1, 2010.

8. Report of the Dietary Guidelines Advisory Committee on the Dietary Guidelines for Americans, 1990, Letter to the Secretary of Agriculture and the Secretary of Health and Human Services. Center for Nutrition Policy and Promotion Web site. www.cnpp.usda.gov/DGAs1990Guidelines.htm. Published May 14, 1990. Accessed August 25, 2010.

9. Williams C. Report of the Dietary Guidelines Advisory Committee on the Dietary Guidelines for Americans, 2010: Resource 1: Children's dietary intakes. US Department of Agriculture, Center for Nutrition Policy and Promotion Web site. www.dietaryguidelines.gov. Accessed October 20, 2010.

10. Reedy J, Krebs-Smith SM. Dietary sources of energy, solid fats, and added sugars among children and adolescents in the United States. J Am Diet Assoc. 2010;110(10):1477–1484.

11. US Department of Agriculture. What we eat in America, NHANES 2007–2008: Snacks: Distribution of snack occasions, by gender and age. Agricultural Research Service Web site. www.ars.usda.gov/ba/bhnrc/fsrg. Published 2010. Accessed October 15, 2010.

12. US Department of Agriculture. Beltsville Human Nutrition Research Center. Food Surveys Research

Group Dietary Data Brief. Snacking patterns of US adolescents: What we eat in America, NHANES 2005–2006. agricultural Research Service Web site. http://ars.usda.gov/Services/docs.htm?docid-19476. Published 2010. Accessed October 18,2010.

13. Ogden CL, Carroll MD, Curtin LR, Lamb MM, Flegal KM. Prevalence of high body mass index in US children and adolescents, 2007–2008. *JAMA.* 2010;303:242–249.

14. Ogden CL, Carroll MD, Flegal KM. High body mass index for age among US children and adolescents, 2003–2006. *JAMA.* 2008;299(20):2401–2405.

15. US Departments of Agriculture and Health and Human Services. Nutrition and your health: *Dietary Guidelines for Americans, 1980.* Center for Nutrition Policy and Promotion Web site. www.cnpp.usda.gov/DGAs1980Guidelines.htm. Accessed September 1, 2010.

16. Report of the Dietary Guidelines Advisory Committee on the *Dietary Guidelines for Americans, 1990,* to the Secretary of Agriculture and the Secretary of Health and Human Services. Center for Nutrition Policy and Promotion Web site. www.cnpp.usda.gov/DGAs1990Guidelines.htm. Published May 14, 1990. Accessed August 25, 2010.

17. Report of the Dietary Guidelines Advisory Committee on the *Dietary Guidelines for Americans, 2010.* Part D. Section 2: Nutrient Adequacy. Center for Nutrition Policy and Promotion Web site. www.cnpp.usda.gov/DGAs2010-DGACReport.htm. Published June 15, 2010. Accessed September 2, 2010.

18. US Department of Agriculture. What we eat in America, NHANES 2007–2008: Nutrient intakes from food: Mean amounts consumed per individual, by family income (in dollars) and age. Agricultural Research Service Web site. http://www.ars.usda.gov/ba/bhnrc/fsrg. Published 2010. Accessed October 10, 2010.

19. Eaton D, Kann L, Kinchen S, Shanklin S, Ross J, Hawkins J, Harris W, Lowry R, McMahnus T, Chyen D, Lim C, Whittle L, Brener N, Wechsler H. Youth risk behavior surveillance - United States, 2009. *MMWR* 2010;59(SS-5):1–142.

20. MEE Productions, Juzang I, Moag-Stahlberg A, Ellis K. Multi-cultural audience research. Copyright National Dairy Council, 2009. Published MEE Productions, May 2009. Philadelphia, PA.

21. Report of the Dietary Guidelines Advisory Committee on the Dietary Guidelines for Americans, 2010. Part D. Section 2: Nutrient adequacy. Center for Nutrition Policy and Promotion Web site. www.cnpp.usda.gov/DGAs2010-DGACReport.htm. Accessed August 22, 2010.

22. US Department of Agriculture. What we eat in America, NHANES 2007–2008: Nutrient intakes from food: Mean amounts consumed per individual, by family income (in dollars) and age. Agricultural Research Service Web site. www.ars.usda.gov/ba/bhnrc/fsrg. Published 2010. Accessed October 10, 2010.

23. Report of the Dietary Guidelines Advisory Committee on the *Dietary Guidelines for Americans, 2005,* Part

D: Science base. US Department of Health and Human Services Web site. www.health.gov/dietaryguidelines/dga2005/report/default.htm. Accessed August 25, 2010.

24. Report of the Dietary Guidelines Advisory Committee on the *Dietary Guidelines for Americans, 2000.* Center for Nutrition Policy and Promotion Web site. www.cnpp.usda.gov/DGAs2000Guidelines.htm. Accessed August 25, 2010.

25. Taras H. Nutrition and student performance at school. *J School Health.* 2005;75(6):199–213.

26. Taras H, Potts-Datema W. Obesity and student performance at school. *J School Health.* 2005;75(8):291–295.

27. Bryan J, Osendarp S, Hughes D, Calvaresi E, Baghurst K, van Klinken JW. Nutrients for cognitive development in schoolaged children. *Nutrition Reviews.* 2004;62(8):295–306.

28. Basch CE. Healthier students are better learners: A missing link in school reform to close achievement gap. *Equity Matters: Research Review* 2010 Mar;6A. www.equitycampaign.org/i/a/document/12557_EquityMattersVol6_Web03082010.pdf. Accessed September 30, 2010.

29. Black M. The evidence linking zinc deficiency with children's cognitive and motor functioning. *Journal of Nutrition.* 2003;133(5)(Supp.1):1473S-6S.

30. Action for Healthy Kids. The learning connection: The value of improving nutrition and physical activity in our schools. Action for Healthy Kids Web site. www.actionforhealthykids.org/resources/learningconnection. Published 2004. Accessed June 2, 2010.

31. Fryar C, Ogden C. Prevalence of underweight among children and adolescents: United States, 2007–2008. *NCHS Health EStat* 2010 Oct. National Center for Health Statistics Web site. www.cdc.gov/nchs/data/hestat/underweight_child_07_08/underweight_child_07_08.htm. Accessed October 25, 2010.

32. Sources of calories from added sugars among the US population, 2005-06: Mean intakes and percentage contribution of foods among children and adolescents. Applied Research Program. National Cancer Institute. Risk Factor Monitoring and Methods Branch Applied Research Program Web site. http://riskfactor.cancer.gov/diet/foodsources/added_sugars/. Accessed August 22, 2010.

33. Epstein LH, Paluch RA, Beecher MD, Roemmich JN. Increasing healthy eating vs. reducing high energy-dense foods to treat pediatric obesity. *Obesity.* 2008;16:318–326.

34. Centers for Disease Control and Prevention. Student health and academic achievement: The association between school-based physical activity, including physical education, and academic performance. National Center for Chronic Disease Prevention and Health Promotion Web site. www.cdc.gov/HealthyYouth/health_and_academics/index.htm. Published 2010. Accessed August 22, 2010.

35. McCormack Brown K, Alfonso ML, Bryant CA. *Obesity Prevention Coordinators' Social Marketing Guidebook.* Tampa, FL: Florida Prevention Research Center at the University of South Florida; 2004.

36. Huang TT, Drewnowski A, Kumanyika SK, Glass TA. A systems-oriented multilevel framework for addressing obesity in the 21st century. *Prev Chronic Dis.* 2009;6(3). www.cdc.gov/pcd/issues/2009/jul/09_0013.htm. Accessed May 10, 2010.

37. Glanz K, Rimer BK. *Theory at a Glance: A Guide for Health Promotion Practice.* 2nd ed. National Institutes of Health, U.S. Department of Health and Human Services. National Cancer Institute Web site. www.cancer.gov/PDF/481f5d53-63df-41bc-bfaf-5aa48ee1da4d/TAAG3.pdf. Published 2005. Accessed August 12, 2010.

38. Chen AY, Escarce JJ. Family structure and childhood obesity, Early Childhood Longitudinal Study–Kindergarten Cohort. Prev Chronic Dis. 2010;7(3). www.cdc.gov/pcd/issues/2010/may/09_0156.htm. Accessed July 15, 2010.

39. Rhee K. Childhood overweight and the relationship between parent behaviors, parenting style, and family functioning. *The ANNALS of the American Academy of Political and Social Science.* 2008;615:11.

40. Patrick H, Nicklas TA. A review of family and social determinants of children's eating patterns and diet quality. *Journal of the American College of Nutrition.* 2005;24(2):83–92.

41. Parenting and Family Life: A National Profile. Child and Adolescent Health Measurement Initiative, 2007. National Survey of Children's Health, Data Resource Center for Child and Adolescent Health. Published October 2009.

42. Rollins BY, Belue RZ, Francis LA. The beneficial effect of family meals on obesity differs by race, sex, and household education: The National Survey of Children's Health, 2003–2004. *J Am Diet Assoc.* 2010;110:1335–1339.

43. Boutelle KN, Birkeland RW, Hannan PJ, Story M, Neumark-Sztainer D. Associations between maternal concern for healthful eating and maternal eating behaviors, home food availability, and adolescent eating behaviors. *J Nutr Educ Behav.* 2007;39:248–256.

44. Cason KL. Family mealtimes: More than just eating together. *J Am Diet Assoc.* 2006;106(4):532–533.

45. Mancino, L, Todd JE, Guthrie J, Lin B-H. How food away from home affects children's diet quality. US Department of Agriculture, Economic Research Service Web site. www.ers.usda.gov/publications/err104/. Published October 2010. Accessed October 25, 2010.

46. Dickstein S. Family routines and rituals–the importance of family functioning. *Journal of Family Psychology.* 2002;16(4): 441–444.

47. Denham SA. Relationships between family rituals, family routines, and health. *Journal of Family Nursing.* 2003;9(3):305–330.

48. Befort C, Kaur H, Nollen N, Sullivan DK, Nazir N, Choi WS, Hornberger L, Ahluwalia JS. Fruit, vegetable, and fat intake among non-Hispanic black and non-Hispanic white adolescents: Associations with home availability and food consumption settings. *J Am Diet Assoc.* 2006;106:367–373.

49. Boutelle KN, Lytle LA, Murray DM, Birnbaum AS, Story M. Perceptions of the family mealtime environment and adolescent mealtime behavior: Do adults and adolescents agree? *Journal of Nutrition Education.* 2001;33:128–133.

50. Feldman S, Eisenberg ME, Neumark-Sztainer D, Story M. Associations between watching TV during family meals and dietary intake among adolescents. *J Nutr Educ Behav.* 2007;39:257–263.

51. Guthrie J, McClelland K. Working parents outsource children's meals. *Amber Waves.* 2009;7(1):5. www.ers.usda.gov/AmberWaves. Accessed August 15, 2010.

52. Heymann SJ, Earle A. The impact of parental working conditions on school-age children: The case of evening work. *Community, Work & Family.* 2001;4(3):305325.

53. US Department of Agriculture. Economic Research Service. Food and Nutrition Assistance Research Program. Parental time, role strain, and children's fat intake and obesity-related outcomes. Contractor and Cooperator Report No. 19. June 2006.

54. Sebastian RS, Enns CW, Goldman JD. US adolescents and MyPyramid: Association between fast-food consumption and lower likelihood of meeting recommendations. *J Am Diet Assoc.* 2009;109(2):226–235.

55. Manchino L, Newman C. Who has time to cook? How family resources influence food preparation. US Department of Agriculture, Economic Research Service Web site. www.ers.usda.gov/Publications/ERR40/. Published May 2007. Accessed October 1, 2010.

56. US Department of Agriculture. What we eat in America, NHANES 2007–2008: Away from home: Percentages of selected nutrients contributed by foods eaten away from home, by family income (in dollars) and age. Agricultural Research Service Web site, www.ars.usda.gov/ba/bhnrc/fsrg. Accessed October 15, 2010.

57. Hair E, Ling T, Wandner L. School food unwrapped: What's available and what our kids actually are eating. *Child Trends Research Brief.* 2008(Nov). www.childtrends.org/Files//Child_Trends-2008_11_17_RB_SchoolFoodPolicy.pdf. Accessed August 29, 2010.

58. Rampersaud GC, Pereira MA, Girard BL, Adams J, Metzl JD. Breakfast habits, nutritional status, body weight, and academic performance in children and adolescents. *J Am Diet Assoc.* 2005;105(5):743–760.

59. Murphy JM, Pagano M, Nachmani J, Sperling P, Kane S, Kleinman R. The relationship of school breakfast to psychosocial and academic functioning: Cross-sectional

ANNUAL EDITIONS

and longitudinal observations in an inner-city sample. *Archives of Pediatric and Adolescent Medicine.* 1998;152:89–907.

60. Wesnes KA, Pincock C, Richardson D, Helm G, Hails S. Breakfast reduces declines in attention and memory over the morning in schoolchildren. *Appetite.* 2003;41(3):329–331.

61. Affenito SG, Thompson DR, Barton BA, Franko DL, Daniels SR, Obarzanek E, Schreiber GB, Striegel-Moore RH. Breakfast consumption by African-American and white adolescent girls correlates positively with calcium and fiber intake and negatively with body mass index. *J Am Diet Assoc.* 2005;105:938–945.

62. American Dietetic Association. Position of the American Dietetic Association: Total diet approach to communicating food and nutrition information. *J Am Diet Assoc.* 2007;107:1224–1232.

Critical Thinking

1. What is meant by "quality calories"?
2. Based on data from NHANES 1977–1978 and 200–2002, describe the major changes in dietary intake of children between these two time periods.
3. Identify the foods that provide the most calories from saturated fat in children's diet. What is the percentage of calories from solid fat for each of these foods?
4. Identify the nutrients that are inadequate in the typical child's diet.

Acknowledgments—This report outlines the premise behind *Kids Eat Right,* the first joint effort of the American Dietetic Association and American Dietetic Association Foundation. The *Kids Eat Right* initiative is the result of a year-long process that included discussions with ADA volunteer leadership, diverse groups of members and ADA-ADAF staff, survey of members' interests, data collection from published research and gleaning of members' food and nutrition expertise. *Kids Eat Right*—whose public education campaign elements include the 2003 and 2010 ADAF *Family Nutrition and Physical Activity Survey* and subsequent report on "The State of Family Nutrition and Physical Activity: Are We Making Progress?"—would not have been possible without the many leading registered dietitians who have generously contributed their knowledge and time to the effort.

It is with much gratitude that I thank all who have contributed to the development of Kids Eat Right. *Many ADA members were especially helpful in creating the foundational elements of* Kids Eat Right *and this touchstone report.*

With regard and esteem, Alicia Moag-Stahlberg, MS, RD, LD, Consultant, Campaign Director, Kids Eat Right

Underage, Overweight

The federal government needs to halt the marketing of unhealthy foods to kids.

SCIENTIFIC AMERICAN

The statistic is hard to swallow: in the U.S., nearly one in three children under the age of 18 is overweight or obese, making being over-weight the most common childhood medical condition. These youngsters are likely to become heavy adults, putting them at increased risk of developing cardiovascular disease, type 2 diabetes and other chronic ailments. In February First Lady Michelle Obama announced a campaign to fight childhood obesity. Helping parents and schools to instill healthier habits in kids is an important strategy in this battle. But the government must take further steps to solve the problem.

In an ideal world, adults would teach children how to eat healthily and would lead by example. But in reality, two thirds of U.S. adults are themselves overweight or obese. Moreover, the food and beverage industry markets sugar- and fat-laden goods to kids directly—through commercials on television, product placement in movies and video games, and other media. Its considerable efforts—nearly $1.7 billion worth in 2007—have met with sickening success: a recent study conducted by researchers at the University of California, Los Angeles, found that children who see more television ads tend to become fatter. You might expect that watching TV, being a sedentary activity is responsible for obesity but the study found that obesity is correlated not with television per se but with advertising. The more commercial programming children watched, the fatter they got compared with those who watched a comparable amount of public television or DVDs. The majority of products marketed during children's programming are foods.

As nutritionist Marion Nestle of New York University has written, society needs to "create a food environment that makes it easier for parents and everyone else to make better food choices." Protecting children from junk-food marketing would help create conditions conducive to achieving a healthy weight.

Unfortunately like the tobacco industry before it, the food industry cannot be trusted to self-regulate in this regard. In a study published in the March *Pediatrics,* investigators looked at the prevalence of food and beverage brands in movies released between 1996 and 2005. They noted, for instance, that although Coca-Cola and PepsiCo have pledged to not advertise during children's television programming, their products routinely appear in movies aimed at kids.

Likewise, in the March *Public Health Nutrition,* researchers reported a 78 percent increase from 2006 to 2008 in the use of cartoon characters, toys and other child-oriented cross promotions on food packaging—much of it for nutritionally bereft foods. A whopping 55 percent of these cross promotions came from food manufacturers that have opted into the Children's Food and Beverage Advertising Initiative, sponsored by the Council of Better Business Bureaus, which promises to limit advertising to kids but allows participants to decide for themselves whether to restrict in-store marketing. Such examples of ineffectual commitments on the part of the food industry abound.

In December a group of U.S. agencies—the Federal Trade Commission, the Centers for Disease Control and Prevention the Food and Drug Administration, and the Department of Agriculture—proposed standards for foods and beverages that are marketed to children between the ages of two and 17. The agencies sensibly recommended that such foods must provide a meaningful contribution to a healthy diet by meeting specified requirements; that the amounts of saturated fat, trans fat, sugar and salt in these foods must not exceed limits set by the group; and that certain clearly healthy foods-such as those that are 100 percent fruits, vegetables or whole grains—may be marketed to kids without meeting the other two standards.

The interagency working group is due to submit a report containing its final recommendations to Congress by July 15. The standards are worthy but have one problem: as they stand, they would be voluntary. They should be mandatory, not optional, and the FDA should implement and enforce them.

The estimated cost of treating obesity-related ailments in adults was $147 billion for 2009. With the health care system already faltering, allowing companies to decide for themselves whether to peddle junk food to kids is a fox-and-henhouse policy this country simply cannot afford any longer.

Critical Thinking

1. Which nutrients are being targeted by the Federal Trade Commission, the Centers for Disease Control, and Food and Drug Administration as being unhealthy for children and, thus, should not be marketed to kids between the ages of 2 to 17?

2. From 2006 to 2008, what percentage increase was observed in the use of cartoon characters, toys, and kid-oriented promotion on food packaging?

3. How have Coca-Cola and PepsiCo addressed the popular opinion to decrease marketing of unhealthy products to kids?

The Impact of Teachers and Families on Young Children's Eating Behaviors

Erin K. Eliassen

Young children depend on their families and teachers to support their well-being and promote positive development, including eating behaviors. Children's food preferences and willingness to try new foods are influenced by the people around them (Bellows & Anderson 2006).

The eating behaviors children practice early in life affect their health and nutrition—significant factors in childhood overweight and obesity (Clark et al., 2007)—and may continue to shape food attitudes and eating patterns through adulthood (Birch 1999; Campbell & Crawford 2001; Westenhoefer 2002). Eating environments—mealtime and snack—that make food fun, offer new foods and a variety, and encourage children to taste and choose the foods they want let children develop food attitudes and dietary practices that ultimately support good health (Campbell & Crawford 2001).

Developing Eating Behaviors

The development of eating behaviors is a dynamic process that begins in infancy and continues throughout life. In this article, *eating behaviors* refers to food preferences, patterns of food acceptance and rejection, and the types and amounts of food a person eats. Genetics and the contexts in which foods are presented are two key factors that underpin the development of eating behaviors. Although parents provide a child's biological predisposition, which may affect factors like taste perception, they are not the only adults influencing the development of a child's eating behaviors. Every family member and caregiver interacting with a child at meals or snacks has the potential to do so.

In center- and home-based child care settings, teachers and family child care providers influence children's eating behaviors by the foods they offer, the behaviors they model, and their social interactions with children at snack and mealtimes (Savage, Fisher, & Birch 2007). Here are a few examples of how these factors influence eating behaviors.

Repeated exposure to a new food reduces a child's fear of the food and helps increase acceptance. Observing families and teachers eating and enjoying a variety of foods makes these foods more appealing to children. In contrast, children who are pressured to eat specific foods learn to dislike them. Restricted access to some foods, such as cookies or potato chips, often results in overconsumption of those foods when children are free to choose them (Savage, Fisher, & Birch 2007).

Educators and Families are Role Models

Based on research, the following six subsections discuss food fears, care environments, food behavior models, food restriction, pressures to eat, and food as a reward or celebration. Each area offers suggestions for educators and families to help children develop positive, early eating behaviors.

Food Fears

Most children naturally demonstrate fears of new foods. Neophobia, or fear of the new, is a protective behavior observed in omnivores, including humans, that helps prevent consumption of harmful substances (Birch 1999). Teachers help decrease children's fears by creating supportive environments with enjoyable, nutritious, and fun early food experiences.

For example, teachers could involve families by encouraging each family to bring every child a tasting sample of a unique food their child enjoys (or the teacher may offer suggestions of foods to taste). The teacher can arrange a tasting schedule, with a different family sharing a food tasting each week. Once every family has had an opportunity to share, host a classroom tasting party with all of the foods and invite parents to enjoy the event with their children. Although experiments vary, researchers tell us that offering a food 10 to 15 times appears necessary to increase a child's food acceptance (Savage, Fisher, & Birch 2007). Activities like tasting parties expose children to foods from different cultures and provide opportunities to learn more about their friends.

Researchers tell us that offering a food 10 to 15 times appears necessary to increase a child's food acceptance.

The acceptance of new foods is a slow process. Particularly through the ages 2 to 5, persistence is essential (Birch 1999; Satter 2008). A teacher/caregiver may think it is best to hold off on introducing food variety until children's fearful responses decrease. Instead, it is important to continue introducing a variety of foods throughout early childhood. Although children are skeptical of many foods during these early years, the variety of foods they accept is greater in this developmental phase than it is in later childhood (Skinner et al., 2002).

Enjoyable or satisfying experiences with a food highly influence a child's subsequent selection of the food on given occasions or its adoption into his or her regular diet. These experiences are as simple as frequent family meals during which the television is off and parents or caregivers are tuned in to the mealtime experience by talking and enjoying the foods themselves. Positive exposure to multiple foods helps children develop a taste for more foods, choose them as regular mealtime selections, and have needed dietary variety—whole grains, fruits, and vegetables. Many children lack opportunities to taste a variety of healthful foods, compared to the numerous chances our culture makes available for tasting high-fat, calorie-dense foods (Savage, Fisher, & Birch 2007).

Care Environments

Child care settings foster positive development of eating behaviors for 2- to 5-year-olds. Caregivers introduce variety in the foods served at meals and snacks and encourage families to do the same when they send lunches from home. Programs can guide parents by sharing comprehensive lists of foods that present a variety of grains, fruits, vegetables, nuts and seeds, and meats and beans, and an illustration of their nutritional value. For instance, using MyPyramid (www.mypyramid.gov) food groups helps families categorize foods and prepare lunches with variety and nutritional balance. Teachers can share examples of simple, creative lunches with variety in color, texture, and taste to appeal to young children.

Being persistent and providing repeated exposures to foods is important for both teachers and families. Avoid temptations to remove healthy foods from the program's meal or snack menus just because children reject them. Support families in continuing to offer lunch items even if their child does not consume the food on a given day. When serving a new item such as snap peas at snack time, include it two or three times a month and encourage children to look, smell, touch, and taste the new food. It is perfectly acceptable for a child to avoid a new vegetable the first several times it is offered. Inviting children to touch and smell the food helps them take small steps toward tasting. Encouraging rather than requiring children to eat a food is the key objective.

Food Behavior Models

Families are typically children's first significant models of eating behavior (Golan & Weizman 2001). Child care providers also are early role models. Positive role modeling correlates with an increased interest in food and less food fussiness among children (Gregory, Paxton, & Borzovic 2010). Poor role

Ten Steps to Positive Eating Behaviors

1. Provide a variety of foods at meals and snacks, especially whole grains, vegetables, and fruits.
2. Offer repeated opportunities to taste new foods.
3. Share with families nutrition resources, such as lists of foods (by category) to guide their food selections and offer new ideas for meals sent from home.
4. Apply the same guidelines to food selections in teachers' lunches brought from home.
5. Sit with children at meals, and enjoy conversation. Talk about the taste, texture, appearance, and healthful aspects of foods.
6. Plan adequate time for all children to finish eating.
7. Respect a child's expression of satiety or sense of being full.
8. Develop a routine for serving snacks, applying the same rules whether offering carrots, crackers, or cookies.
9. Wash hands before snack and mealtime; encourage touching and smelling a food as a step toward tasting.
10. Find alternatives to using food as a reward or serving foods high in fat, sugar, or salt as part of a celebration.

models influence children's perceptions of foods and mealtimes (Matheson, Spranger, & Saxe 2002). For example, negative comments about the taste or texture of a food will make a child less willing to try it. On the other hand, a child is more likely to try a food if he or she observes an adult enjoying it.

Teachers and caregivers become role models by engaging with children at mealtime and sitting down and eating with them. This practice is often called family-style dining. When early childhood programs provide meals, teachers and staff can model healthy eating behaviors by eating the same foods the children eat.

Staff who bring their lunches can model the same kinds of healthy eating as described in the guidelines the program suggests for families who send lunches with their children. For example, if parents send a fruit and a vegetable item, then teachers can include both of these items in their lunches. If children have milk, water, or 100 percent fruit juice as a beverage, teachers should drink these same beverages.

Interesting and engaging mealtime conversations create greater food enjoyment (Hughes et al., 2007). Adults can talk positively about the foods they are eating and also invite the children to describe colors, tastes (sweet, sour, salty), and textures (crunchy, smooth, stringy). However, the conversation should not be about the food alone. Also engage children in conversation about other appropriate topics, such as animals or family activities. Too much emphasis on the foods may decrease the children's interest.

Teachers and care-givers become role models by engaging with children at meal-time and sitting down and eating with them.

Food Restriction

Many well-meaning adults try to control the way children eat. They may believe that restricting or forbidding unhealthy foods will decrease children's preference for them, but the opposite is true (Satter 2008). Pressuring a child to eat one type of food (such as fruit or vegetables) leads to resistance. When an adult restricts access to certain foods (such as sweets or french fries), a child may become preoccupied with the restricted food.

A study on the effect of restricted access to foods among a population of 3- to 6-year-olds (Fisher & Birch 1999) found that the children focused great attention on the visible but inaccessible food through spontaneous clapping and chanting. In a similar study (Fisher & Birch 1999), restricting a desired, palatable snack food substantially increased children's selection of that food compared to times when both it and similar foods were freely available.

Avoid making comments about children's frequency or quantity consumption of a given food. For example, when serving cookies for snack, offer them as all other snacks are served. Their quantity should not be restricted unless the quantity of all snack foods is restricted. Early childhood educators can develop routines for offering all snacks, both unfamiliar and favorite foods, in the same unbiased way.

Pressure to Eat

When families or teachers pressure children to eat at mealtimes, the practice negatively influences a child's food intake as well as attitude toward food (Galloway et al., 2006). Gregory, Paxton, and Brozovic (2010) report that children pressured to eat were less interested in food over time; whereas, when parents modeled healthy eating, the children expressed greater interest in food and less food fussiness. Coercion to eat specific quantities or types of foods may mean that children eat more at the given meal, but over time they will likely avoid the targeted food (Satter 2008).

In a study involving adults, Batsell and colleagues (2002) traced common food dislikes to the adults' childhood experiences in being pressured to consume certain foods. Galloway and colleagues (2006) learned that refraining from the use of pressure and simply eating with and talking to the children had a more positive impact on children's attitude toward the food offered.

While pressure to eat contributes to a dislike of certain foods, emphasis on having a "clean plate" may hinder children's recognition of the internal cues of hunger and satiety and contribute to overeating (Satter 2008). It is important for adults to respect the child's expression of food preference and fullness (particularly if the child tastes a food) and to follow a schedule that gives children enough time to eat.

Food as a Reward or Celebration

Food as reward or celebration is common in some early childhood settings. Such practices may be well intentioned but can have negative consequences and impact long-term eating behaviors (Birch 1999; Brown & Ogden 2004). Food rewards or party treats are often sweets or other "desired" snack items. Giving a desired food as a reward enhances a child's preference for the food (Puhl & Schwartz 2003).

By establishing guidelines for the use of food in the classroom, early childhood programs encourage families to provide alternatives to fast-food lunch parties or cupcake celebrations and to bring instead, for example, fruits or muffins. Class celebrations or everyday activities also give young children opportunities to prepare their own foods in the classroom. Children enjoy making edible art fruit or vegetable skewers, or snacks resembling animals.

Alternative practices for recognition and celebration are growing in variety in early childhood settings. Instead of food, teachers recognize children by giving them special opportunities, such as selecting a song for the group to listen or dance to, choosing a game to play with friends, or having first choice of equipment for gross motor play. Non-food-related activities, like bringing a favorite book or game to class to read or share with friends, are other ways to acknowledge individuals.

Conclusion

Early childhood educators who understand the importance of their role in the development of children's healthful eating behaviors can help improve the lifelong health of the children they serve. They can offer meaningful, positive experiences with food, including growing, preparing, and eating foods with children. Regardless of the foods offered at home, the early childhood educator has the opportunity to model selection and enjoyment of a variety of foods. Food in the program should be associated with opportunities and fun experiences rather than rules and restrictions. Tasting activities help children learn about foods, manners, and even other cultures.

Everyone caring for children needs to be aware that some food strategies have negative effects on the development of eating behaviors. Food practices involving pressure and restriction may not only affect childhood health but also have long-lasting implications, such as problematic behaviors of binge eating and dietary restraint among adults (Puhl & Schwartz 2003).

Regardless of the foods offered at home, the early childhood educator has the opportunity to model selection and enjoyment of a variety of foods.

A supportive, caring early childhood environment offers guidance through adult modeling, serving a variety of nutritious foods at meals and snacks, and exposing children to new foods in the classroom. These practices encourage children's development of healthy eating attitudes and behaviors and promote positive long-term health outcomes.

References

Batsell, R., A. Brown, M. Ansfield, & G. Paschall. 2002. "You Will Eat All of That! A Retrospective Analysis of Forced Consumption Episodes." *Appetite* 38 (3): 211–19.

Bellows, L., & J. Anderson. 2006. "The Food Friends: Encouraging Preschoolers to Try New Foods." *Young Children* 61 (3): 37–39. www.naeyc.org/yc/pastissues/2006/may.

Birch, L. 1999. "Development of Food Preferences." *Annual Reviews of Nutrition* 19 (1): 41–62.

Brown, R., & J. Ogden. 2004. "Children's Eating Attitudes and Behaviour: A Study of the Modeling and Control Theories of Parental Influence." *Health Education Research* 19 (3): 261–71.

Campbell, K., & D. Crawford 2001. "Family Food Environments as Determinants of Preschool-Aged Children's Eating Behaviors: Implications for Obesity Prevention Policy. A Review." *Australian Journal of Nutrition and Dietetics* 58 (1): 19–25.

Clark, H., E. Goyder, P. Bissel, L. Blank, & J. Peters. 2007. "How Do Parents' Child-Feeding Behaviours Influence Child Weight? Implications for Childhood Obesity Policy." *Journal of Public Health* 29 (2): 132–41.

Fisher, J., & L. Birch. 1999. "Restricting Access to Palatable Foods Affects Children's Behavioral Response, Food Selection, and Intake." *American Journal of Clinical Nutrition* 69 (6): 1264–72.

Galloway, A., L. Fiorito, L. Francis, & L. Birch. 2006. "'Finish Your Soup': Counterproductive Effects of Pressuring Children to Eat on Intake and Affect." *Appetite* 46 (3): 318–23.

Golan, M., & A. Weizman. 2001. "Familial Approach to the Treatment of Childhood Obesity." *Journal of Nutrition Education* 33 (2): 102–07.

Gregory, J., S. Paxton, & A. Brozovic. 2010. "Maternal Feeding Practices, Child Eating Behavior and Body Mass Index in Preschool-Aged Children: A Prospective Analysis." *The International Journal of Behavioral Nutrition and Physical Activity* 7: 55–65.

Hughes, S., H. Patrick, T. Power, J. Fisher, C. Anderson, & T. Nicklas. 2007. "The Impact of Child Care Providers' Feeding on Children's Food Consumption." *Journal of Development & Behavioral Pediatrics* 28 (2): 100–07.

Matheson, D., K. Spranger, & A. Saxe. 2002. "Preschool Children's Perceptions of Food and Their Food Experiences." *Journal of Nutrition Education and Behavior* 34 (2): 85–92.

Puhl, R., & M. Schwartz. 2003. "If You Are Good You Can Have a Cookie: How Memories of Childhood Food Rules Link to Adult Eating Behaviors." *Eating Behaviors* 4 (3): 283–93. www.faeriefilms.com/images/Schwartz_-_If_You_Are_Good.pdf.

Satter, E. 2008. *Secrets of Feeding a Healthy Family.* Madison, WI: Kelcy Press.

Savage, J., J.O. Fisher, & L. Birch. 2007. "Parental Influence on Eating Behavior: Conception to Adolescence." *Journal of Law, Medicine & Ethics* 35 (1): 22–34.

Skinner, J., B. Carruth, W. Bounds, & P. Ziegler. 2002. "Children's Food Preferences: A Longitudinal Analysis." *Journal of the American Dietetic Association* 102 (11): 1638–47.

Westenhoefer, J. 2002. "Establishing Dietary Habits During Childhood for Long-Term Weight Control." *Annals of Nutrition & Metabolism* 46 (supplement): 18–23.

Critical Thinking

1. Describe how families and teachers can improve food behavior of children during lunch or snack time.

2. Critique common practices in U.S. homes and schools that negate acceptance of consuming a variety of healthy foods.

2. Explain how food restriction affects eating behavior.

ERIN K. ELIASSEN, EdD, RD, LD, is an assistant professor in the Department of Family and Consumer Sciences at Eastern Kentucky University in Richmond. As a registered dietitian, she provides education and training on the topic of child feeding to health care providers, educators, and parents of young children.

Engaging Families in the Fight against the Overweight Epidemic among Children

Mick Coleman, Charlotte Wallinga, and Diane Bales

"Epidemic!" "Alarming!" "A threatening storm!" These powerful descriptors have been used by the Centers for Disease Control and Prevention (CDC) (Polhamus et al., 2004), the American Academy of Pediatrics (Committee on Nutrition, 2003; Council on Sports Medicine and Fitness and Council on School Health, 2006), and other medical professionals (Olshansky et al., 2005) to describe the increase in the number of U.S. children who are overweight. Indeed, data compiled from the National Health and Nutrition Examination Survey by the CDC (2007) show that the prevalence of overweight preschool-age children, 2 to 5 years old, increased from 5% in the period 1971–74 to 13.9% in the period 2003–04. During the same time periods, the prevalence of overweight 6- to 11-year-olds increased from 4% to 18.8% and the prevalence of overweight 12- to 19-year-olds increased from 6.1% to 17.4%. Across age groups, the prevalence of overweight children remains higher among low-income and minority groups than among children as a whole (Anderson & Butcher, 2006).

In this article, we provide an update on the overweight epidemic with early childhood educators in mind. We begin with information about the consequences of being overweight for children's health. We then examine the multiple factors that contribute to the overweight epidemic. Next, we look at the case for involving families in the fight against the overweight epidemic among children. Finally, we share three principles and associated strategies that early childhood educators can use to help families guide their children toward a healthy lifestyle.

Consequences Associated with Children Being Overweight

Cardiovascular Disease. It is estimated that a majority (61%) of overweight children from 5 to 10 years old have one or more cardiovascular risk factors (Freedman, Dietz, Srinivasan, & Berenson, 1999), such as high blood pressure, high cholesterol, and hardening of the arteries (Daniels, 2006; Freedman et al., 1999). While these biological processes can take decades to progress to a stroke or heart attack, it is feared that becoming overweight during childhood may accelerate their impact and lead to an early death (Daniels, 2006).

Diabetes

Diabetes in children also is attributed to the increased incidence of children being overweight (Daniels, 2006; Ludwig & Ebbeling, 2001). Diabetes, in turn, can lead to blindness, heart disease, kidney disease, and loss of limbs (The Center for Health and Health Care in Schools, 2005).

Asthma

The risk of asthma is higher among children who are overweight (Gilliland et al., 2003). In addition, overweight children with asthma have been found to use more medicine, make more visits to the emergency room, and spend more days wheezing than non-overweight children with asthma (Belamarich et al., 2000).

Sleep Apnea

Being overweight carries a higher risk of sleep apnea, an abnormal collapse of the airway during sleep, both in adults and children (Daniels, 2006). As a result, overweight children may exhibit daytime sleepiness, which, in turn, can lead to a decrease in physical activity and further heighten the risk for being overweight (Daniels, 2006). In addition, daytime sleepiness can negatively impact children's classroom performance. Over the long term, sleep apnea also can increase blood pressure, further raising the risk of heart disease.

Quality and Length of Life

Overweight children and their parents report significantly lower quality of life scores for physical, emotional, social, and school functioning than do families with children diagnosed as "healthy" (Schwimmer, Burwinkle, & Varni, 2003). Perhaps more alarming, because of the increased incidence of childhood overweight, young children today may live less healthy and shorter lives than their parents (Olshansky et al., 2005). Should this occur, being overweight would indeed prove to be the "threatening storm" that reverses the steady rise in life expectancy observed during previous centuries.

Factors Contributing to the Overweight Epidemic among Children

Children become overweight when they eat too many calories and do not get enough physical activity to burn off those calories (Anderson & Butcher, 2006; U.S. Department of Health and Human Services, 2001). Although genetics and body metabolism both contribute to this imbalance, certain lifestyle factors also must be considered (Anderson & Butcher, 2006; Council on Sports Medicine and Fitness and Council on School Health, 2006).

The Food Environment

Children in the United States have an overwhelming abundance of food choices. Unfortunately, not all foods found in grocery stores are healthy, few fast food meals are healthy, and pre-packaged foods and soft drinks are often high in fat, sugar, and calories. Advertisements also can be confusing and sometimes misleading. For example, although many prepackaged foods are advertised as healthy (e.g., "reduced fat"), they may contain as many or more calories than the foods they are designed to replace (CDC, 2005a). We only need to look at the vending machines at our work sites to realize that milk, juices, and healthy snacks are far less available than their less healthy counterparts. Unfortunately, vending machines and food advertising through television programming remain a fact of life in too many elementary and middle schools, perhaps, in part, because of the added income they bring to schools (Anderson & Butcher, 2006; Cawley, 2006).

Portion Sizes

Yet another factor contributing to the confusing food environment is portion size (Cawley, 2006). Food manufacturers began producing larger portion sizes in the 1970s and continued to do so at an increasing rate through the 1980s and 1990s, leading children and adults to eat more and take in more calories during meals and snacks (CDC, 2005a; Young & Nestle, 2002). It easy to understand why children have difficulty establishing healthy eating patterns.

Schedules

Skipping breakfast and eating fast food are characteristics of a national mindset in which food quantity and convenience override considerations of food quality and health. Even though many ready-to-eat healthy foods are available (e.g., fruits), families often prefer prepackaged foods because they have

longer shelf lives, do not require cleaning, and appeal to the tastes of children. Nevertheless, results from research suggest that eating food away from home, especially at fast food establishments, contributes to children becoming overweight (Davis et al., 2007). Likewise, skipping breakfast is a risk factor for becoming overweight (Davis et al., 2007).

Technological Advances and Urban Design

While technology has contributed to the quality of our lives, it also has reduced our level of physical activity. For example, as children spend more time watching television, they spend less time engaged in outdoor physical activities. Likewise, many families live in communities designed more for vehicles than for walking and biking (Fierro, 2002). Urban sprawl, combined with inadequate sidewalks and heavy traffic, prevents children from walking or riding bikes to school and parks (Anderson & Butcher, 2006).

Play and Physical Education

Recess and time for free play have been eliminated or shortened in many school systems (U.S. Department of Health and Human Services, 2004). In addition, rules regarding physical education for elementary school children vary widely (National Conference of State Legislatures, 2005). These changes have come about at least in part due to the increased concern over preparing children to meet mandated test scores (Anderson & Butcher, 2006). In response, such groups as the American Association for the Child's Right to Play (www.ipausa.org) are advocating for the 60 minutes of daily physical activities often recommended by the medical profession (Council on Sports Medicine and Fitness and Council on School Health, 2006; Davis et al., 2007).

The Case for Engaging Families as Health Educators

Increasingly, families are being viewed as essential in the fight against the overweight epidemic among children. Families, more than any other social institution, serve as both mediators and monitors of children's health behaviors.

Families as Mediators

Families mediate their children's eating behaviors through their choice and preparation of snacks and meals, as well as through their decisions of where to eat when outside the home. Families serve as mediators of children's physical activities through the rules they set regarding the amount of time children spend watching television and playing computer games. Likewise, families determine the degree to which children are involved in such physical activities as games, recreational pursuits, home chores, and yardwork.

Families as Monitors

Families also serve as monitors of their children's eating and physical activity patterns. Although some families appear to

Table 1 Families as Health Educators: Guides for Developing Healthy Lifestyle Activities for Families

Family-based Activities. In order to make healthy living truly a family affair, strive to develop activities that involve all family members in a household and not just a child or a parent-child dyad. Otherwise, efforts to fight family overeating and inactivity may not be successful.

Time Efficiency. Because families lead busy lives, develop family involvement activities that can be incorporated into their usual routines (e.g., dinner, bedtime, housework). Families are more likely to try healthy lifestyle activities if they fit into their daily schedules.

Simplicity. The fewer materials and directions needed to complete an activity, the better. Families may not bother to attempt a healthy lifestyle activity if that activity involves numerous materials and directions.

Clarity. Check all printed materials for clarity. If doubt remains about certain words or phrases, ask a few families to read the materials and provide you with feedback. Identify volunteers to translate printed materials into the languages represented in your classroom.

Fun. No one wants to eat bland food or engage in boring or unpleasant physical activities. Use your creativity and consult with community nutritionists and recreation specialists to develop fun and creative activities that reinforce healthy eating and exercise.

Encourage Rather Than Preach. Avoid a "preaching" stance by acknowledging that we all have a right to watch television, play video games, and eat a piece of cake. Disallowing these things altogether will only serve to sabotage families' efforts. Note the importance of moderation, not total elimination, when suggesting activities that help move families toward a more active and healthy lifestyle.

have difficulty recognizing the potential health risks associated with being overweight (Young-Hyman, Herman, Scott, & Schlundt, 2000), a number of family-based intervention programs have achieved success in lowering the weight of overweight children (see Epstein, Valoski, Wing, & McCurley, 1994; Golan & Crow, 2004; Golan, Weizman, Apter, & Fainaru, 1998; Harvey-Berino & Rourke, 2003; Lindsay, Sussner, Kim, & Gortmaker, 2006). Indeed, one of the most basic ways that parents can monitor and contribute to their children's development of healthy eating patterns is by establishing a family rule about eating dinner together (Lindsay et al., 2006).

The importance of a family-based approach to addressing the overweight epidemic becomes even clearer when we consider how families must juggle multiple schedules and unique demands, which can interfere with their ability to serve as effective monitors of their children's eating patterns and exercise activities. As a result, consideration must be given to respecting the realities of family life when planning family activities to promote healthy eating and exercise. Table 1 presents guides that we have followed in carrying out training related to healthy living. These guides also were the foundation for our development of the activity ideas found in Table 2 and Figure 1.

Involving Families in the Fight against the Overweight Epidemic

Early childhood educators have the expertise to bridge the gap between factual health information and the application of family involvement practices to promote family-oriented healthy eating and exercise. Three recommendations from the CDC (2005b) for involving families in promoting a healthy approach to eating and physical activity are especially relevant to early childhood teachers' work with families.

Guide 1. Encourage Families to Serve as Role Models

A family-based approach to fighting against the factors contributing to children being overweight is in keeping with current recommendations that recognize the importance of parents as children's most important role models in adapting a healthy lifestyle (Council on Sports Medicine and Fitness and Council on School Health, 2006; Davis et al., 2007; Lindsay et al., 2006). Families that model healthy eating patterns, regularly participate in physical activities, and talk about the benefits associated with a healthy lifestyle set an example for children to follow. Younger children, in particular, are more likely to mimic the behavior of important adults like parents and guardians. Some ideas to share with families to help them model healthy living habits can be found in Table 2.

Guide 2. Encourage Families to Engage in Healthy Activities in Different Settings

Help families discover practical ways to eat healthy meals and exercise throughout the week. Family activity calendars, like the one presented in Figure 1 for families of preschool and kindergarten children, can provide the encouragement families need to work toward a healthy lifestyle within and outside the home.

Guide 3. Advocate for Quality School and Community Physical Activity Programs

Families may not always see themselves as having the knowledge or skills needed to serve as health advocates for their children. Help promote families' knowledge, confidence, and skills in the following ways:

Figure 1   Themes and Ideas for an Activity Calendar

Theme	Mon	Tue	Wed	Thu	Fri
Practice Fundamental Motor Skills	*Trapping.* Sit on the floor and roll a large ball back and forth. Roll it to one side, then the other side. Roll it slowly, then quickly.	*Catching.* Help your child practice catching a large ball by rolling it down a slide or chute. Then, toss the ball back and forth to each other.	*Hopping.* Hop like a rabbit or grasshopper. See how long you can hop on one foot.	*Weaving.* Weave through an obstacle course of chairs or sheets hung over an outdoor line.	*Throwing.* Practice throwing a ball through a hula hoop from different distances and angles.
Encourage Creative Movement	Attach a large scarf to your child's pants or around her waist. Do the same for yourself. Pretend you have been swept up by the wind and are floating in the sky. What do you see below?	Observe how bugs move on the ground. Take turns making up your own creative bug movements.	Use ribbons attached to your wrists as butterfly wings. Fly around and visit your favorite flowers and plants.	Some communities have free introductory dance classes. Take your family to different classes. Which ones do family members enjoy the most?	Put on a fast song. Everyone make up a silly dance, the sillier the better.
Family Relaxation and Recreation	As a family, take a stroll around the neighborhood after dinner. Using hints, play a game of "guess what I see."	As a family, color and decorate heavy paper plates. Use them as frisbees. Aim for a tree or play toss and catch.	Read a book with or to your child. Make up a story together. Be sure to write it down and draw pictures so you can enjoy it again later.	Use the Internet or library to look up dances from different cultures. Try a new dance each week.	As a family, bowl, play a round of miniature golf, ride bikes, dance, etc. Don't make it competitive. Just have fun.
Movement Games	Try walking in a straight line while balancing a balloon or foam ball in your hand. Repeat, this time walking in a circle or along a winding path.	Play "Simon Says" by directing your child to move in different ways. Repeat, with your preschooler giving you directions.	Make up your own family movement game. Remember to keep it simple so everyone can play and have fun.	Divide into pairs and play a game of opposites. If your partner hops forward, you hop backward. If you partner crouches on her knees, you jump up in the air.	As a family, form a line and play a movement game of follow the leader. Take turns being the leader.

Table 2 Ideas for Helping Families Become Healthy Role Models

Incorporate the following ideas into classroom newsletters, family workshops, and parent-teacher conferences to help families become healthy role models for their children.

Starting Smart: Teaching Young Children About Healthy Foods While Grocery Shopping

1. Help your child name the different types of vegetables and fruits on display in the produce section. Note that these foods are good for our bodies. When passing by the cookie and candy aisles, note that we should eat only a little of these items, and only occasionally. Help reinforce this message by "skipping" past these aisles with your child as you move on to more healthy foods.

2. Make a shopping list using pictures of healthy foods. Help your child cut out and paste the pictures onto sheets of paper. As your child decorates each page, note that the foods in the pictures are good for our bodies because they give us energy and help our bodies stay strong and healthy. Arrange the pictures in an order that reflects the layout of your grocery store. Hand your child a few pictures of the healthy food you are shopping for before entering each aisle. Your child can use the pictures to help you look for the healthy food. This game will also help distract him from looking for less healthy foods.

3. Point out the different colors, shapes, and textures associated with such foods as bell peppers, apples, onions, grapes, tomatoes, nuts, and lettuces. Help your child pick foods with the colors, shapes, or textures she would like to try in a snack or meal.

Eating In, Eating Out: Managing the Food Environment

1. Make sure that fresh and dried fruit, juice, milk, and water are readily available and easily accessible to everyone in the family. Putting juice and water in colorful pitchers will help catch your child's attention. Ask your child to draw pictures of his favorite fruits. Paste the pictures onto serving bowls to encourage him to go to those bowls for his snacks.

2. Ask your child to name her favorite healthy foods and write these on a large sheet of paper. Work with your child to write her own recipe, using some of the foods from her list. Use the recipe when preparing a family snack or meal.

3. When eating out, help your child find and make healthy choices by limiting your and his choices to only healthy items. Share the healthy choice you have made and repeat the healthy choices available to your child.

Serve as an Exercise Role Model

1. Take your child shopping for your exercise clothing and equipment. Talk about why you wear these clothes and how you use the equipment.

2. When dressing for exercise, talk to your child about why you are stretching, drinking water, and dressing in certain types of clothes. After exercising, talk to your child about how you feel.

3. Allow your child to play with your exercise equipment in a supervised and safe environment. Do not try to teach athletic skills. Instead, let her experiment with different movements.

Exceptions to the Rule

1. Practice moderation, not elimination. Allow your child to eat sweets now and then, explaining the importance of not making them a part of our daily diet. Repeating this message will help your child develop the mindset needed to follow a balanced diet.

2. At the end of holiday celebrations, help your child divide the candy he received into small portions and put them into individual sandwich bags. Give him two bags each week. One can serve as a special snack for the week. Encourage him to share the other bag with a family member. Serve something healthy (milk, water, or an apple) to drink or eat with the candy.

Practices to Avoid

1. Avoid the mindset of "Do as I say, not as I do," as it strikes children as being unfair. When they see adults eating candy or fast food, they have a difficult time understanding why they cannot do the same. Eating healthy is a family affair. Everyone should follow the same rules.

2. Avoid forcing your child to eat foods she does not like. Instead, use a "try me" approach to encourage your child to try new foods. Visit the following United States Department of Agriculture website to learn about the variety of foods you can serve that have similar nutritional qualities: www.mypyramid.gov/pyramid/index.html

3. Avoid using food as a reward. Such rewards often consist of unhealthy sweets, and this can promote unhealthy food choices and eating patterns.

4. Avoid placing your child on a strict diet. This will only interfere with her ability to develop the knowledge, skills, and motivation needed to follow a balanced diet. If you believe your child is overweight, consult with a nutritionist or your family physician to develop a plan of action that addresses both eating and physical activity patterns of behavior.

Television and Electronic Games

1. Follow the recommendation of the Council on Sports Medicine and Fitness and the Council on School Health (2006) of limiting your child's television viewing to no more than 2 hours per day. Help remind your child of this family rule by monitoring his television viewing and using the hands of a clock to show how much time he has left to watch television before it is turned off for the day.

(continued)

Table 2   Ideas for Helping Families Become Healthy Role Models *(continued)*

2. Take inventory of the number of electronic games in your home versus games and materials that promote physical activity, such as bikes, badminton sets, jump ropes, balls, and rackets and bats. Are your purchases more heavily weighted toward sedentary electronic games? If so, make a concentrated effort to balance out your purchases when selecting gifts for your child during the holidays and on her birthday.

3. Take television shows and electronic games outside. Work with your child to plan a version of her favorite television show or an electronic game that can be played outside. Follow two rules. First, the game must be safe and nonviolent. Second, it must involve movement. For example, you may plan a game called the human pinball machine. Friends and family members can take turns serving as stationary "bumpers" located at arm's length from each other (the bumpers cannot move from their spot) and "balls." Each "ball" attempts to run through the pinball machine without being touched by the stationary "bumpers."

- *Note how your center or school promotes healthy eating and physical activity.* Point out classroom menus and outdoor play equipment to families when conducting registration and orientations. Explain how menus and physical activities are developed. Encourage dialogue by asking families about their children's favorite foods and physical activities.

- *Make health part of parent-teacher conferences.* Address children's nutritional habits and physical activities that you have observed in the classroom. Compare your observations to those made by families in the home environment. Provide families with a list of community youth groups that offer free or inexpensive age-appropriate activities, like dance and swimming. Visit with a local school nutritionist or your local cooperative extension agent to gather ideas for quick and healthy snacks for families to try at home. Invite these experts to conduct family night workshops on such topics as childhood nutrition, reading and understanding food labels, using the food pyramid, and identifying misleading food advertisements. Invite professionals from your local department of recreation to demonstrate noncompetitive games that families can play at home, as well as fun activities that promote children's fundamental motor skills, like those presented in Figure 1.

- *Encourage families to share.* Inviting family members to the classroom to share their recreational hobbies is an inexpensive way to introduce children to a variety of physical activities. If children do engage in the activity being demonstrated, pair the visiting parent with an early childhood physical education teacher to ensure that developmentally appropriate practices are followed.

- *Engage families in the learning process.* Recruit families to work with children in growing a garden of herbs and vegetables in pots or raised beds. Families that are unable to come to the classroom can be provided with tip sheets on how to grow herbs and vegetables at home. Invite families to help children prepare healthy salads and other dishes using the herbs and vegetables they harvest.

Conclusion

There are no easy solutions to addressing the epidemic of children who are overweight. The authors hope that the information and ideas presented in this article will help early childhood educators play an active role in working with families to help children develop the eating and activity patterns needed for a healthy lifestyle.

References

Anderson, P. M., & Butcher, K. F. (2006). Childhood obesity: Trends and potential causes. *The Future of Children: Childhood Obesity, 16*(1), 19–45.

Belamarich, P. F., Luder, E., Kattan, M., Mitchell, H., Islam, S., Lynn, H., & Crain, E. F. (2000). Do obese inner-city children with asthma have more symptoms than nonobese children with asthma? *Pediatrics, 106*(6), 1436–1441.

Cawley, J. (2006). Markets and childhood obesity policy. *The Future of Children: Childhood Obesity, 16*(1), 69–88.

Center for Health and Health Care in Schools. (2005). *Childhood overweight: What the research tells us.* School of Public Health and Health Services, The Georgia Washington University Medical Center. Retrieved June 29, 2008, from www.healthinschools.org/~/media/Files/obesityfs.ashx.

Centers for Disease Control and Prevention. (2005a). *Overweight and obesity: Contributing factors.* Retrieved June 29, 2008, from cdc.gov/nccdphp/dnpa/obesity/contributing_factors.htm.

Centers for Disease Control and Prevention. (2005b). *Healthy youth! Promoting better health strategies.* Retrieved June 29, 2008, from www.cdc.gov/HealthyYouth/physicalactivity/promoting_health/strategies/families.htm.

Centers for Disease Control and Prevention. (2007, May 22). *Overweight prevalence.* Retrieved June 29, 2008, from www.cdc.gov/print.do?url=http%3A%2F%2Fwww.cdc.gov%2Fnccdphp%2Fdnpa%.

Committee on Nutrition. (2003). Prevention of pediatric overweight and obesity. *Pediatrics, 112*(2), 424–430.

Council on Sports Medicine and Fitness and Council on School Health. (2006). Active healthy living: Prevention of childhood obesity through increased physical activity. *Pediatrics, 117*(5), 1834–1842.

Daniels, S. R. (2006). The consequences of childhood overweight and obesity. *The Future of Children: Childhood Obesity, 16*(1), 47–67.

Davis, M. M., Gance-Cleveland, B., Hassink, S., Johnson, R., Paradis, G., & Resnicow, K. (2007). Recommendations for prevention of childhood obesity. *Pediatrics, 120* (Supplement 4), S229–S253.

Epstein, L. H., Valoski, A., Wing, R. R., & McCurley, J. (1994). Ten-year outcomes of behavioral family-based treatment for childhood obesity. *Health Psychology, 13*(5), 373–383.

Fierro, M. P. (2002). *The obesity epidemic—How states can trim the fat. Issue Brief.* National Governors Association Center for Best Practices. Online: www.nga.org/portal/site/nga.

Freedman, D. S., Dietz, W. H., Srinivasan, S. R., & Berenson, G. S. (1999). The relation of overweight to cardiovascular risk factors among children and adolescents: The Bogalusa heart study. *Pediatrics, 103*(6), 1175–1182.

Gilliland, F. D., Berhane, K., Islam, T., McConnell, R., Gauderman, W. J., Gilliland, S., Avol, E., & Peters, J. M. (2003). Obesity and the risk of newly diagnosed asthma in school-age children. *American Journal of Epidemiology, 158*(5), 406–415.

Golan, M., & Crow, S. (2004). Targeting parents exclusively in the treatment of childhood obesity: Long-term results. *Obesity Research, 12*(2), 357–361.

Golan, M. A., Weizman, A., Apter, A., & Fainaru, M. (1998). Parents as the exclusive agents of change in the treatment of childhood obesity. *American Journal of Clinical Nutrition, 67*(6), 1130–1135.

Harvey-Berino, J., & Rourke, J. (2003). Obesity prevention in preschool Native-American children: A pilot study using home visiting. *Obesity Research, 11*(5), 606–611.

Lindsay, A. C., Sussner, K. M., Kim, J., & Gortmaker, S. (2006). The role of parents in preventing childhood obesity. *The Future of Children: Childhood Obesity, 16*(1), 169–186.

Ludwig, D. S., & Ebbeling, T. B. (2001). Type 2 diabetes mellitus in children: Primary care and public health considerations. *Journal of the American Medical Association, 286*(12), 1427–1430.

National Conference of State Legislatures. (2005). *Childhood obesity: An overview of policy options in legislation for 2003–2004.* Online: www.ncsl.org/programs/health/childhoodobesity.htm.

Olshansky, S. J., Passaro, D. J., Hershow, J. L., Carnes, B. A., Brody, J., Hayflick, L., Butler, R. N., Allision, D. B., & Ludwig. D. S. (2005). A potential decline in life expectancy in the United States in the 21st century. *New England Journal of Medicine, 253*(11), 1138–1145.

Polhamus, B., Dalenius, K., Thompson, D., Scanlon, K., Borland, E., Smith, B., & Grummer-Strawn, L. (2004). *Pediatric nutrition surveillance 2002 report.* Atlanta, GA: U.S. Department of Health and Human Services, Centers for Disease Control and Prevention.

Schwimmer, J. B., Burwinkle, T. M., & Varni, J. W. (2003). Health-related quality of life of severely obese children and adolescents. *Journal of the American Medical Association, 289*(14), 1813–1819.

U.S. Department of Health and Human Services. (2001). *The surgeon general's call to action to prevent and decrease overweight and obesity.* Rockville, MD: Public Health Service, Office of the Surgeon General.

U.S. Department of Health and Human Services. (2004). *Healthy People 2010 Progress Review: Nutrition and overweight.* Online: www.healthypeople.gov/data/2010prog/focus19/default.htm.

Young, L. R., & Nestle, M. (2002). The contribution of expanding portion sizes to the U.S. obesity epidemic. *American Journal of Public Health, 92*(2), 246–249.

Young-Hyman, D., Herman, L., Scott, D. L., & Schlundt, D. G. (2000). Care giver perception of children's obesity-related health risk: A study of African-American families. *Obesity Research, 8*(3), 241–248.

Critical Thinking

1. What percentage of overweight children, 5–10 years old, have high blood pressure, high cholesterol, and/or hardening of the arteries?

2. What are the six health-related consequences associated with children being overweight?

3. What are three examples of how families can serve as positive role models for overweight kids?

MICK COLEMAN is Professor, **CHARLOTTE WALLINGA** is Associate Professor, and **DIANE BALES** is Associate Professor, Department of Child and Family Development, University of Georgia, Athens.

Do Organics Promote Children's Health?

Research Shows Pesticides May Cause Neurological Disorders.

CAROL ANN BRANNON

The Choose MyPlate message is concise and colorful: "Make half your plate fruits and vegetables." While the health benefits of a diet rich in fruits and vegetables is well documented, there's increasing concern about the safety of exposure to agricultural pesticide residues on produce, especially for pregnant women and young children. The emerging research linking pesticide exposure to childhood neurobehavioral disorders has captured parents' attention.

As often happens, commercial promotion, hearsay, and rumors have clouded the issue and confused consumers. Dietitians should anticipate parents' most frequently asked questions about pesticides, organic foods, and the potential link to attention, behavioral, and cognitive problems in children and offer personalized, practical, budget-friendly options for purchasing organic foods. This continuing education activity will review current studies on organophosphate (OP) pesticides and their potential to impair neurodevelopment and cause neurobehavioral disorders in children, and provide dietitians with practical tips for counseling clients.

Do Pesticides Cause ADHD in Children?

Recent studies linking ADHD and pesticide exposure have made headlines and prompted parental questions about the possible connection between children's diets and their attention, cognition, behavior, and sensory issues as well as their overall health.

Their questions include: Is there a connection between the increased incidence of neurobehavioral disorders like ADHD and learning differences and the increased use of agricultural pesticides? How safe is conventionally grown produce for pregnant women, infants, and young children? Do the health benefits of a diet rich in conventionally grown fruits and vegetables outweigh the risks of pesticide exposure? How can organic produce be incorporated into a family's food budget?

The percentage of children with learning and developmental disabilities (LDDs), including ADHD and autism spectrum disorder, as well as food allergies and autoimmune-related disease, has increased steadily over the past 40 years. ADHD is the most prevalent and researched pediatric psychiatric disorder, with an estimated 8.7% of U.S. children aged 8 to 15 meeting the diagnostic criteria. The fourth edition of the ***Diagnostic Statistical Manual of Mental Disorders*** of the American Psychiatric Association defines ADHD as a neurobiological disorder characterized by hyperactivity-impulsiveness and inattention or the inability to sustain attention or concentration in developmentally appropriate ways. ADHD is classified into two categories, poor sustained attention and hyperactivity-impulsiveness, and three subcategories, predominantly inattentive, predominantly hyperactive-impulsive, and combined types.

ADHD can cause academic, social, and psychological problems, adversely affecting a child's self-esteem and ability to reach his or her full potential. Studies have shown that without treatment, children with ADHD are at an increased risk of lower academic achievement, injuries, alcohol or substance abuse, and early pregnancy.

Learning Objectives

After completing this continuing education activity, nutrition professionals should be better able to:

1. Evaluate several reasons children are at greater risk of harm from pesticide exposure than adults.
2. Distinguish the signs of ADHD.
3. Examine the association between pesticide exposure and neurobehavioral conditions in children.
4. Illustrate the process for evaluating and regulating the safety of chemicals in the United States.
5. Provide dietary and budgetary guidance to consumers regarding the purchase of organic produce and foods.

The precise etiology of LDDs is unknown, but many factors (eg, genetics, environmental toxins, nutrition) are implicated. More research continues to focus on the impact of environmental neurotoxins on brain development and function, including attention, learning, and behavior. Neurotoxins can damage, destroy, or impair nerve tissue; interfere with brain development; and disrupt the endocrine (hormone) system.

Pesticide Use on the Rise

In the past 50 years, the use of agricultural pesticides has increased significantly as large-scale commercial farms have replaced family-operated farms. Pesticides are neurotoxins developed to kill pests (eg, rodents, insects, weeds, fungi) that hinder crop growth. The generous use of pesticides, synthetic fertilizers, hormones, and antibiotics has become routine to ensure optimal crop yield.

In 1939, the organochlorine called dichlorodiphenyltrichloroethane (DDT) was discovered as an inexpensive and effective pesticide. DDT was widely used until the early 1970s when harmful environmental effects couldn't be ignored. In 2004, more than 100 countries signed the Stockholm Convention on Persistent Organic Pollutants, banning the use of DDT and other pesticides. However, DDT is still used to kill mosquitoes in several southern African and Asian countries where malaria is endemic. Experts reason that malaria is a greater threat to health and life than DDT exposure. More than 700,000 African children die yearly from malaria.

Despite being banned 40 years ago, DDT and its residues remain in our environment and the adipose tissue of a large population of humans today. DDT and its metabolite dichlorodiphenyldichloroethylene (DDE) are classified as endocrine disruptors. Evidence suggests there's an association between long-term DDT and DDE exposure and preterm birth and low birth weight; growth reduction in boys; earlier puberty in girls; adverse pregnancies; endocrine disorders, including diabetes; breast cancer in women; reduction in semen quality in men; and risk of cancer. The Environmental Protection Agency (EPA) considers DDT a probable carcinogen, while the U.S. National Toxicology Program states DDT is "reasonably anticipated" to be a human carcinogen. A 2007 study concluded that American women exposed to high levels of DDT before midadolescence had a five-fold increase in the risk of developing breast cancer.

Still, the OP class of pesticides is the most common and heavily used in the United States, widely applied to crops of corn, soy, wheat, and various fruits and vegetables. As of 2010, the EPA had registered 32 OP pesticides. The EPA considers residue in food and drinking water, as well as residential pesticide use, important sources of exposure. The Centers for Disease Control and Prevention regards diet as the major source of pesticide exposure for infants and children.

Children at Risk

A fundamental principle in pediatric medicine and nutrition is that "children are not little adults." This observation is especially relevant regarding children and neurotoxin exposure. The EPA and the National Academy of Sciences report that "standard chemicals are up to ten times more toxic to children than to adults, depending on body weight."

At conception, children are more vulnerable to harm from toxic chemical exposure than adults. Immediately after conception, cells begin rapidly dividing as the brain and organ systems develop. Even a tiny dose of a neurotoxic chemical early in the prenatal period can interfere with or impair healthy brain development. The fetus, depending on the stage of development, is selectively sensitive to particular neurotoxins. Two birth cohort studies suggest that increased levels of OP exposure in utero resulted in greater numbers of abnormal reflexes in newborns. A study of 329 California 7-year-olds, primarily children of Latino farm workers, found an association between prenatal exposure to OP pesticides and lower IQ scores.

Exposure to OP pesticides may initially occur in utero, but as infants and children grow, their exposure is likely to increase through diet and outdoor activities. Infants take more breaths per minute and have more skin surface relative to their body weight than adults; therefore, their exposure to pesticides is greater than adults. Infants and young children engage in hand-to-mouth behaviors that can increase their risk of environmental exposure. Children live and play closer to the ground than adults, so their risk of exposure to volatile pesticide vapors is greater. In addition, children, more often than adults, eat and drink relative to their body weight, which can lead to higher exposures of pesticide residue per pound of body weight.

Even chronic low-level neurotoxin exposure can be harmful because children's immune systems are immature, and the activity and expression of detoxifying enzymes is reduced. The potential for harm exists into late adolescence as the brain continues to develop.

Neurotoxic Properties and Effects

OP pesticides act by impairing acetylcholinesterase, the enzyme responsible for the degradation of acetylcholine, a neurotransmitter. Acetylcholine is essential to skeletal-muscle motor neurons, peripheral parasympathetic and sympathetic neurons, and multiple fibers in the central nervous system, including those that assist in regulating memory acquisition. Impairment of acetylcholinesterase causes an accumulation of acetylcholine, or choleric excess, in the central and peripheral nervous systems. This choleric excess results in continued stimulation followed by suppression of neurotransmission—it's this effect that kills pests.

There's strong toxicological evidence demonstrating that repeated low-level exposure to OP pesticides adversely affects neurodevelopment and growth in developing animals. The findings from animal studies demonstrate a link between OP pesticide exposure in utero and impaired maze performance, locomotion, and balance postpartum.

OP pesticides are harmful to humans as well. In the body, pesticides are broken down into compounds including dialkyl phosphate (DK) and dimethyl alkylphosphate (DMAP), which are detectable and measurable in urine. The harm caused in adults and children can vary depending on dose and length of exposure. Acute high-level OP pesticide exposure and poisoning is more likely to occur in an occupational or agricultural setting. The signs and symptoms of acute OP pesticide poisoning caused by cholinergic excess include copious respiratory and oral secretions, diarrhea, vomiting, sweating, altered mental status, autonomic instability, and generalized weakness.

However, the signs and symptoms of chronic low-level OP exposure are subtler, and the lag time between exposure and manifestation of signs and symptoms varies (see below). With repeated exposure, even in small amounts, pesticides can build up in body tissue stores.

Pesticides and Neurobehavioral Disorders

Emerging studies suggest a connection between OP pesticide exposure and the development of various neurobehavioral disorders, particularly ADHD. Kofman and colleagues found a link between an OP pesticide and delays in learning rates, reduced physical coordination, and behavioral problems, especially in children with ADHD. Two separate studies, both conducted in agricultural areas (one in Mexico and one in California's Central Valley), have suggested a tie between increased levels of OP pesticides in children and a rise in maternally reported pervasive developmental disorder, an umbrella term for a group of disorders that includes autism and Asperger's syndrome.

Perhaps the most notable study to date was conducted by Bouchard and colleagues.[4] This study, which caught the media's attention and was widely reported, examined health data from 2000 to 2004 of 1,139 children aged 8 to 15 that was representative of the U.S. population. Children in this study who had higher urinary levels of the OP metabolites DK and DMAP were more likely to meet the diagnostic criteria for ADHD.

While this study couldn't and doesn't prove that pesticides cause ADHD, it demonstrates a possible association between pesticide exposure and the risk of developing ADHD. Experts agree this research is persuasive, but more prospective studies are needed for clarification. This study was unique because it demonstrated that even in the smallest amounts, pesticides might affect neurotransmitters and brain and neurobehavioral development (eg, inattention, impulsivity, hyperactivity, learning difficulties).

U.S. Pesticide Monitoring

The EPA is responsible for regulating pesticides under the Federal Insecticide, Fungicide, and Rodenticide Act (FIFRA) and the Food Quality Protection Act of 1996 (FQPA). In 1991, the Pesticide Data Program (PDP) was initiated for the purpose of pesticide data collection. The PDP plays an important role in administrating the FQPA, which mandates that pesticide residue data must be collected from the foods infants and children most frequently consume. The EPA uses PDP data to assess pesticide

safety and tolerances (maximum residue limits). The EPA has maximum safety tolerance levels for some pesticides, and no tolerance safety levels for other pesticides. A no-tolerance level means there should be no detectable pesticide residues on produce. The EPA, the USDA, and the FDA are involved in the regulation, use, and safety of agricultural pesticides.

Before pesticides are distributed, sold, or used, they must go through the EPA registration process, which can last as long as nine years and cost millions of dollars. A company seeking pesticide registration must provide data from various short-term and long-term tests performed according to EPA guidelines to evaluate the pesticide's potential to cause harm. Criteria include cancer and reproductive system disorders in humans, wildlife, fish, and plants, including endangered species and nontarget organisms. In addition, possible contamination of surface or ground water from leaching, runoff, and spray drift is assessed.

A pesticide becomes registered when the EPA determines that the highest possible dose, either as a single exposure or chronic exposure, has a no-observable adverse effect level in experimental animals. The EPA then determines the reference dose (RD), the amount of a pesticide residue a person can consume daily for 70 years without any expected health-related problems. The RD is used as the toxicological indicator when pesticide residues are tested on foods designated for human consumption. A chemical classified as having no observable adverse effects differs from a chemical "proven safe" or secure from risk or harm.

Most conventionally grown produce contains residues that are within the EPA allowable limits. Some produce may have residues from multiple pesticides. The U.S. Pesticide Residue Program Report (2008) found that 28% of frozen blueberries, 25% of strawberries, and 19% of celery samples had detectable concentrations of malathion, an OP pesticide, but residue amounts were within EPA safety levels. Malathion has been widely used since 1956 to eradicate mosquitoes, boll weevils, and fruit flies that threaten crop yields and transmit harmful viruses, pathogens, and diseases.

Do pesticides pose a health risk at low levels of exposure that were once considered insignificant? A growing number of experts question the current acceptable "toxic threshold" level—the lowest exposure thought to be harmful.

Biological monitoring in the United States indicates that pesticides and other contaminants are more prevalent than originally thought, with higher levels seen in some subpopulations. In a study of low-income pregnant women and newborns in New York City, detectable levels of OP pesticides were found in 70% of the women, and the cord-blood samples of 64% of newborns had detectable levels.

Organic Foods Reduce Exposure

A 2003 study by Curl and colleagues reported that children aged 2 to 5 who ate conventionally grown foods had six times more urinary OP pesticide metabolites (DK and DMAP) than children who ate organic foods. Another study published in

2008 by Lu and colleagues involved 23 children aged 3 to 11 who consumed only conventional diets. During the one-year study, the children consumed conventionally grown foods but were switched to organic diets for five consecutive days in the summer and fall. Investigators obtained urine samples twice daily for seven, 12, or 15 consecutive days during each season of the year. They measured specific urinary metabolites of malathion, chlorpyrifos, and other OP pesticides. Concentrations of OP-specific metabolites were reported and classified into one of three categories: detectable, detectable but not quantifiable, or undetectable. Researchers found that children who switched from eating conventionally grown produce to eating organic produce had either undetectable or detectable but not quantifiable levels of urinary pesticide metabolites.

Seven Frequently Asked Questions

The definition of organic has become clearer with the establishment of specific standards for growing and processing produce. But as you know, parents still ask dietitians for the definition of organic and guidance on purchasing these food items. Here are some of the questions parents often ask and answers you can provide:

1. **How is organic produce different from conventionally grown produce?** The philosophy of organic farming is the preservation of the cycle of life by utilizing food waste and manure to rebuild the soil for future food production. The primary goal of organic farming is to sustain ecological harmony and interdependence between soil, plants, animals, and humans.

   The USDA defines organic as produce that's grown without the use of most conventional pesticides, fertilizers made with synthetic ingredients or sewage sludge, bioengineering, or ionizing radiation. Organic crops must be grown on soil free of prohibited substances for three years before they're classified as organic.

   Organic farmers use renewable resources and value soil and water conservation. In contrast to long-lasting synthetic pesticides, botanical or nonsynthetic pesticides used in organic farming are quickly broken down by sunlight and oxygen. However, an estimated 10% to 25% of organic fruits and vegetables contain some residues of synthetic pesticides due to polluted groundwater and rain but in amounts significantly lower than conventional produce.

   Organically produced whole foods will have a green and white organic seal on the label, indicating compliance to strict USDA organic standards and inspection. Packaged or commercially prepared foods that are labeled 100% organic have no synthetic ingredients, while foods containing a minimum of 95% organic ingredients are eligible to use the USDA organic seal. A packaged or commercially prepared food that's labeled "made with organic ingredients" must contain at least 70% organic ingredients but cannot use the USDA seal.

New ADHD Diagnosis Guidelines for Kids

On October 16, the American Academy of Pediatrics (AAP), at their annual national meeting and conference in Boston, released expanded guidelines for the diagnosis and management of ADHD in preschool children aged 4 and older. The previous AAP guidelines, issued 10 years ago, were written for the diagnosis and treatment of ADHD in children aged 6 to 12. This updated report, "ADHD: Clinical Practice Guidelines for the Diagnosis, Evaluation, and Treatment of Attention-Deficit/Hyperactivity Disorder in Children and Adolescents," was published in the November issue of *Pediatrics.*

2. **What's different about organically produced meat, poultry, eggs, and dairy foods?** Organic meat, poultry, eggs, and dairy foods come from animals that don't receive antibiotics or growth hormones. The philosophy of organic livestock production is to provide conditions that meet the health needs and natural behavior of the animal. Organic livestock must be given access to the outdoors, fresh air, water, sunshine, grass, and pasture. Organic livestock must be fed 100% organic feed that's free of any animal by-products, hormones, antibiotics, or other animal drugs. If an organic animal gets sick and receives antibiotics, it's not considered organic any longer. Certified organic farmers must keep extensive records to trace the animal from birth to the market. Meat labeled organic is 100% organic—there's no "partially organic" category.

3. **Are organic foods safer?** If safer means free from bacterial contamination and other harmful organisms, the answer is no. The USDA makes no claims that organic foods are safer to eat than conventional foods. The Organic Trade Association says organic products are as safe as conventionally produced foods. Because certified organic farmers adhere to strict guidelines for safe and hygienic food production and comply with all local, state, and federal health standards, one can infer that their products are grown and handled with care and may be less likely to become contaminated. However, any produce—organic and nonorganic—can become contaminated with harmful bacteria. To ensure food safety, one should follow proper hand- and produce-washing procedures as well as safe food storage and cooking practices.

4. **Are organic foods more nutritious?** There's an ongoing debate about whether organic foods are superior to conventional foods in nutrient content. The USDA makes no claims that organic foods are more nutritious than conventional foods. A systematic evaluation of 162

studies, of which 55 were considered of satisfactory quality and extensively analyzed, found that conventionally produced crops had a significantly higher content of nitrogen, while organically produced crops had a significantly higher content of phosphorus and higher titratable acidity. The investigators concluded that the small differences detected in nutrient content were biologically plausible and most likely related to differences in production methods. However, it's important to note that investigators of this systematic review didn't consider the presence of contaminants (pesticides or other possible environmental toxins) as a factor in assessing nutritional value or safety.

Designing a scientific study to investigate and compare the nutrient content of organic and conventionally produced foods is a challenge, as it requires controlling for all variables (soil quality and condition and maturity at harvest) that could influence nutrient content. Despite the challenges of research design, a small number of studies indicate that organic produce has a greater mineral content than conventional produce. This higher mineral content is most likely due to the use of organic fertilizers (compost or manure). Diversity in local soil conditions is an important variable in nutrient content.

However, organic products may offer health benefits beyond mineral content. Some organic fruits and vegetables may have higher levels of phytochemicals compared with those conventionally grown. The use of organic fertilizers in organic farming results in plants with lower levels of nitrogen and nitrate. Dietary nitrate can be metabolized to nitrite and then converted in the presence of stomach acid to nitrosamines, which are linked to cancer development in animals and potentially humans. Much more research is needed in this area.

5. **Do organic foods taste better?** There's no clear scientific evidence to prove that organic produce tastes better; however, consumers of organics are adamant that the flavor and freshness of organic foods, especially locally grown produce, is superior to conventional foods. Taste is subjective and personal, and the power of suggestion may be at work here.

Possible Health Effects of OP Exposure

- Runny nose
- Chest tightness
- Shortness of breath
- Sweating
- Nausea
- Vomiting
- Stomach cramps
- Muscle twitching
- Confusion
- Seizures
- Paralysis
- Coma
- Death

6. **Is natural the same as organic?** No. The terms "free range," "hormone free," or "natural" aren't synonymous with organic. The term "natural" broadly refers to minimally processed foods that are free of synthetic preservatives, artificial additives, hydrogenated oils, stabilizers, and emulsifiers. Natural food products aren't regulated; however, the USDA allows meat and poultry to use this term for products that have been minimally processed, that don't differ fundamentally from the raw product, and that contain no artificial ingredients, such as carrageenan or monosodium glutamate. The majority of raw meat and poultry found in grocery stores fits this definition. Natural doesn't mean hormone or antibiotic free.

7. **Are organics worth the price?** That's an individual decision. While most parents probably would prefer to purchase organic foods, the higher cost of organics is an obstacle. Organic foods cost an average of 50% more than conventionally grown produce. Nonetheless, organic food sales are increasing and are no longer just available in health food stores. Advocates of localism (the preference for food produced close to its market, usually on small farms) say reduced transport and storage costs can make these foods more reasonably priced.

Dirty Dozen

(highest in pesticide residue)

Fruits: peaches, apples, nectarines (imported), strawberries, blueberries (domestic), grapes (imported)

Vegetables: sweet bell peppers, celery, spinach, lettuce, potatoes, kale/collard greens

Not-So-Dirty Dozen

(lowest in pesticide residue)

Fruits: watermelon, grapefruit, kiwifruit, mangoes, pineapple

Vegetables: eggplant, cabbage, sweet peas, asparagus, sweet corn, avocados, onions

Source: Environmental Working Group (www.ewg.org/foodnews/summary)

Buying Organics on a Shoestring

Here's what you can suggest to clients who wish to buy organic produce but are concerned about the cost:

- **Make a grocery list based on planned menus.** Suggest clients make a shopping list and stick to it. That way they'll resist impulse purchases and allocate more grocery dollars for organic foods. Advise them to shop the perimeter of the store, since the most expensive processed foods are located in the interior aisles.
- **Shop for seasonal produce.** Seasonal produce is less expensive. Buy in bulk and freeze or can certain items to use later.
- **Buy from local farmers' markets and/or join a community co-op.** It isn't necessary to become a strict locavore, but if clients do a little research, they can identify nearby organic growers who can and will sell in bulk. Farmers' markets are great places to meet fellow organic shoppers. And for a small monthly or annual fee, they can join a community co-op to get reasonably priced organic and local produce.
- **Join a community-supported agriculture program.** Members pay a weekly fee and in return receive a set amount of seasonal organic produce at reasonable prices. Generally, there's a designated weekly pick-up location.
- **Purchase frozen organic foods.** Frozen organics can be found in most supermarket freezer sections and are usually less expensive than fresh organics.
- **Buy generic or store brand organics.** Many chain stores are offering their own brands of certified organic canned or frozen foods.
- **Clip coupons.** Suggest clients visit www.organiccoupons.com, a website that provides money-saving coupons for organic products.
- **Prioritize purchases.** It's possible to become fixated on purity at any price. However, not all conventionally grown produce is created equal. Some are less contaminated with pesticide residues than others. See the chart above for a list of fruits that contain the highest and lowest amounts of pesticides. Clients can purchase organic varieties of those

foods that have the most pesticide residues and buy the conventionally grown produce that has the least.

- **Wash produce thoroughly to remove any lingering dirt, pesticide residue, and bacteria.** The USDA advises consumers to wash fruits and vegetables (including produce with inedible skin) under cold running water. Clients can scrub fruits and vegetables if the outer surface or skin is firm. Don't use soap since the FDA hasn't approved the use of soap products on foods; consumers can ingest soap or detergent residues the produce absorbs. In addition, clients should remove any damaged or bruised parts on fruits and vegetables because potentially harmful bacteria can thrive in these nooks and crannies. And they should remove and discard the outer leaves of leafy vegetables, then wash the remaining leaves.
- **Trim visible fat and skin from meat and poultry.** Pesticide residues can collect in fat.
- **Plant an organic garden.** If planting a full-size garden seems overwhelming for clients, they can start with container gardening. Container gardens will enable clients to grow plants exclusively in containers instead of in the ground. They're ideal for people living in apartments or urban areas or for those unable to plant a traditional in-ground garden. Moreover, working in the garden is a valuable opportunity for parent-child bonding and nutrition education.

Critical Thinking

1. Justify three reasons children are at greater risk of harm from exposure to agricultural chemicals.
2. Critique the proposed link between pesticide exposure and neurobehavioral conditions (ie, ADHD).
3. Describe how the Environmental Protection Agency determines the safe dose of a pesticide.

CAROL ANN BRANNON, specializes in nutrition and feeding therapy for children and adults with developmental and learning differences in her private practice in metro Atlanta.

From *Today's Dietitian*, December, 2011. Copyright © 2011 by Today's Dietitian. Reprinted by permission.

Ultimate Food Fight Erupts as Feds Recook School Lunch Rules

Nirvi Shah

Across the country, school cafeteria managers, farm lobbyists, food companies, celebrity chefs, students, and parents have started the ultimate food fight.

The skirmish is over the U.S. Department of Agriculture's efforts, prompted by the recent passage of the Healthy, Hunger-Free Kids Act, to rewrite the rules about meals served through the National School Lunch and Breakfast programs. At stake is what will and won't be offered in the breakfasts and lunches schools serve millions of children every weekday.

"It's not your grandmother's school lunch anymore," Nancy Rice, the head of the School Nutrition Association, said at one of the advocacy group's gatherings last month.

The first rewrite of school-meal rules in 15 years, the proposed standards aim to cut sodium, boost the amount and types of fruits and vegetables students are offered, cut saturated fat, increase whole grains, and for the first time, limit calories. (The new proposed standards don't set limits on or address sugar, in part because sugar wasn't addressed in school meal requirements created by the Institute of Medicine. The USDA based its proposal largely on the Institute's recommendations.) The proposed rules, intended to simultaneously combat childhood obesity and malnutrition, have drawn thousands of emails, letters, and drawings that voice opinions about the proposed nutrition standards for school meals. And some of the interest has been high-profile, including school food activist Jamie Oliver, also known as "The Naked Chef," who has thrown his support behind the changes; the Berkeley, Calif.-based organic and natural foods company Annie's Homegrown, which created a website devoted to sending thank-you notes to the USDA for adding more vegetables to school meals; and the Washington-based National Potato Council, which also has a new website pushing for more potatoes to be allowed in school meals.

The proposed rules were published in January and comments are expected to roll in until the April 13 deadline. It may be next year before the rules are final, giving schools until at least the 2012–13 school year to put the new standards into practice. But stakeholders are asking for many concessions, saying some of the requirements would be impossible or have already proved so in school cafeterias.

"It is difficult to have one-size-fits-all," Agriculture Secretary Tom Vilsack told school nutrition directors in March. "I feel your pain. The trick is doing the balancing act . . . between what is appropriate . . . and fiscally responsible."

One of the biggest concerns is the expected cost to school districts: $6.8 billion over five years on food and labor. Some districts would have to buy new kitchen equipment, too.

The New Menu for Cafeterias

The nutrition standards for school meals would change dramatically under the new Healthy, Hunger-Free Kids Act. Among the proposed changes:

All Meals

- Milk: One-cup servings of unflavored milk must be 1 percent milk-fat or fat-free, and one-cup servings of flavored milk must be fat-free.
- At first, half of bread products served must be made with at least 51 percent whole grains. Two years after the USDA implements the nutrition regulations, all breads served must be at least 51 percent whole grain.

Breakfast

- Students must be offered one full cup of fruit at breakfast. Only half a cup could be juice, and that would have to be 100 percent fruit juice. Fruit could be replaced with vegetables.
- A meat or meat alternative, such as eggs, yogurt, or cheese, would have to be served every day. Tofu is not an approved meat alternative.
- The calorie range is 350 to 500 for elementary students, 400 to 550 for middle schoolers, and 450 to 600 for high schoolers.

- No starchy vegetables—potatoes, corn, peas, or lima beans—are allowed.
- Over the course of 10 years, schools must reduce sodium to 430 milligrams or less per breakfast for elementary students, 470 milligrams or less for middle schoolers, and 500 milligrams or less for high schoolers.

Lunch

- Elementary and middle students must be offered a one-half cup serving of fruit every day. High school students must be offered a cup every day.
- The calorie range is 550 to 650 in elementary school, 600 to 700 in the middle grades, and 750 to 850 in high school.
- Elementary and middle school students must be offered at least one ¾-cup serving of vegetables every day; one cup for high school students.
- Starchy vegetables must be limited to a one-cup serving a week.
- A one-half-cup serving of dark-green vegetables must be offered at least once a week.
- A one-half-cup serving of orange vegetables must be offered at least once a week.
- A one-half-cup serving of legumes—black beans, black-eyed peas, garbanzo beans, green peas, kidney beans, lentils, lima beans, soy beans, split peas, and white beans—must be served once a week.
- Over 10 years, schools must reduce sodium to 430 milligrams or less per lunch in elementary school, 470 milligrams or less in middle school, and 500 milligrams or less in high school.

The price tag was a main reason the American Association of School Administrators, the National School Boards Association, and the Council of the Great City Schools lobbied against the law. Because of the cost, the state of the economy, and the possibility that additional federal money per meal to meet the requirements may not materialize until after they go into effect, the Arlington, Va.-based AASA, in its comments, said districts need more time to put the final regulations into practice. The School Nutrition Association, a group of 55,000 school nutrition directors based in National Harbor, Md., also wants more time, in part because some foods required aren't available in some regions.

Adding more fresh fruits and vegetables this year to school meals in Norfolk, Va., cost about $500,000, said Helen Phillips, the school district's senior director of school nutrition and president-elect of the School Nutrition Association. But at least in her district, changes in anticipation of the federal regulations have been put in over time, allowing her to space out the added costs. For districts with less progressive menus, costs could shoot upward more quickly.

"The cost is big anyway," Ms. Phillips said. But compounding the change, "food costs are at an all time high."

But Margo G. Wootan, the director of nutrition policy at the Center for Science in the Public Interest in Washington, which lobbied for the law, finds neither the timeline nor the costs insurmountable.

"There are lots of school districts that are serving healthy meals under the current reimbursement rate," Ms. Wootan said, referring to how much school districts are paid by the USDA per meal.

The federal agency has suggested districts raise prices, if necessary, to offset costs, although school nutrition directors fear that could turn off some students.

Whole-Grain Everything

Aside from cost, there are concerns about nearly every part of the regulations. One proposed rule requires schools to switch all breads—tortillas, pizza crust, pancakes—to whole grains. At first, half of all bread products must be whole-grain rich, or made with at least 51 percent whole grains. Two years after the rules are final, all grains served would have to be whole-grain rich.

In the Sioux Falls, S.D., schools, Child Nutrition Supervisor Joni Davis said her 21,500-student district is halfway there.

"We've been talking to vendors, and they're listening," Ms. Davis said, although at first, they thought she was "a little bit crazy" for asking for whole-grain breading on chicken patties.

But the Anne Arundel County schools in Maryland abandoned a yearlong effort to switch to whole grains for some lunch items, said Jodi Risse, the supervisor of food and nutrition services in the 75,000-student district. While students didn't seem to notice the change in breakfast breads, they quickly learned to avoid pizza and egg rolls made with whole grains. "We couldn't tell as adults," Ms. Risse said, but for students, "over a few months we saw the consumption of egg rolls just go away. They probably don't eat it that way anywhere else." And there can be a tradeoff when adding whole grains: more sugar. For example, when the Schwan Food Co. of Marshall, Minn., reformulated the pizza it makes for schools to increase whole grains, it added sugar, a comparison of the printed nutrition facts for the two products shows. The USDA said it hopes that calorie requirements will keep sugar levels in check.

'Bok Choy? Watercress?'

In the Burlington, Vt., schools, Food Service Director Doug Davis said his 4,000-student district has easily incorporated orange and dark-green vegetables into menus, in part because of a farm-to-school program that emphasizes local produce.

Lunch Letters

In letters to the Agriculture Department, children thank the federal agency for the proposed nutrition rules:

"Those are the kinds of things that grow best for us," Mr. Davis said, so students are used to eating kale and butternut squash. The proposed rules require at least one half-cup serving each of dark-green and orange vegetables a week.

They include bok choy, broccoli, collard greens, dark green leafy lettuce, kale, mustard greens, romaine lettuce, spinach, turnip greens, and watercress, and acorn squash, butternut squash, carrots, pumpkin, and sweet potatoes.

Burlington students eat vegetables, including zucchini and carrots, in breakfast breads, too.

But back in Sioux Falls, Ms. Davis said her district hasn't been big on squash and pumpkin, and including dark-green vegetables, other than broccoli, may be tricky.

"Bok choy? Watercress? That's going to be different. Can you put broccoli on your menu every week as your dark green?" she said. "When we think of kids trying new vegetables, the first time they look at it. The second time they smell it. And the fourth, maybe, they eat it."

Besides the challenge of adding new items is the required serving size, said Bob Bloomer, a regional vice president for Chartwells-Thompson Hospitality of Charlotte, N.C., which provides meals for about 470 Chicago public schools. The proposed regulations would require a minimum of one cup of fruit at breakfast for all students, only half of which may be 100 percent fruit juice. For elementary and middle school students, another half cup of fruit and a ¾-cup serving of vegetables would be offered at lunch, when high schoolers get a full cup each of fruits and vegetables.

"A cup of vegetables? No high school student is going to take a cup of vegetables," Mr. Bloomer said. He and others worry much of the additional produce will end up in the garbage instead of students' stomachs.

Potato Pushback

While children must be served more veggies, the proposal also says cafeterias must reduce starchy items. Potatoes, corn, green peas, and fresh lima beans—those that weren't picked dry off the plant—would be limited to one cup total per week at lunch. Sweet potatoes aren't considered a starchy vegetable in the proposal.

"It doesn't make any sense at a time when you're telling kids to consume more vegetables," said John Keeling, the executive vice president and chief executive officer of the National Potato Council. He said the bad rap on french fries has tainted the popular, cheap tuber, which is high in fiber and potassium and low in calories.

Many schools serve "fries" that are actually baked in the oven, he said. His organization recommends allowing four half-cup servings of spuds a week, plus a serving of another starchy vegetable, and allowing potatoes at breakfast. The School Nutrition Association goes further: They asked for four half-cup servings of potatoes a week in elementary school, and no limits on the number of days those half-cup servings are offered in middle and high school per week—as long as kids can't take seconds and neither potatoes nor any other vegetable could be fried.

The recommendation isn't because cutting back on potatoes isn't impossible, said Ms. Phillips, of the SNA. In her menus in Norfolk, Va., there are weeks when potatoes aren't offered at all. But other districts may rely more heavily on potatoes. "It goes back to where districts are currently," she said, and "a concern . . . that we do have for children. Some of their favorite vegetables are starchy vegetables. To limit them to just that to one cup a week might discourage them from eating vegetables at all."

But Ms. Wootan of the Center for Science in the Public Interest, said the problem with potatoes isn't whether they are fried or roasted.

"It's just the variety," she said. "If kids were eating carrots as their only vegetable at every meal, that wouldn't be a good thing either."

Got (Fat-Free Chocolate) Milk?

The National Dairy Council worries that chocolate milk, long the dairy king among students, may be less inviting in fat-free form. Flavored milks that are anything but fat-free wouldn't be allowed under the new guidelines, although schools could serve unflavored milk with up to 1 percent milk-fat. "We want to make sure there are not unintended consequences," said Ann Marie Krautheim, senior vice president of nutrition affairs of the Council, based in Rosemont, Ill. In other words, if students dislike fat-free flavored milk, they might not drink milk at all.

But in Anne Arundel, students never noticed the switch to skim chocolate and strawberry milk this school year, Ms. Risse said. To make up for the missing fat, the milk has a little more sugar and flavoring, but the district's milk consumption is virtually unchanged. For some districts, however, including Norfolk and Burlington, fat-free flavored milk isn't available from the closest dairies, one reason the School Nutrition Association wants more time before the regulations take effect.

"We need to get the standards out there, let industry meet the standards, and then have time to bid those items," Ms. Phillips said.

Districts do have 10 years to cut back on sodium. While that's enough time for manufacturers to reformulate recipes and for districts to develop spice blends to compensate for the reduced salt, the sodium requirements are unrealistic, said the School Nutrition Association, adding that they are so low they're less than what a hospital might serve a patient on a low-sodium diet.

"School food will taste so dramatically different from what a child would eat at home and at a restaurant that participation will drop," Ms. Phillips said. The association endorses only the first two phases of sodium reduction, but not the final limits. She pointed out that a cup of milk has 120 milligrams of sodium naturally, or about 1/5 of what will be allowed.

In Chicago, the district has already cut sodium to the level required in the first phase of the reductions. Mr. Bloomer said he has been hounding food manufacturers to cut sodium further in processed foods they supply to the district. And district policy doesn't allow added salt on vegetables, to which a blend of spices is now added. Some kids haven't been impressed.

"No matter how good a fresh vegetable is, it needs a little bit of something," he said, which his district adds in the form of spices and herbs.

Whether it's no-salt-added vegetables, roasted butternut squash, or fat-free chocolate milk, by far the biggest challenge for school districts will be to convince kids to eat what will be offered after all the meticulous meal planning and calorie counting.

David Just, a professor at Cornell University in Ithaca, N.Y., and co-director of the school's Center for Behavioral Economics in Child Nutrition Programs, works on ways to get students to eat healthier at lunch through the placement of items, renaming foods, and other subtle measures.

"It isn't nutrition until it's eaten," he said.

Critical Thinking

1. Describe the nutrition standards set by the Healthy, Hunger-Free Kids Act for meals served in the National School and Breakfast programs.

2. Explain why sugar is not addressed in the Healthy, Hunger-Free Kids Act.

3. Critique the breakfast and lunch standards. What do you think will be the most challenging standards to meet?

4. How will these new standards impact food suppliers and food companies?

From *Edweek*, April, 2011. Copyright © 2011 by Editorial Projects in Education. Reprinted by permission.

Junk Food-Free Vending Machines Go to School

Nick Leiber

Jeff Lowell, an assistant principal at Interlake High School in Bellevue, Wash., normally dismisses the e-mails he gets from businesses trying to sell to his 1,500 students. He was intrigued, however, by the pitch he received in September from **Fresh Healthy Vending,** a San Diego franchise operaton that offers vending machines stocked with snacks and drinks it touts as alternatives to junk food. "Everybody [understands] what eating right does for you and how much it ends up affecting your ability to think," Lowell says. "We decided we wanted to try it."

Lowell signed a one-year contract allowing Fresh Healthy to park its machines near Interlake's gym in exchange for 15 percent of profits. In late November, Fresh Healthy installed three machines, featuring goodies such as Kashi granola bars and Stonyfield Farm fruit smoothies, next to older machines that sell Powerade and Dasani water—though no soda—through a long-standing agreement with **Coca-Cola Enterprises.** The top seller in the new machines so far: Pirate's Booty cheese puffs.

Fresh Healthy is one of more than a dozen small companies that aim to bring healthier fare to school vending machines. To do so they must navigate a tangle of rules created in the wake of 2004 federal law that required school districts to establish local policies aimed at improving student nutrition and reducing childhood obesity. Those rules prompted the bulk of the 10,500 U.S. vending machine companies to avoid schools. "There were fewer and fewer operators handling school accounts because it was a tough process to find products that met the patchwork of school guidelines," says Ned Monroe, senior vice-president for government affairs for the National Automatic Merchandising Assn. The trade group estimates that just 10 percent of its vending operator members sell in schools now, down from about 25 percent a decade ago.

1500—Schools with Fresh Healthy's vending machines

The hodgepodge of local policies will soon be replaced. Under a law that regulates schools participating in the federal school lunch program, which President Barack Obama signed on Dec. 13, the U.S. Agriculture Dept. now can impose nutritional standards on all snacks and refreshments sold in schools. The national guidelines will make it easier for vending companies to sell to many local districts. Producers are likely to be more willing to make foods suitable for vending machines if they know what requirements they must meet. "Food companies [are] trying to be ahead of the game and have products in the marketplace available to meet those standards as soon as they're published," says Diane Pratt-Heavner, a spokeswoman for the School Nutrition Assn., a trade group of food companies and school cafeteria managers.

Small vending machine operators that specialize in healthy snacks are confident the new law will boost their business. "I can't even tell you the response we're getting since this latest piece of legislation passed," says Fresh Healthy founder Jolly Backer, who launched the company in May to sell and supply franchises. He charges franchisees about $11,000 per machine, which they then manage, ordering from Fresh Healthy online and restocking once or twice a week. Fresh Healthy has machines in more than 2,000 locations, about three-quarters of them schools. "Our race is to get space," says Backer, 55. "A lot of schools would just as soon get rid of vending programs because they haven't found out about healthy options yet." He expects revenue at the 22-employee company to at least double this year, to more than $10 million.

Sean Kelly, the 27-year-old chief executive of **Human Healthy Vending** in Los Angeles, says the new law will help him expand from 300 machines to perhaps 1,500 by yearend. He hopes to convince schools that the vending machine business isn't "synonymous with scam" and that it sells more than junk food. Kelly expects revenue to triple this year to more than $9 million. "We see tons of opportunity," he says.

The biggest U.S. vending machine operators—**Canteen, Sodexo,** and **Aramark**—have started offering healthier food in recent years. Canteen has a fledgling operation of about 200 machines (out of a total of 300,000) selling vegan foods and local fare. Since 2003, 15 percent of the products in its company-owned machines have met Canteen's reduced fat and sugar criteria. In 2001, Sodexo introduced a similar program for 20 percent of its products. The company says it plans to increase healthy choices to 30 percent by April. Aramark followed suit in 2005 with a labeling program showing nutritional values for products in its machines.

The new entrants say they aren't worried about industry giants muscling in on their niche. "I don't get that concerned about it because of the uniqueness of what we do," says William H. Carpenter Jr., president of **Vend Natural** in Annapolis, Md., which counts USDA headquarters among the locations for its 535 healthy vending machines. He says the company's revenue, "well north of $10 million," is on track to increase by more than 25 percent this year. "The growth is just so huge," Carpenter says, "not only because of what's happening under the current Administration but just how people want to eat."

Critical Thinking

1. Describe the effects of the federal law passed in 2004 regarding vending in schools.

2. How did the 2004 school vending law impact the number of vending companies that sell to schools?

3. Evaluate whether the law passed on December 13, 2010 will impact vending in schools. Explain your reasoning.

4. Defend the statement regarding the December 2010 school vending law, "Producers are likely to be more willing to make foods suitable for vending machines if they know what requirements must be met."

From *Bloomberg BusinessWeek*, January 17–23, 2011. Copyright © Bloomberg 2011 by Bloomberg BusinessWeek. Reprinted by permission of Bloomberg LP via YGS Group.

The School Lunch Wars

Sixty-five years ago, the federal school lunch program was created to make American schoolchildren healthier. Today, it's helping to make them fatter. Will a new law change the diets of millions of kids raised on French fries and chicken nuggets?

KRISTEN HINMAN

When Colombia native Beatriz Zuluaga, a professional cook for 20 years, became the admissions director at CentroNía's DC Bilingual Public Charter School in 2007, she thought she was leaving her old career far behind. Then she laid eyes on the trays in the lunchroom. Mashed potatoes from a box, chicken nuggets, chocolate milk—to Zuluaga, the processed fare didn't look fit for growing kids. At her last job, Zuluaga had cooked for 450 people a day. Surely she could take over the school's kitchen, no?

She unpacked her knives and started whipping up from-scratch dishes: lasagna with lentils, peppers stuffed with barley and turkey, roasted beets. The reformation did not go over well. One offense after another set the tongues of parents and teachers wagging. *What is that? How can you serve that to children? Why are you trying to turn my kid into a vegetarian?*

Three years later, Zuluaga has given up on the beets. But American cheese has been scrapped for calcium-rich provolone. White flour has been swapped for whole wheat in pizza crust. Fruit juice, high in sugar, is out. The school nurse is reporting fewer sick kids, and Zuluaga has chuckled at least once when a parent remarked on the new efficacy of her child's bowel movements. More than a third of parents have participated in the school's nutrition workshops.

But when I visited the school last fall, all Zuluaga had to do to temper her optimism was walk into a DC Bilingual lunchroom and discover a chubby, misbehaving fourth grader relegated to a table facing the wall and going to town on his brown-bag lunch: an Oscar Mayer Lunchables "pizza." As the boy perched a piece of pepperoni and some shredded cheese atop a cracker, Zuluaga picked up the packaging to inspect its long ingredient list, then put it back down, crossed her arms, and frowned. I expected her to seize the opportunity for a teachable moment, but she was silent. Later she explained, "He didn't go to the grocery store and buy that."

Zuluaga's education, as it were, mirrors what's occurring in schools across America as proponents of whole—that is, minimally processed—foods try to introduce children to more nutritious diets through the $9.8 billion federal school lunch program, which feeds about 32 million of America's 50 million schoolchildren every school day. One in three American children and teenagers today is overweight or obese. Last year, in a report titled *Too Fat to Fight,* a group of retired military brass blamed school lunches for the fact that an estimated 27 percent of American youth are too overweight to serve in the armed forces. A study of Michigan sixth graders published in December found that regularly consuming school lunches was a greater risk factor for obesity than spending two or more hours a day watching television or playing video games.

First lady Michelle Obama, a former hospital executive, has made the war on obesity her defining cause, and put the school lunch program in her crosshairs. In December, thanks in part to her lobbying, Congress passed the Healthy, Hunger-Free Kids Act, which awards schools that meet certain nutritional guidelines an extra six cents per student meal. The extra pennies increase federal reimbursements for lunches above the rate of inflation for the first time in three decades. The law, which cuts funds from future federal food-stamp benefits to cover the reimbursement hike, also grants the U.S. Department of Agriculture (USDA) more power to police what's served in school cafeterias. In reality, though, the battle over school lunches is just beginning, as educators confront a culture that prizes its hamburgers and French fries.

How did a program that was designed to improve the nutrition of the nation's children become a culprit in the scourge of childhood obesity?

As early as the 19th century, some American schools operated their own school lunch programs, often with the help of volunteers. In the 1930s, in the midst of the Great Depression, the federal government began providing some funds for school lunches on an ad hoc basis. But many children still didn't get enough to eat. The problem was thrown into stark relief during World War II, when it was discovered that half of all draftees who were deemed unfit for service were rejected because of malnutrition. In 1946, Congress passed the National School Lunch Act "as a measure of national security." The law guaranteed a free or subsidized midday meal for millions of needy children. It was also intended to teach America what to eat. "Not only is the child taught what a good diet consists of," noted a congressional agriculture committee report, "but his parents and family likewise are indirectly instructed."

During the Depression, when farmers were surrounded by mountains of unsold commodities and schools were full of hungry children, New Deal politicos had used the USDA to funnel surpluses to school cafeterias. Thus, when it came time to designate an authority for the new national lunch program, the USDA seemed a natural choice. Schools would receive subsidized commodities and cash reimbursements in exchange for feeding low-income children lunches that met USDA nutrition standards. And so the same law that was supposed to ensure a nutritious midday meal for millions of kids also created an enduring market for American farmers.

It was up to state officials to administer the federal funds. For the first two decades student participation was low, partly because many schools lacked adequate facilities but also because local authorities often established the eligibility threshold with little regard for students' actual need. The poor results prompted Congress in the 1960s to establish a federal eligibility standard linked to the poverty level.

Today, students from families with incomes below 130 percent of the poverty level ($28,665 for a family of four) eat for free. The school receives a federal subsidy of $2.72 per meal. Children from families earning up to 185 percent of the poverty level pay 40 cents per meal, and the subsidy is correspondingly reduced. Other students pay the "full" price, an average of $1.60. The government also provides a small subsidy for these meals, on the principle that child nutrition contributes to national security. (Even so, schools often are not able to cover the production cost of the "full" price meals and essentially make up the difference from the subsidies meant for lower-income kids. A controversial provision of the new law will rectify that by requiring some districts to charge more for full-pay lunches.)

Student participation doubled within the first few years after the federal eligibility standards were set. Educators suddenly found themselves in the food business. Poorer districts, particularly, didn't have functioning kitchens, or the money to improve them. It became standard practice for cafeteria staff to purchase ready-made heat-and-eat meals, whose less-than-palatable qualities made headlines once it was learned that much of the food was being thrown out. These reports, along with the fact that the government was subsidizing lunches for middle-income families that could afford to pay full price, caught the attention of Ronald Reagan's cost-conscious administration. Among the resulting USDA proposals was the reclassification of ketchup as a vegetable—on the theory that replacing broccoli and lima beans with cheap condiments would reduce so-called plate waste. That idea caused a political uproar and was never carried out, but in 1981 Congress slashed school lunch reimbursement rates by a third and eliminated money for equipment.

Already making do with slim resources and now facing more budget pressures, some schools turned to professional vendors to replace the cafeteria ladies of old. At the same time,

many schools added "à la carte" items that could be sold to anyone who could pay. Since the government didn't reimburse for à la carte fare, and thus didn't regulate its nutritional content, school officials were free to offer French fries, nachos, and pizza. Some items were branded by fast-food companies such as Domino's Pizza and Taco Bell. Many schools also allowed companies to install vending machines that dispensed snack foods, candy, and soda, from which the schools kept a portion of the sales.

Consumption of government-subsidized school lunches began to fall off because of the "needy" stigma associated with the reimbursable meals. Kids who had once purchased meals at full price switched to the more tempting à la carte line. Some lower-income students simply went without. In response, cafeteria managers goosed the offerings to make them more enticing. Out went baked chicken, in came chicken nuggets; roasted potatoes gave way to Tater Tots. Cheap commodities were available from the government, in all the processed forms kids were believed to covet. USDA nutrition standards were lax enough that it was possible to satisfy the grain and protein requirements with, say, breaded and fried fish sticks, or the fruit requirement with sugar-laced canned peaches.

In 1990, only one percent of schools were serving meals that met the USDA's dietary guidelines for percentage of calories from fat.

In 1990, the USDA commissioned a comprehensive analysis of the school lunch program to see how it stacked up against the agency's Dietary Guidelines for Americans. In yet another bureaucratic oddity of the program, schools had to meet a different, and looser, set of nutrition standards. "The results were disturbing," recounts sociologist Janet Poppendieck in *Free for All* (2010), a survey of the politics surrounding school lunch programs. "On average, school lunches were deriving not [the recommended] 30 but 38 percent of calories from fats, not [the recommended] 10 but 15 percent from saturated fats. The meals were also found to be high in sodium. . . . Only one percent of schools were serving, on average, meals that complied with the dietary guidelines for percentage of calories from fat—one percent!"

Without allocating more money, Congress in 1994 required that school menus meet the USDA's Dietary Guidelines for Americans. But what was on the plate changed very little. Today, less than 20 percent of schools cook lunch from scratch. Eighty percent of schools exceed the fat allowance per meal. The average high school lunch has 1,600 milligrams of sodium—100 milligrams more than the daily amount deemed within healthy limits for children.

In the late 1990s, some school districts around the country quietly began removing vending machines or putting the kibosh on minimally nutritious à la carte programs. But the reformers who eventually drew national attention were two chefs who had far more ambitious goals. Alice Waters, whose Berkeley restaurant Chez Panisse was in the vanguard in serving seasonal and local cuisine, won over the California state superintendent of education with Edible Schoolyard, a garden project at a Berkeley middle school. By 2002, produce gardens had been established in more than 2,000 of California's 9,000 schools. The same year, Waters convinced the Berkeley Unified School District to hire Ann Cooper, who became known as "the Renegade Lunch Lady," to revamp its food service program with whole foods. (Cooper has since gone to work for the Boulder Valley School District in Colorado.)

To the California duo, the biggest culprit in the child nutrition crisis is the transformation of agriculture since World War II and the rise of agribusiness. Livestock is raised in mechanized indoor facilities rather than pastures, cash-crop monoculture has replaced the diversified family farm, and the food industry has undergone far-reaching consolidation. Today, only two percent of Americans—supported by government subsidies—produce food, and they do so at prices so low that the other 98 percent don't have much incentive to question the system. Pervasive marketing by fast-food companies pitching cheap children's "Happy Meals" and other convenience foods to working parents has helped establish a drive-through culture. The eat-your-vegetables ethos has given way to an emphasis on food that can be put on the table quickly (if it's consumed at a table at all) and that children will eat without a battle royale every evening.

The view that poor-quality school lunches are the result of a broken food system has led food activists to see the USDA as part of the problem. How, they ask, can an authority responsible for helping agribusiness produce and market its output also be an effective nutrition watchdog in school cafeterias?

In 2009, two months after moving into 1600 Pennsylvania Avenue, Michelle Obama planted an organic kitchen garden on the White House lawn, a step of both symbolic and practical significance. With her backing, the USDA dusted off projects that promote local and regional food systems, rolling out a local-foods marketing campaign called "Know Your Farmer, Know Your Food." Another initiative aims to help small and medium-size farms sell their products to schools.

What elevated Obama's whole foods advocacy above the charges of impracticality and foodie snobbery leveled at Waters and Cooper was the rollout last February of a campaign dubbed "Let's Move" that puts the focus squarely on health—and on those responsible for the well-being of children. "Our kids didn't do this to themselves," Obama said when she announced the wellness plan. "Our kids don't decide what's served to them at school or whether there's time for gym class or recess. Our kids don't choose to make food products with tons of sugar and sodium in supersized portions, and then to have those products marketed to them everywhere they turn. And no matter how much they beg for pizza, fries, and candy, ultimately they are not, and should not be, the ones calling the shots at dinnertime. We're in charge. We make these decisions."

In placing the blame for the obesity epidemic on corporate food processors, educators, and parents, Obama picked the

right targets. Conventional agriculture isn't the main problem. If there were greater demand for less-processed ingredients, agribusiness companies could produce them. Nor is the USDA's jurisdiction of the program a real obstacle to reform. In the 1970s and again in 2001, the department pressed Congress for more regulatory authority over à la carte and vending machine offerings—only to come up short against the soft drink and snack food lobbies. The real problem—and the solution—is a lot closer to the school lunch lines than Washington, or America's feedlots and farm fields.

About five years ago Linda Henke, superintendent of the Maplewood–Richmond Heights School District in suburban St. Louis, decided to start mingling with her high schoolers in the lunchroom. When she saw the array of Pop-Tarts, candy, and "cheese fries" that had been mainstays on the à la carte menu for years, she was disgusted. "It was the fish not seeing the water," she says of her years-long inattention to what her students were eating. She started to lay the groundwork for some drastic changes.

Three years ago, with the help of her congressman, Russ Carnahan, a local university, and a group of family farmers desperate for new markets, Henke began making over the district's food program. She prohibited candy and chips in the cafeterias and had all vending machines but one removed. She required that all the starches come from whole grain sources and banned the purchase of chicken patties and nuggets—processed chicken, period. Whenever possible, ingredients were to be Missouri grass-fed beef and pesticide-free produce. Local sourcing would allow the staff to order whole foods, which is not always an option when purchases are made through the USDA or a distributor. This way, the district could prepare the foods as desired—apples for applesauce, tomatoes for marinara and salsa, for example—while controlling for calorie, fat, and sodium content. An à la carte line was preserved at the high school, but it no longer serves cheese fries and other junk food.

When I visited last fall, I was struck by the positive vibe around the revamped program. A teacher said he'd lost seven pounds by eating in the high school cafeteria every school day for the previous three months. A senior girl who had embraced the changes from the beginning observed that even she was surprised when football players started eating salads. The elementary school's cook of 14 years told me her job is now harder, but it's rewarding. She recounted a recent visit to the school her sister's kids attend in Indiana. "They had all this processed food that we don't serve anymore, and I was thinking, 'This is farm country! If we're city people and we can cook, why can't they?'"

These reforms have not come cheaply. The meals cost from $3.75 to $4.25 apiece to prepare. Henke's board of education has allowed her to run the program at a deficit equal to roughly one teacher's salary. But if she wants to keep using local food sources, she has to convince a consortium of schools to buy in. The farms that have been supplying Maplewood–Richmond Heights on an experimental basis need to sell their food at great volumes to turn a profit. One of Henke's selling points to other school officials? Her cafeterias are selling 10 percent more lunches.

Administrators such as Henke, Beatriz Zuluaga, and others in Kentucky, Wisconsin, and Texas have revealed some important principles. It takes a tough-minded school leader to assert that nutrient-rich food is the right choice for kids—and that it's an appropriate use of government dollars. Kids will complain initially but will come around. And a number of collateral benefits follow when students eat well. Anecdotal reports from schools with healthful and flavorful food indicate that teachers have started eating with students, attendance rates are higher, and fewer students fall asleep in class or commit vandalism and violence at school.

So far, these cafeteria visionaries are the exception. Since 2004, the USDA has administered the HealthierUS School Challenge, awarding distinction, but no money, to schools that voluntarily improve the healthfulness of their meals. By last fall, only a paltry 841 of the 101,000 schools in the National School Lunch Program (less than one percent) had received awards. That leaves a lot of schools that are still promoting Tater Tot Day and reheating frozen pizzas.

Food activists hope that the passage of the Healthy, Hunger-Free Kids Act will make a big difference. More money will buy better ingredients and pay for more staff to prepare foods from scratch. At least as important is the USDA's increased authority over the nutrition standards of all food served in schools, and the department's proposal to establish more rigorous standards,

including two vegetables per meal, strict sodium limits, and, for the first time, maximum calorie counts.

It could take another generation to see meaningful change in the waistlines of American children. Yes, reform will require more government money. But at least as important is a stomachs-and-minds campaign aimed at the nation's adults: food service directors who cling to the argument that a child won't drink low-fat milk, so cookies 'n' cream–flavored milk is better than no calcium at all; parents who ask, *Why do you want to turn my kid into a vegetarian?;* and teachers who snort, *How can you serve beets to students?*

Critical Thinking

1. How much does the federal school lunch program cost the U.S. government? How many children are fed every day by this program?

2. Describe the Healthy, Hunger-Free Kids Act. How is the increased reimbursement going to be funded?

3. Explain why school lunches have changed from scratch-made food to processed, easy-to-prepare foods.

4. Compare the amount of reimbursement schools receive from the federal government with the costs of buying lunch in a restaurant.

KRISTEN HINMAN is a journalist based in Washington, D.C., who writes frequently about food. Her work has been published in *The Atlantic, The Washington Post,* and *Slate.*

From *The Wilson Quarterly,* May 19, 2011, pp. 16–21. Copyright © 2011 by The Wilson Quarterly. Reprinted by permission of Kristen Hinman and Woodrow Wilson International Center for Scholars.

UNIT 3
Nutrients

Unit Selections

Learning Outcomes

After reading this unit, you will be able to:

- Describe the health benefits of potassium, vitamin D, magnesium, and B-12.

- Defend the concept that consuming certain nutrients from foods is better than consuming them from supplements or fortified foods.

- Critique the proposed negative effects of folic acid fortification of U.S. cereal grains with the positive effect.

- Explain why the type of research that is conducted is the most important consideration when reviewing information about research on nutrients.

- Compare and contrast epidemiological or observational studies with randomized intervention-based clinical trials.

- Identify the four groups that should pay particular attention to sodium content of foods and consume no more than 1,500 mg of sodium per day, as recommended in the Dietary Guidelines for Americans.

- Describe the characteristics that salt brings to manufactured and mass-produced food.

- Identify the challenges of conducting a large clinical trial on high salt and low salt diets.

- Discuss why female athletes are at higher risk of iron deficiency.

- Determine the best way to increase iron intake in female athletes.

Student Website
www.mhhe.com/cls

Internet References

Dietary Supplement Fact Sheet: Vitamin D
http://ods.od.nih.gov/factsheets/vitamind.asp
Food and Nutrition Information Center
www.nal.usda.gov/fnic
Nutritionalsupplements.com
www.nutritionalsupplements.com
Office of Dietary Supplements: Health Information
http://ods.od.nih.gov/Health_Information/Health_Information.aspx
U.S. National Library of Medicine
www.nlm.nih.gov

Nutrition is a young and evolving science. Early research into nutrients began in the mid-18th century with investigations into how the body requires and uses calories from the macronutrients (carbohydrates, protein, and fats). It wasn't until the early 20th century that scientists began to discover, investigate, and identify the micronutrients and their effect on human health. The fundamentals of nutrition were discovered just over 100 years ago. From a perspective of scientifically confirming results, this is a short amount of time. A vast amount of knowledge about nutrients has been discovered, and scientists continue to investigate the best way for these nutrients to be provided—safely and in proper amounts to facilitate optimal functioning of the human body.

The articles of this unit have been selected to present current knowledge about macronutrients and micronutrients, with particular interest in the nutrients of concern as indicated in the 2010 U.S. Dietary Guidelines: vitamin D, calcium, potassium, sodium, and "good fats."

One of the current challenges in evaluating nutrition science is translating and applying the results to improvements in human health. The golden standard for research is the randomized clinical trial; however, there are weaknesses in clinical trials designs with a nutrition focus, for example, the controversy regarding vitamin D research. In the article "Which Pills Work?" Melinda Moyer discusses the current controversy over recommendations for vitamin D intake and supplementation.

Too often the resounding message about nutrition and our diets is that we eat too much of the "bad stuff." An important message that is underpublished is that our diets commonly lack certain vitamins and minerals that are beneficial. In the first article, "Getting Enough, What You Don't Eat Can Hurt You," Bonnie Liebman sheds light on the nutrients that are commonly deficient in the U.S. diet: potassium, vitamin D, magnesium, and vitamin B-12.

The USDA and HHS are now recommending that all American adults strive to consume 1,500 mg of sodium rather than the previously recommended 2,300 mg. The reasoning for lowering the recommended amount across the board is that over 70 percent of the population fit into groups that are at high risk for developing hypertension, stroke, and heart disease. The challenge with meeting this guideline is that it will be difficult to consume processed foods or eat in restaurants in the United States. A proposed next step of the USDA is to address the amount of sodium in the processed foods, which is the main source of sodium in the U.S. diet. "Keeping a Lid on Salt: Not So Easy" by Nanci Hellmich covers many of these challenges with restricting sodium in the current U.S. food environment.

Sports nutrition and nutrition to improve physical performance are popular topics among the general population and within the profession of dietetics. More Americans are increasing their activity level to meet or exceed the exercise recommendations published in the Dietary Guidelines. As a result, more people are exercising at the level of "athlete" rather than occasional exerciser. The article by Ellen Coleman addresses how to properly fuel and hydrate for optimal athletic conditioning.

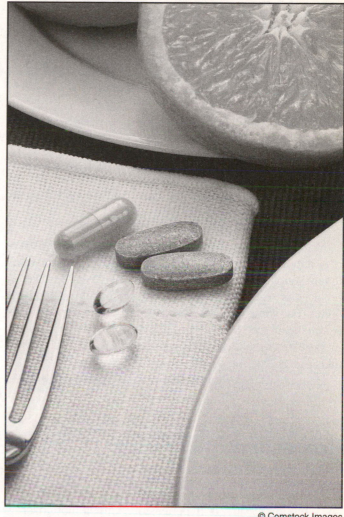

© Comstock Images

Iron deficiency is the most prevalent micronutrient deficiency in the world. It is estimated that 12% of 20- to 49-year-old females are iron deficient. Female athletes are at higher risk for iron deficiency. Sports anemia was first reported in male athletes more than 40 years ago. Iron deficiency in female athletes has been the target of recent research. The proposed contributing factors are inadequate intake of iron rich foods and the physiologic losses of iron during physical activity. Consumption of iron supplements and foods fortified with iron are recommended techniques to improve the iron status of physically active women. The article review by Bass and McClung explores recent research on the efficacy of supplementation and fortification of iron to improve the iron status of female athletes.

The articles selected for Unit 3 will provide additional information to the micronutrient sections of a general nutrition course. Several of the articles also address the challenges of interpreting and evaluating scientific nutrition research.

Getting Enough?

What You Don't Eat Can *Hurt You*

BONNIE LIEBMAN

Too much sugar. Too much salt. Too much saturated fat. We eat too much of all three. And we eat too much, period.

Yet we also eat too little.

Many Americans fall short of the recommended intakes of a handful of nutrients. Several key players—potassium, magnesium, vitamin D, and vitamin B-12—may make or break your risk of high blood pressure, diabetes, and brittle bones. For some of those nutrients, only foods—not pills—can make up the shortfall. For others, only a pill will do.

Here's why and how to get the nutrients you may be missing.

Here are four key nutrients you may lack—and where to get them.

Potassium

The numbers are staggering:

- One in three adults in the United States has high blood pressure, or hypertension. Among those over 65, it's two out of three. And another one out of four adults has pre-hypertension.

- Of the 74.5 million Americans with hypertension, 56 percent don't have it under control. That includes 22 percent who don't even know they have it.

- Roughly three out of four people who suffer a stroke, a heart attack, or congestive heart failure have hypertension.

Too much salt, too much weight, too little exercise, too much alcohol, and other risk factors can raise blood pressure. Potassium can trim it.

"It's absolutely clear that potassium can lower blood pressure," says Frank Sacks, professor of cardiovascular disease prevention at the Harvard School of Public Health in Boston.

In 1988, the INTERSALT study of 52 large populations reported that people with higher potassium intakes had lower blood pressures.[1] By 1997, a meta-analysis of 33 studies found that potassium supplements (2,300 milligrams a day) lowered systolic blood pressure by an average of 3.3 points.[2] (Systolic pressure is the higher of the two blood pressure numbers.)

"That meta-analysis conclusively showed that potassium supplements reduce blood pressure," says Lydia Bazzano, assistant professor of epidemiology at the Tulane School of Public Health in New Orleans.

In animal studies, potassium protects rats from stroke.[3] "And in human population studies, low potassium is a predictor for stroke," adds Sacks.

For example, in a study that tracked 43,000 men for eight years, those who consumed the most potassium (4,300 mg a day) were 38 percent less likely to suffer a stroke than those who consumed the least (2,400 mg a day).[4]

Potassium matters because it seems to counter the damage caused by sodium. "If people are eating high amounts of sodium, potassium will lower blood pressure more," explains Sacks. "The higher the sodium, the more potassium helps."

And when researchers tracked 2,275 participants in the Trials of Hypertension Prevention for 10 to 15 years, they found that the risk of heart attack or stroke depended more on potassium *and* sodium than on either one alone.[5]

Even without berries, half a cantaloupe has 16 percent of a day's potassium and only 90 calories. Mmm.

Scientists aren't sure exactly how potassium lowers blood pressure. Among the possibilities: it makes the larger blood vessels more flexible.[6]

"The flexibility of the big arteries like the aorta or carotid arteries is very important in maintaining a nice, lower, youthful blood pressure," explains Sacks. "In older people, arteries are less elastic." And that boosts blood pressure.

The Bottom Line

Whether it's blood pressure, stones, or bones you're worried about, the message is clear: "Eat potassium-rich fruits and vegetables like you'd get in a DASH diet," says Tulane's Lydia Bazzano.

Potassium may also lower blood pressure by dilating the small blood vessels.[6] "You don't want the tiny vessels clenched," says Sacks. "Resistance to blood flow will increase blood pressure."

What's clear is that a healthy, potassium-rich diet can revitalize arteries, big or small. "Conditions we thought were permanent with age can be reversed in four weeks," says Sacks. "Four weeks of a lower-sodium, potassium-rich DASH diet completely reverses the effect of age on blood pressure."

A DASH (Dietary Approaches to Stop Hypertension) diet is rich in potassium, thanks to 11 (modest) servings a day of fruits and vegetables, with two servings of low-fat dairy foods, and with low levels of saturated fat, added sugars, and refined flour.

"Potassium may account for half of the effect of the overall DASH diet," says Sacks.

The citrate that's usually bound to the potassium in fruits and vegetables could also help. Potassium citrate lowers blood pressure more than the potassium chloride that is in some salt substitutes, supplements, and potassium-fortified foods.[7]

Another reason to get potassium from food: high-dose potassium supplements—far more than the amounts that occur naturally in food—can be hazardous.

"If you have kidney disease and don't know it, you could potentially end up with too much potassium in your blood, and that's life-threatening," explains Bazzano. "It can stop your heart."

Bonus: getting potassium citrate from fruits and vegetables may prevent kidney stones.

In the Health Professionals Follow-Up Study of more than 45,000 men, those who consumed the most potassium (about 4,300 mg a day) had roughly half the risk of kidney stones over 14 years of those who ate the least (roughly 2,700 mg).[8]

"If you eat more fruits and vegetables, your urine citrate goes up, and that should reduce the risk of kidney stones," says study coauthor Gary Curhan, associate professor of epidemiology at the Harvard School of Public Health.

"But it's probably the citrate or some other alkali, not the potassium."

How does citrate prevent kidney stones?

"It forms soluble complexes with calcium, so it keeps the calcium from sticking to oxalate or phosphate," says

Potassium on Tap

If you're like 90 percent of men and 99 percent of women, you get less potassium than experts recommend (4,700 mg a day). Go for fruits and vegetables so you can eat bigger servings—these are small—without piling on calories.

Potassium	Calories	% IOM*
Clams (4 oz. cooked)	170	15
Beet greens (½ cup cooked)	20	14
Yellowfin tuna or Halibut (4 oz. cooked)	160	14
Pacific cod (4 oz. cooked)	120	12
Non-fat or Low-fat plain yogurt (8 oz.)	135	12
Swiss chard (½ cup cooked)	20	10
Acorn squash (½ cup cooked)	55	10
Sweet potato with skin (½ cup cooked)	90	10
Lima beans (½ cup cooked)	110	10
Edamame, shelled (½ cup cooked)	130	10
Wild Coho salmon (4 oz. cooked)	160	10
Spinach (½ cup cooked)	20	9
Tomato sauce (½ cup)	30	9
Banana (1)	105	9
Orange juice (1 cup)	120	9
Low-fat fruit yogurt (8 oz.)	225	9
Farmed Atlantic salmon (4 oz. cooked)	235	9
Cantaloupe (¼)	45	8
Dried apricots (¼ cup)	80	8
Non-fat or Low-fat milk (1 cup)	90	8
Kidney beans or Lentils (½ cup cooked)	115	8
Avocado (½ cup)	120	8
Navy or Pinto beans (½ cup cooked)	125	8
Tomato paste (2 Tbs.)	25	7
Baked potato with skin (½ cup cooked)	55	7
Great Northern beans (½ cup cooked)	105	7
Prunes (¼ cup)	105	7
Pistachios (¼ cup)	180	7
Tomato (1)	20	6
Beets (½ cup cooked)	35	6
Butternut squash (½ cup cooked)	40	6
Peach or Nectarine (1)	60	6
Raisins (¼ cup)	110	6
Brussels sprouts (½ cup cooked)	30	5
Artichoke hearts (½ cup cooked)	45	5
Spinach (¼ cup raw)	5	4
Grapes (1 cup)	60	4
Apple (1)	95	4
Boston or Romaine lettuce (1 cup raw)	10	3

*Percent of the daily intake (4,700 milligrams) recommended by the Institute of Medicine (IOM).

Sources: USDA and manufacturers. Chart compiled by Amy Ramsay, Danielle Hazard, and Melissa Pryputniewicz.

Curhan. "So it's less likely that oxalate or phosphate crystals will form."

Preventing calcium oxalate crystals is key. "More than 80 percent of kidney stones are made of calcium oxalate," says Curhan.

And there may be a bonus for bones, he adds. "Citrate should reduce urine calcium excretion as well."

Scientists used to think that potassium could lower the risk of osteoporosis, but no longer.

"Potassium isn't the key to bone health," says Bess Dawson-Hughes, director of the Bone Metabolism Laboratory at the Jean Mayer U.S. Department of Agriculture Human Nutrition Research Center on Aging at Tufts University in Boston. "It's the alkaline accompaniment of potassium that's good."

Vitamin D

Osteoporosis, or brittle bones, takes a huge toll on the public's health:

- One in two women and one in four men over age 50 will break a bone because of osteoporosis.[9]
- Osteoporosis caused more than 2 million fractures in 2005, including roughly 297,000 hip fractures, 547,000 spine fractures, 397,000 wrist fractures, 135,000 pelvic fractures, and 675,000 fractures at other sites.
- Half of all women and 30 percent of all men over 50 have osteopenia (low bone mass) in their hips, which often leads to osteoporosis.[10]
- Six months after a hip fracture, only 15 percent of patients can walk across a room without help.

If you ask people how to strengthen bones, the nutrient they're most likely to mention is calcium. But, in fact, average calcium intakes are now close to the recommended levels, in part because 43 percent of Americans get some calcium from a supplement.[11]

What many people don't know is that calcium may not prevent fractures if you don't get enough vitamin D, which helps the body absorb calcium.

"It's looking like the combination of calcium and vitamin D is effective," says Tufts' Bess Dawson-Hughes.

In a 2007 meta-analysis, calcium supplements alone didn't lower the risk of fractures.[12]

"But when you look at calcium plus vitamin D, the risk reduction was significant," says Dawson-Hughes. "So we should absolutely aim for the recommended levels of both."

Calcium plus D could also protect young bones. In a study of 3,700 young female U.S. Navy recruits, those who were given calcium (2,000 mg a day) and vitamin D (800 IU a day) were 20 percent less likely to be diagnosed with stress fractures during eight weeks of training than those who got a placebo.[13]

How much vitamin D is enough?

The Bottom Line

Shoot for 800 to 1,000 IU of vitamin D a day from foods and supplements if you're over 60, and 400 IU a day if you're younger. Shoot for 1,200 mg of calcium a day from food and supplements if you're over 50, and 1,000 mg a day if you're a younger adult.

"My interpretation of current evidence is that our blood levels should not be lower than 30 nanograms per milliliter," says Dawson-Hughes. "If you look at data from the National Health and Nutrition Examination Survey, about 70 percent of older adult men and women were lower than that."

To reach adequate blood levels, most older people need more vitamin D than is now recommended (400 IU a day from age 51 to 70, and 600 IU over 70).

"The vast majority of the older global population would need 800 to 1,000 units of vitamin D a day," from food or a supplement, explains Dawson-Hughes. She led a group of experts who came up with new guidelines for the International Osteoporosis Foundation.[14]

"And high-risk older people—those who have no effective sun exposure or don't absorb vitamin D well or who have very dark skin or osteoporosis—would need more than 800 to 1,000 units a day to get to desired serum levels," she adds.

It's tough to get even 800 IU of vitamin D from foods. A cup of milk is fortified with only 100 IU, and a tablespoon of fortified margarine has 60 IU. Unless you eat fish like red salmon (800 IU per 3 oz. of cooked fish) almost every day, you won't reach those levels.

Getting enough vitamin D may protect more than bones. Evidence suggests that it may lower the risk of colon cancer, heart attacks, stroke, Type 2 diabetes, falls, and some autoimmune diseases.

And a 2007 meta-analysis of 18 trials found a 7 percent lower risk of dying over six months to seven years when people were given vitamin D (usually to reduce the risk of bone fractures).[15]

However, a recent study raised the possibility that high blood levels of vitamin D could increase the risk of pancreatic cancer.[16] The higher risk was only seen in people from states with low sun exposure (Michigan, Minnesota, and Wisconsin, in this study), and it wasn't linked to how much vitamin D people were getting from supplements, so it's somewhat of a mystery.

"The government has funded a huge vitamin D intervention trial giving people 2,000 IU a day or a placebo," says Dawson-Hughes. "So that will give us more information."

(Most women over 65 or men over 60 are eligible to join the VITAL trial, which is also testing fish oil. If you're interested, call 1-800-388-3963 or go to vitalstudy.org.)

"We're looking at cancer, heart disease, stroke, diabetes, high blood pressure, vision, bone density, memory loss, depression, and autoimmune outcomes," says JoAnn Manson, a professor of medicine at the Harvard Medical School who is leading the trial.

Too much calcium without vitamin D may also pose a risk. In July, British researchers reported that high doses of calcium from supplements—1,000 mg a day in most cases—*without* vitamin D raised the risk of heart attacks, but only in people who were already getting more than 800 mg of calcium from food.[17] (The average adult gets 1,000 to 1,200 mg of calcium a day from foods and supplements combined.[11])

Beans are rich in magnesium, not to mention fiber, folate, protein, and potassium. Such a bargain!

"I would not go a whole lot above the recommended intake because it adds no value and could be adding risk," says Dawson-Hughes. (The researchers didn't look at people who were given calcium plus vitamin D, citing evidence that vitamin D would lower death rates.)

Magnesium

An estimated 23.6 million Americans—including one out of four people aged 60 or older—have Type 2 diabetes. Roughly 5.7 million of them don't know it. And 57 million others have pre-diabetes.

The disease takes a heavy toll:

- Adults with diabetes are two to four times more likely than others to have a stroke or to die of heart disease.
- Diabetes is the leading cause of new cases of blindness among people 20 to 74 and the leading cause of kidney failure.
- More than 60 percent of people with diabetes have nervous system damage.
- Each year, about 70,000 Americans with diabetes have a foot or leg amputated.[18]

Type I diabetes, which typically strikes in childhood, occurs when the body's immune system destroys beta-cells in the pancreas that make insulin, the hormone that controls blood sugar levels. Type 1 accounts for 5 to 10 percent of diabetes cases.

In Type 2 diabetes (which this article will refer to simply as "diabetes"), the body's cells don't use insulin properly. As the need for insulin rises, the pancreas gradually loses its ability to make enough, and blood sugar levels climb.

What causes diabetes?

Extra pounds are by far the biggest risk factor. Genes, lack of exercise, and diet also play a role. Whole grains,

A Mouthful of Magnesium

A typical woman gets 250 milligrams of magnesium a day, but should get 320 mg. A typical man gets 335 mg, but should get 420 mg. The Daily Value (DV) is 400 mg. Here's how to get more magnesium without overdoing the calories.

Magnesium	Calories	% DV*
Pumpkin seed kernels (¼ cup)	170	41
Brazil nuts (¼ cup)	220	31
Halibut (4 oz. cooked)	160	30
Kellogg's Original All-Bran cereal (½ cup)	80	25
Almonds (¼ cup)	205	25
Cashews (¼ cup)	195	22
Spinach (½ cup cooked)	20	20
Swiss chard (½ cup cooked)	20	19
Soybeans (½ cup cooked)	150	19
Yellowfin tuna (4 oz. cooked)	160	18
Lima beans (½ cup cooked)	105	16
Quinoa (½ cup cooked)	110	15
Black beans (½ cup cooked)	115	15
Dark chocolate (1.4 oz.)	220	15
Haddock (4 oz. cooked)	125	14
Peanuts (¼ cup) or Peanut butter (2 Tbs.)	195	14
Hazelnuts (¼ cup)	210	14
Beet greens (½ cup cooked)	20	12
Okra (½ cup cooked)	25	12
Black-eyed peas (½ cup cooked)	100	12
Navy beans (½ cup cooked)	125	12
Semisweet chocolate (1.4 oz.)	190	12
Walnuts (½ cup)	195	12
Oat bran (½ cup cooked)	45	11
Great Northern beans (½ cup cooked)	105	11
Kidney or Pinto beans (½ cup cooked)	115	11
Non-fat plain yogurt (8 oz.)	125	11
Brown rice or Lentils (¼ cup cooked)	110	10
Garbanzo beans (¼ cup cooked)	135	10
Low-fat plain yogurt (8 oz.)	145	10
Sunflower seed kernels (¼ cup)	190	10
Tofu (½ cup raw)	95	9
Pistachios (¼ cup)	175	9
Oatmeal (½ cup cooked)	85	8
Post Original Shredded Wheat (½ cup)	85	8
Canned light tuna in water (4 oz.)	130	8
Low-fat fruit yogurt (8 oz.)	225	8
Bulgur (½ cup cooked)	75	7
Non-fat milk (1 cup)	85	7
Spinach (1 cup raw)	5	6
Whole wheat bread (1 slice, 1 oz.)	70	6

*Percent of the Daily Value (400 milligrams).

Sources: USDA and manufacturers. Chart compiled by Amy Ramsay, Danielle Hazard, and Melissa Pryputniewicz.

fiber-rich foods, and coffee (decaf or regular) seem to lower the risk. Sugar-sweetened beverages, processed meats, and white potatoes seem to raise it.

One nutrient that often gets overlooked: magnesium.

"We have a lot of evidence from observational studies that magnesium is beneficial for preventing Type 2 diabetes," says Yiqing Song, an associate epidemiologist at Brigham & Women's Hospital in Boston.

For example, when researchers tracked more than 85,000 women in the Nurses' Health Study for 18 years and 42,000 men in the Health Professionals Follow-Up Study for 12 years, those who consumed the most magnesium (about 375 mg a day for women and 450 mg a day for men) had a 27 percent lower risk of diabetes than those who consumed the least magnesium (about 200 mg a day for women and 270 mg a day for men).[19]

The Iowa Women's Health Study and the Women's Health Study came up with similar results.[20,21]

"In the Women's Health Study, we found an association between a low magnesium intake and an increased risk of diabetes only among overweight women," says Song.

"Magnesium may be more beneficial for overweight women because they are more likely to be at high risk for diabetes," he notes.

In some studies, women with higher magnesium intakes—no matter what their weight—had lower fasting insulin levels.[21,22] That may mean a lower risk of diabetes.

What's more, in the Nurses' Health Study and the Women's Health Initiative Observational Study, those who consumed more magnesium had lower levels of c-reactive protein and other signs of chronic low-level inflammation.[23,24]

"Chronic inflammation may be the link between obesity and Type 2 diabetes," explains Song. "Obesity can cause chronic inflammation.

"The two major features of diabetes are insulin resistance and beta-cell dysfunction," he notes.

"Chronic inflammation may cause insulin resistance in peripheral tissues, and it may damage the beta-cells in the pancreas that secrete insulin."

Still, adds Song, "Observational studies can't show cause and effect. We need direct evidence from a large, long-term clinical trial before we can make any conclusive statements for magnesium and Type 2 diabetes."

The first step: a small pilot trial giving magnesium to people for a few months. "We're going to assess the direct effects of oral magnesium supplements on insulin sensitivity and insulin secretion in obese individuals because they are at high risk for diabetes," says Song.

A trial is critical because it could be something other than the magnesium in magnesium-rich foods that protects against the disease.

"Fiber, folic acid, potassium, and magnesium are all correlated together," says Song. "But for magnesium, we also have evidence from animal studies. There's no evidence from animal studies that fiber, potassium, or folic acid reduces the risk of diabetes. So if you consider all the evidence, we think magnesium is an important factor."

Vitamin B-12

"Low vitamin B-12 status is very common in older people," notes Martha Morris of the USDA Human Nutrition Research Center on Aging at Tufts University.

Vitamin B-12 is found in animal foods, including dairy, eggs, fish, poultry, and meat. But most people with low B-12 don't run short because they lack those foods.

"Low B-12 status occurs because of how our digestive systems age," says Morris. "Some people lose the ability to extract vitamin B-12 from food protein."

In about 30 percent of older people, the lining of the stomach starts to wither, so it doesn't secrete enough gastric acid to release vitamin B-12 from food.

That's why the Institute of Medicine recommends that anyone over age 50 get at least 2.4 micrograms of B-12 a day from a fortified food or supplement. Even without stomach acid, you can still absorb the crystalline form of B-12 they contain.

Roughly one out of five Americans aged 60 or older has low B-12 status.[25] "These people don't feel like they have anything wrong with them," notes Morris. But they're more likely to do poorly on tests of memory and mental ability.[26]

"We found cognitive impairment was almost twice as common in people with low B-12 status," she adds.

And in the Chicago Health and Aging Project and the Oxford Healthy Ageing Project in England, seniors who entered the studies with low B-12 status were more likely to show a drop in cognitive test scores six to ten years later.[27,28]

"This association suggests that low B-12 status contributes to cognitive impairment in the elderly," says Morris. She uses the word "suggests" because these types of studies can't prove cause and effect.

So far, studies that have given people high doses of vitamin B-12 (often with other B vitamins) for up to six months haven't found improved test scores.[29] (And B vitamins don't slow memory loss in people who already have Alzheimer's disease.[30])

However, in the Women's Antioxidant and Folic Acid Cardiovascular Study, which tested high doses of B vitamins on 2,000 women aged 65 or older who were at high risk

The Bottom Line

If you're over 50, make sure your multivitamin contains at least 100 percent of the Daily Value (DV) for vitamin B-12 (6 micrograms).

If you don't take a multi, take a B-12 supplement (the lowest dose available may be 100 mcg, which is okay). A month's supply of a store brand shouldn't cost more than about $1.50.

To play it safe, don't take a daily multivitamin with 100 percent of the DV for folic acid *and* eat a breakfast cereal (or other food) every day that contains more than 25 percent of the DV. Don't worry about fruits, vegetables, or other foods that are rich in naturally occurring folate.

for heart disease, the vitamins seemed to help women who entered the trial with low B-vitamin intakes. Those women were less likely to decline on memory and other cognitive tests over five years if they got B vitamins than if they got a placebo.[31]

But if too little B-12 is a problem, simply getting more from a multivitamin or breakfast cereal may not be the answer.

"Among people with low B-12 status, high folic acid status is strongly associated with cognitive impairment," says Morris.

The folate that occurs naturally in food isn't a problem. "The normal circulating form of folate—methylfolate—was not related to cognitive impairment at all," says Morris. "Only unmetabolized folic acid was."[32]

Unmetabolized folic acid comes from vitamin supplements or from grain foods—breads, cereals, pasta, rice, and tortillas—that are made with "enriched" flour. In 1998, the Food and Drug Administration added folic acid to the other B vitamins and iron that companies are required to add to refined flour and white rice. The folic acid lowered rates of spina bifida and other neural tube birth defects by 26 percent.[33]

If you're taking a multi with 100 percent of a day's folic acid, look for a cereal with no more than 25 percent of a day's worth. Unsweetened shredded wheat has no added folic acid.

But no one expected fortification to lead to unmetabolized folic acid.

"When the FDA decided to fortify the food supply with folic acid, scientists assumed that all the folic acid would be converted to natural folate on the way through the digestive tract," says Morris.

"But we're finding folic acid in body tissues. In a recent paper, we found that a third of seniors have circulating unmetabolized folic acid."

Older people with unmetabolized folic acid are more likely to take supplements and eat fortified foods, but that doesn't completely explain why they have higher levels than others.[34] Genetics may affect what happens to folic acid once it's in your body.

But the link with cognitive decline in people with too little B-12 and too much folic acid is worrisome. "Something is going on in the brain with unmetabolized folic acid, and we don't know what it is," says Morris.

And that makes it tricky to get more B-12. "I can't say take a multivitamin or fortified breakfast cereal because it would also give you a lot of folic acid," she adds. "If you're taking a multi, you're getting a full day's supply." That's 400 micrograms.

"Then you may be getting 100 mcg from fortified grain foods. And if you eat certain breakfast cereals, you'll get another 400 mcg, so you're getting more than two full days' supply. You really have to read cereal boxes."

To complicate matters, getting a blood test for vitamin B-12 may not tell you much. "The test is very insensitive," says Morris.

A more sensitive test is for methylmalonic acid, which goes up when you get too little B-12. (Levels over 210 mmol/L can mean low B-12 status.) But it's more expensive.

References

1. *BMJ 297:* 319, 1988.
2. *JAMA 277:* 1624, 1997.
3. *Hypertension 7:* 110, 1985.
4. *Circulation 98:* 1198, 1998.
5. *Arch. Intern. Med. 169:* 32, 2009.
6. *Hypertension 55:* 681, 2010.
7. *Hypertension 45:* 571, 2005.
8. *J. Am. Soc. Nephrol. 15:* 3225, 2004.
9. nof.org/osteoporosis/diseasefacts.htm
10. *J. Bone Miner. Res. 25:* 64, 2010.
11. *J. Nutr. 140:* 817, 2010.
12. *Lancet 370:* 657, 2007.
13. *J. Bone Min. Res. 23:* 741, 2008.
14. *Osteoporosis Internal. 21:* 1151, 2010.
15. *Arch. Intern. Med. 167:* 1730, 2007.
16. *Cancer Res. 69:* 1439, 2009.
17. *BMJ 341:* c3691, 2010.
18. cdc.gov/diabetes/pubs/factsheet07.htm
19. *Diabetes Care 27:* 134, 2004.
20. *Am. J. Clin. Nutr. 71:* 921, 2000.
21. *Diabetes Care 27:* 59, 2004.
22. *J. Am. Coll. Nutr. 22:* 533, 2003.
23. *Am. J. Clin. Nutr. 85:* 1068, 2007.
24. *Diabetes Care 33:* 304, 2010.
25. *Am. J. Clin. Nutr. 89:* 693S, 2009.
26. *Am. J. Clin. Nutr. 89:* 702S, 2009.
27. *Neurology 72:* 361, 2009.

28. *Am. J. Clin. Nutr. 86:* 1384, 2007.
29. *Arch. Intern. Med. 167:* 21, 2007.
30. *JAMA 300:* 1774, 2008.
31. *Am. J. Clin. Nutr. 88:* 1602, 2008.
32. *Am. J. Clin. Nutr. 91:* 1733, 2010.
33. *MMWR 53:* 362, 2004.
34. *Am. J. Clin. Nutr. 92:* 383, 2010.

Critical Thinking

1. Describe the health benefits of potassium, vitamin D, magnesium, and vitamin B-12

2. Compare the amount of potassium recommended by the Institutes of Medicine with the RDA for potassium.

3. Defend the premise that it is better to consume potassium-rich foods than to take potassium chloride in supplements.

4. Explain why researchers cannot definitively say that magnesium intake is linked to type 2 diabetes even though there are several epidemiological studies that support the claim.

From *Nutrition Action HealthLetter,* September 2010, pp. 2–8. Copyright © 2010 by Center for Science in the Public Interest. Reprinted by permission.

Vitamins, Supplements

New Evidence Shows They Can't Compete with Mother Nature

Americans want to believe in vitamin and mineral pills: We spent an estimated $10 billion on them in 2008, according to the Nutrition Business Journal. But recent studies undertaken to assess their benefits have delivered a flurry of disappointing results. The supplements failed to prevent Alzheimer's disease, cancer, heart attacks, strokes, type 2 diabetes, and premature death.

"We have yet to see well-conducted research that categorically supports the use of vitamin and mineral supplements," says Linda Van Horn, PhD, a professor of preventive medicine at Northwestern University's Feinberg School of Medicine in Chicago. "Most studies show no benefit, or actual harm."

The Power of Food

While some people may need supplements at certain stages of their lives, nutritional deficiencies are uncommon in the U.S. "Almost all of us get or can get the vitamins and minerals we need from our diet," says Paul M. Coates, PhD., director of the Office of Dietary Supplements at the National Institutes of Health (NIH).

Major health organizations for cancer, diabetes, and heart disease all advise against supplements in favor of a healthful diet rich in fruits, vegetables, whole grains, and legumes. Unlike pills, those foods contain fiber plus thousands of health-protective substances that seem to work together more powerfully than any single ingredient can work alone. "That's why it's dangerous to say, 'I know I don't eat well, but if I pop my vitamins, I'm covered,'" says Karen Collins, RD, nutrition adviser to the American Institute for Cancer Research. "We now know that you're not covered."

Too Much Can Harm

Another concern is that some vitamin pills can be toxic if taken in high doses for a long time. Studies show that beta-carotene pills, for example, can increase the risk of lung cancer in smokers, and a 2008 review suggests that the pills, plus supplemental doses of the vitamins A and E, may increase the risk of premature death. In addition, a government survey found that more than 11 percent of adults take at least 400 international units of vitamin E a day, a dose that has been linked to heart failure, strokes, and an increased risk of death.

People are also apt to combine vitamin tablets and fortified foods, which can cause problems. For instance, too much folic acid—added to wheat products in this country—can mask vitamin B12 deficiency. Untreated, that can lead to irreversible nerve damage. In addition, high doses of folic acid may be associated with an increased risk of precancerous colon polyps, according to a trial of some 1,000 people at risk for them. "We're getting several alarming signals that more may not be better," says Susan T. Mayne, PhD., a professor of epidemiology at the Yale School of Public Health.

Yet despite the unfavorable results, vitamin and mineral pills are widely used to fend off diseases. Read on to find our review of the latest evidence on their effects.

Critical Thinking

1. If people choose to consume their nutrient requirements by taking supplements, what nutrients are they not consuming?

2. What type of cancer has been linked to excess intake of folic acid?

3. What nutrient in supplement form has been shown to increase the risk for smokers developing lung cancer?

Which Pills Work?

The recent finding that vitamin D supplements are largely unnecessary exposes a rift among nutrition researchers.

MELINDA WENNER MOYER

Physicians have recommended vitamin D supplements to their patients for a decade, with good reason: dozens of studies have shown a correlation between high intake of vitamin D—far higher than most people would get in a typical diet and from exposure to the sun—and lower rates of chronic diseases, such as cancer and type 1 diabetes. So when the Institute of Medicine, which advises the government on health policy, concluded in November that vitamin D supplements were unnecessary for most Americans and potentially harmful, patients were understandably confused.

The issue exposes a rift among experts over what constitutes valid proof when it comes to nutrition and could affect medical advice on many other supplements. On the one hand are scientists who insist that the only acceptable standard is the randomized clinical trial, which often compares the effects of a medical intervention, such as high intake of vitamin D, with those of a placebo. The scientists who reviewed the vitamin D findings fall heavily into this camp: trials "typically provide the highest level of scientific evidence relevant for dietary reference intake development," they wrote. Their report set intake levels based only on clinical trial data.

The institute panel, however, discarded a raft of observational studies, in which researchers compare the health of populations who take vitamin D supplements with those who do not. In theory, such epidemiological studies are inferior to clinical studies because they rely on observations out in the real world, where it is impossible to control for the variables scientists seek to understand. Researchers compensate for the lack of control by using large sample sizes—some vitamin D studies track 50,000 people—and applying statistical techniques. According to these studies, high levels of vitamin D are generally beneficial.

In the aftermath of the institute report, some physicians are now taking potshots at clinical studies. In nutrition, they say, true placebo groups are hard to maintain—how do you prevent people in a control group from, say, picking up extra vitamin D from sunlight and food, which can lead to underestimating the vitamin's benefits? It is also tough to single out the effect of one vitamin or mineral from others, because many work in tandem. "It is wrong-headed thinking that the only kind of evidence that is reliable is a randomized controlled trial," says Jeffrey Blumberg, a Tufts University pharmacologist.

The next chapter in this debate may come in the spring, when the Endocrine Society releases its own vitamin D guidelines. The organization now recommends higher blood levels of the vitamin than the institute suggested—30 nanograms per milliliter as opposed to 20—which would require supplements. Stay tuned.

Critical Thinking

1. Explain why the IOM concluded that vitamin D supplements are unnecessary and possibly harmful for most Americans.

2. Defend the position of physicians who are opposed to the IOM excluding results from the large observational research studies in favor for the randomized clinical trials only.

3. Differentiate observational research and intervention research.

4. Compare and contrast epidemiological, laboratory, clinical trials, and case study research designs.

Keeping a Lid on Salt: Not So Easy

Known as a silent killer, it's part of how we live.

NANCI HELLMICH

For years, Americans have been advised to consume less sodium, and they've taken that advice with a grain of salt.

Even many health-conscious consumers figured it was the least of their worries, especially compared with limiting their intake of calories, saturated fat, trans fat, cholesterol and sugar.

All that changed last week when a report from the Institute of Medicine urged the government to gradually reduce the maximum amount of sodium that manufacturers and restaurants can add to foods, beverages and meals. The report put a spotlight on what doctors and nutritionists have argued is a major contributor to heart disease and stroke.

More than half of Americans have either high blood pressure or pre-hypertension, says cardiologist Clyde Yancy, president of the American Heart Association and medical director at the Baylor Heart and Vascular Institute in Dallas.

"That puts a lot of us in the bucket of people who need to be on a lower sodium diet. Sodium contributes to most people's high blood pressure, and for some it may be the primary driver."

Cutting back on sodium could save thousands of people from early deaths caused by heart attacks and strokes each year, and it could save billions of dollars in health care costs, he says.

Others second that. "Salt is the single most harmful element in our food supply, silently killing about 100,000 people each year," says Michael Jacobson, executive director of the Washington, D.C.-based Center for Science in the Public Interest. "That's like a crowded jet-liner crashing every single day. But the food industry has fended off government action for more than three decades."

Now salt has our attention.

But reducing it in the American diet is easier said than done. "We have, in essence, ignored the advice because we are driven by convenience, and sodium makes a fast-food lifestyle very easy," Yancy says. "To change, we would need to live and eat differently."

Very differently.

Americans now consume an average of about 3,400 milligrams of sodium a day, or about 1½ teaspoons, government data show. Men consume more than women.

But most adults—including those with high blood pressure, African Americans, the middle-aged and the elderly—should consume no more than 1,500 milligrams a day, according to the dietary guidelines from the U.S. Department of Agriculture. Others should consume less than 2,300 milligrams, or less than a teaspoon, the guidelines say.

And yet it's virtually impossible to limit yourself to such amounts if you often eat processed foods, prepared foods or restaurant fare, including fast food. Most Americans' sodium intake comes from those sources, not the salt shaker on the table.

Some restaurant entrees have 2,000 milligrams or more in one dish. Fast-food burgers can have more than 1,000 milligrams. Many soups are chock-full of sodium. So are many spaghetti sauces, broths, lunch meats, salad dressings, cheeses, crackers and frozen foods.

Can't see it, can't taste it.

Salt serves many functions in products. Besides adding to a food's taste, it is a preservative. "You can't see it," Yancy says. "You can't even taste it because you are so accustomed to it. If you want the freedom to make healthy choices, you are limited by today's foods. That's a problem."

To change that, food companies and restaurants will have to come up with new ways to formulate products and recipes to help consumers gradually lower their salt levels, which would wean them off the taste.

That's a huge challenge, but nutritionists and public health specialists say it can be done and will be worth it. "There is no health benefit to a high-sodium diet, and there is considerable risk," says Linda Van Horn, a professor of preventive medicine at Northwestern University Feinberg School of Medicine.

Even those whose blood pressure is in the normal range should watch their intake, Yancy says. "Here's a wake-up call: Every American who is age 50 or older has a 90% chance of developing hypertension. That increases the risk of heart disease and stroke. This is a preventable process, and it's preventable with sodium reduction, weight control and physical activity."

Why It Can Be Harmful

There are several theories for why sodium increases blood pressure, Yancy says, "but the most obvious one is that it makes us retain fluids, and that retention elevates blood pressure," which injures blood vessels and leads to heart disease and stroke. "It's a connect-the-dots phenomenon."

Some people, especially some African Americans, are more salt-sensitive than others, Yancy says.

"When they are exposed to sodium, they retain more fluid, and because of the way their kidneys handle sodium, they may have a greater proportional rise in blood pressure," he says.

The cost of this damage? An analysis by the Rand Corp. found that if the average sodium intake of Americans was reduced to 2,300 milligrams a day, it might decrease the cases of high blood pressure by 11 million, improve quality of life for millions of people and save about $18 billion in annual health care costs.

The estimated value of improved quality of life and living healthier longer: $32 billion a year. Greater reductions in sodium consumption in the population would save more lives and money, says Roland Sturm, a senior economist with Rand.

Yancy says the country doesn't just need health care reform, "we need health reform. If we don't adjust the demand part of the equation, no system will work. Remarkably, people might be overall healthier by simply reducing sodium."

But Yancy says people need to keep in mind that sodium is just one of the factors that increase the risk of heart disease and stroke. Others include obesity, consuming too much sugar and too few fruits and vegetables, lack of physical activity and smoking.

Salt Industry Disagrees

Leaders in the salt industry say their product is being unfairly maligned. The Institute of Medicine report and the government "are focusing on one small aspect of health, which is a small increase in blood pressure in a small segment of population," says Lori Roman, president of the Salt Institute, an industry group.

Some of the research that ties salt to health risks is based on faulty assumptions and extrapolations, Roman says. She says a recent worldwide study indicated there is no country where people eat an average of less than 1,500 milligrams a day. "That's way below the normal range," Roman says. The Italians eat more sodium than Americans, but their cardiovascular health is better than Americans', and the reason is they eat a lot of fruits and vegetables, she says.

"This is the real story that the government is missing," Roman says. "It is the secret to good health."

She says people may end up following a less healthy diet if they cut back on sodium. "Have you ever bought a can of low-sodium string beans and then tried to season it to taste good? It's impossible," Roman says. "Here's one of the unintended consequences of this recommendation: People will eat fewer vegetables, and by eating fewer vegetables, they will be less healthy."

Yancy says the first step for many people is making the decision to cut back on salt intake. He knows from experience that it can be done.

An African American, Yancy, 52, has high blood pressure and a family history of heart disease and stroke. He's lean and exercises for an hour a day, but still he has to take medication for hypertension. Before he started watching his sodium intake a few years ago, Yancy says, he was consuming more than 4,000 milligrams a day, partly because he grew up in southern Louisiana and was used to a salty, high-fat diet.

But he has weaned himself off the taste. He doesn't have a salt shaker in his house, and he reads the labels on grocery store items and doesn't buy any that have more than 100 milligrams of sodium in a serving.

"I taste the salt in items and put them aside. I find it difficult to enjoy prepared soups. I can taste the salt in prepared meals. I've learned to make my own soups."

When he eats out, he orders salads and asks for his fish and meat to be grilled. "Typically, I eat fish with lemon juice and pepper."

Even so, he believes his sodium intake is probably higher than it should be because he often eats in restaurants and cafeterias, and many foods have hidden sodium.

Changes in food products need to be made over time as the Institute of Medicine report suggests, says Van Horn, a research nutritionist at Northwestern. "If we drop the sodium overnight, people will be desperately seeking salt shakers."

So how hard is it going to be to reduce the salt in processed and prepared foods?

"We've been trying to reduce the sodium in foods for more than 30 years. If this were easy, it would have been accomplished," says Roger Clemens, a professor of pharmacology at the University of Southern California and a spokesman for the Institute of Food Technologists.

The primary dietary source of sodium is sodium chloride, also known as table salt, he says. There are other sodium salts, such as sodium bicarbonate (baking soda) in baking and sodium benzoate (preservative) in bread and beverages. And there are potassium salts that are used in foods—as emulsifiers in cheese and buffers in beverages, he says.

"Salt is a natural preservative. It has been used in the food supply to ensure food safety for centuries," Clemens says. "It's critical for preserving bacon, olives, lunch meats, fish and poultry."

"Some foods, such as cheese, can only be produced with salt. No other compound allows the proteins to knit together to become cheese."

If It Doesn't Taste Good . . .

To make cheese that is lower in sodium, foodmakers must put the cheese through a special procedure that basically extracts some of the sodium. "It's a very long, tedious process," he says.

Salt also is crucial for making most breads. To get dough to rise, manufacturers use sodium chloride and sodium bicarbonate, Clemens says. "If you were to eat a sodium-free product, the texture and flavor would be markedly different. It would be more compressed. I don't think you'd like it at first."

He says some manufacturers have experimented with low-sodium items, and in some cases consumers have turned up their noses. "If it doesn't taste good, consumers won't buy it."

Melissa Musiker, a nutrition spokeswoman for the Grocery Manufacturers Association, agrees. "You can't get ahead of consumers," she says. "You work on the recipes, test them, see how consumers respond and go back and tweak."

There is no one single alternative for replacing it in various foods, she says. "It has to be replaced on an ingredient-by-ingredient basis."

Clemens says food companies will continue to try to develop new technologies to lower the sodium.

"It has taken us 30 years to get this far, and it will probably take us another decade to get a significant difference in the intake. If we can lower sodium in our diet, we'll have a huge health impact on generations to come."

Critical Thinking

1. Identify the four groups of people who should consume less than 1,500 mg of sodium per day, as recommended in the Dietary Guidelines for Americans.

2. What is the largest source of sodium in the typical western diet?

3. How does dietary sodium increase blood pressure in someone who is salt sensitive?

Friend or Foe?

Salt's reputation as a health hazard has recently taken a pounding. Graham Lawton sifts through the evidence.

GRAHAM LAWTON

On my dining table at home sits a container of small, white crystals. One of my daily rituals is to grind some of these crystals onto food; occasionally I dab a finger onto one and pop it into my mouth. They taste metallic and mineral, like the ocean.

Like many people, salt is a routine part of my diet. And yet this mineral that I so casually sprinkle onto my food could kill me. Not immediately, but if I carry on like this, it may well get me in the end.

The World Health Organization says the world is in the grip of a "crisis" of non-infectious diseases. Salt is one of the main culprits because of its effect on blood pressure. Only one substance gives the WHO greater cause for concern, and that is tobacco.

For the past 40 years, doctors around the world have been waging a war on salt. In some places they have been very successful. "All politicians and public health people say we've got to do something about it," says Graham MacGregor, professor of cardiovascular medicine at the Wolfson Institute of Preventive Medicine in London and director of World Action on Salt and Health.

And yet in recent months something has shifted. You might call it a sea change. Headlines have appeared questioning the benefits of eating less salt. Some have claimed salt reduction is positively harmful; even Scientific American declared: "It's time to end the war on salt." What is going on? Can four decades of health advice really be wrong?

Salt - or more accurately its constituent ions sodium and chloride - is a vital nutrient. Sodium and chloride help maintain fluid balance and sodium is one of the ions nerve cells use to create electrical impulses.

The typical food available to our hunter-gatherer ancestors would have been low in salt so we have evolved an exquisite system for detecting it in our diet. One of our five types of taste bud is dedicated to salt, the only one tuned to a single chemical. Unlike energy, our bodies cannot readily store salt and so we are experts at hanging on to it, largely through a recycling unit in the kidneys. It is possible to survive perfectly well on very little salt.

Until recently most humans ate no salt other than what was naturally in their food, amounting to less than half a gram a day.

Pure salt only entered the food chain around 5000 years ago when the Chinese discovered it could be used to preserve food.

Salt has since played a leading role in human history. It assisted the transition to settled communities and became one of the world's most valued commodities.

Although we no longer have to rely on salt to keep food from spoiling our appetite for it is undiminished. Most people eat much more salt than they need. While US dietary guidelines set an adequate intake of 3.75 grams a day, the average westerner eats about 8 grams; in some parts of Asia, 12 is the norm.

Despite a widespread belief that we have an innate liking for salt, this appetite appears to be learned. People living in traditional societies, such as the highlanders of Papua New Guinea, have no access to pure salt and find it repulsive, but if they move to the city they quickly take to it. As with chilli and caffeine, it seems we can learn to love the intrinsically aversive flavour of salt.

And like an addictive drug, the more you eat the more you crave, as salt receptors on the tongue become desensitised by overuse. Once in this habituated state, unsalted foods taste bland and uninteresting. It can take several weeks of salt withdrawal for taste preferences to return to normal.

It doesn't help that today's diet is full of salt. Around three quarters of the salt we eat is added to food before it even reaches our plates, not only in the obvious culprits like cured meat and smoked fish but also concealed in breakfast cereal, biscuits, cheese, yoghurts, cake, soup and sauces. Even bread is surprisingly salty.

There is a multitude of reasons why processed food is so laden with salt. As well as prolonging shelf-life, it makes cheap ingredients taste better and masks the bitter flavours that often result from industrial cooking processes. It can be injected into meat to make it hold more water, thus allowing water to be sold for the price of meat. It improves the appearance, texture and even the smell of the final products. And it makes you thirsty, boosting sales of drinks.

This effortless consumption of salt horrifies doctors. Our kidneys can excrete some excess salt but even so, people who consistently eat more than about half a gram a day-that is, practically all of us-build up excess sodium. To keep fluid concentrations stable, our bodies retain extra water. "We're all sloshing around with a litre or a litre and a half compared with what we would be if we were on our evolutionary salt intake," says MacGregor.

An inevitable consequence of this excess fluid is a rise in blood pressure. Exactly how is not clear. Nor is the reason why some people are more sensitive than others. But the fact that it does is uncontroversial.

It is the effect on blood pressure that causes problems. High blood pressure is one of the main risk factors for cardiovascular disease; even small increases raise your risk of having a stroke. "Everything that lowers blood pressure works. There's no argument," says MacGregor.

For this reason, salt reduction has become one of the most important public health targets in the west. Dietary guidelines vary, but generally recommend eating no more than 5 to 6 grams of salt a day. And these levels are far from ideal—they are merely what is considered realistic in a world awash with salt.

Try calculating your own salt intake and you'll soon learn how hard it is to meet even this modest target. I worked out my daily total and found that I eat around 8 grams a day.

In theory, salt is an easy target for action. If food manufacturers slowly reduced the salt content of their products, everyone would eat less salt and nobody would even notice as their taste buds gradually resensitised.

Staunch Defender

In the UK, this kind of salt reduction was first mooted in 1994 but hastily shelved after protests from food manufacturers. In the intervening years lobbying by scientists, public health groups and bodies such as the Food Standards Agency gradually turned the tide—not least by raising public awareness—and now the industry is broadly reconciled to modest salt reductions. Elsewhere the picture is more mixed, with US manufacturers especially truculent. The most vigorous defender of the status quo is the Salt Institute, a trade body based in Alexandria, Virginia, representing 48 producers and sellers of sodium chloride. The institute has a long history of trumpeting any research that goes against the orthodoxy and picking holes in the evidence against salt.

So what is the evidence? Over the years dozens of studies have been done and while the findings are far from uniform, the general direction of travel is clear.

One approach is to look for a link between how much salt people eat when left to their own devices and their rates of heart attacks and strokes. Over the years many such studies have been done. In 2009, cardiologist Francesco Cappuccio of the University of Warwick, UK, pooled all the data and found a strong relationship between a salty diet and cardiovascular disease (*BMJ*, vol 339, p b4567).

Another way is to intervene directly in people's diets—take two groups of people, get one of them to eat less salt for a while and see what the outcome is. These trials take more work than observational studies but several have been done. The biggest managed to get thousands of people to cut down on salt by about 2 grams a day for up to four years and saw a 25 percent fall in cardiovascular disease (*BMJ*, vol 334, p 885).

Or you can look at whole countries, taking the before-and-after approach. Fifty years ago northern Japan had one of the world's biggest appetites for salt—an average of 18 grams a day per person—and shockingly high numbers of strokes. The government implemented a salt reduction programme and by the late 1960s average salt consumption had fallen by 4 grams a day and stroke deaths were down by 80 percent. Finland, another salt-guzzling nation, achieved similar gains in the 1970s.

However, the evidence is not always so clear. In July the Salt Institute was presented with its biggest PR coup for years when the Cochrane Collaboration, an internationally renowned body dedicated to assessing medical evidence, published a long-awaited study on salt and cardiovascular disease.

As is usual for Cochrane, the study was a "meta-analysis", pooling the results of all the best-designed randomised controlled trials that have been done, the highest standard of proof in medicine. Seven trials met the quality criteria, with over 6000 subjects in total.

The analysis did show that people who cut back on salt have slightly lower blood pressure and are less likely to die from heart attacks and strokes. But, crucially, the effect on deaths wasn't big enough to be statistically significant. The Cochrane team could not rule out the possibility that the reductions had happened by chance.

The research was published simultaneously by Cochrane and the *American Journal of Hypertension* (vol 24, p 843), whose editor-in-chief Michael Alderman is a long-time critic

Well seasoned Typical salt content of some common processed foods. Recommended upper level per day is 5.75 grams in the US

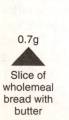   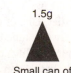 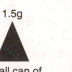

0.7g	0.4g	2.0g	0.5g	2.2g	1.4g	1.5g	1.8g	0.2g
Slice of wholemeal bread with butter	Bowl of cereal with milk	Typical pre-packed sandwich	Bag of ready-salted crisps	Small cheeseburger and fries	Small can of tomato soup	Small can of baked beans	Small pot of yoghurt	Sweet biscuit

of salt reduction. In an accompanying editorial (vol 24, p 854), Alderman, who was once a paid consultant for the Salt Institute, repeated his oft-stated claims that there is not enough evidence for salt reduction. Sensing a story, many newspapers ran with his line.

Is Alderman correct? Not surprisingly, MacGregor thinks not. For one thing, he claims the Cochrane study is flawed. When he reanalysed the same data in a slightly different way, he found a reduction that was statistically significant (The Lancet, vol 378, p 380). Alderman criticises this as "salami epidemiology", but even in the original analysis the link between salt and death rates only just slipped below statistical significance. Far from casting doubt on salt reduction, some argued that the findings supported it.

The Cochrane report wasn't the end of it. Last month Alderman's journal published a further meta-analysis purporting to show that salt reduction could actually be harmful (doi:10.1038/ajh.2011.210). It concluded that while cutting salt lowered blood pressure, blood levels of certain hormones and lipids were increased, which could theoretically raise cardiovascular risk.

But many of the studies included in the analysis lasted just a few days and involved big salt reductions. MacGregor accepts that sudden and steep salt reduction can lead to counterproductive hormonal changes, but says that modest reductions, say from 8 to 6 grams, do not. "There's no evidence whatsoever that a modest reduction does any harm," he says.

One lesson from these latest studies is that headlines can be misleading; the devil is in the detail. That is why the salt reducers talk about the "totality of the evidence". Nutrition science is notoriously hard. You need large numbers of people to detect the outcome of small dietary changes and there are so many confounding factors that sometimes paradoxical results pop up.

"Nutrition is not black and white," says Susan Jebb of the UK Medical Research Council's Human Nutrition Research unit in Cambridge. "It's not about one definitive trial, it's about the totality of the evidence. In this case the balance of evidence strongly supports reductions in salt."

There is one way of settling the debate. Take 30,000 people, put half of them on a high-salt diet and half on a low-salt diet for at least five years and see what happens.

"Try calculating your own salt intake and you'll soon learn how hard it is to meet even modest targets"

Unfortunately, this trial will probably never be done. According to Cappuccio it would be impractically big, prohibitively expensive, and ethically questionable—not to mention hard to achieve in today's salt-saturated world. The salt lobby disagrees. "To say it is too expensive and takes too many people is a bogus argument," says Alderman. "It can be done and it should be done." As for ethics, he asks which is worse: to do the

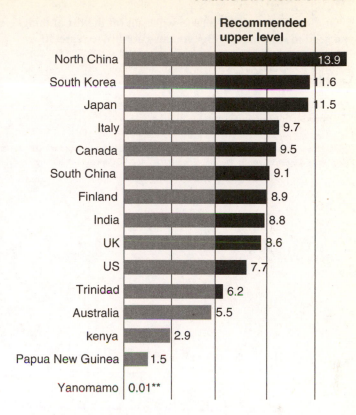

	Recommended upper level
North China	13.9
South Korea	11.6
Japan	11.5
Italy	9.7
Canada	9.5
South China	9.1
Finland	8.9
India	8.8
UK	8.6
US	7.7
Trinidad	6.2
Australia	5.5
kenya	2.9
Papua New Guinea	1.5
Yanomamo	0.01**

** an indigenous people of the Amazon, Brazil/Venezuela border who have the lowest recorded salt intake in the world

An appetite for salt   National average salt intake (grams of salt per day)
Source: Bmj, vol 297,326 (For Australia, World Action on Salt and Health)

experiment, or to foist salt reduction on everyone without being sure it won't do any harm?

But perhaps the salt lobby will be quite happy for the trial never to happen. Demanding definitive proof before taking action sounds reasonable, but if you know that proof will never arrive all you are doing is defending the status quo.

Like the tobacco industry before it, the salt industry inevitably feels threatened by public health campaigns aimed at reducing consumption of its one and only product. And as with tobacco, its best tactic is to spread doubt. "What the Salt Institute wants is the idea that there is disagreement among the experts," says MacGregor. In fact, there are very few independent experts who are against salt reduction.

Even the chief author of the Cochrane study, statistician Rod Taylor at the Peninsula Medical School in Exeter, UK, agrees with MacGregor that the findings lend further support to salt reduction. "Our results do not mean that asking people to reduce their intake of salt is not a good thing," he says.

"We have much stronger evidence for salt than we do for fat, for the benefits of eating fruit and vegetables or losing weight," argues MacGregor. "There has never been a randomised controlled trial of cigarette reduction. Should we not have done anything about cigarettes?"

Of course it would be nice to wipe salt off the list of things you need to worry about. But you may not live to regret it.

Critical Thinking

1. Describe six attributes of adding salt during food production/manufacturing.

2. Examine the position of the Salt Institute lobbyist regarding lower dietary salt recommendations. Expound upon the bias of the position of this lobbyist group.

3. Evaluate the challenges of conducting a large clinical trial on high salt and low salt diets.

GRAHAM LAWTON is deputy editor of *New Scientist*.

From *New Scientist Magazine,* December 3, 2011, pp. 46–49. Copyright © 2011 by Reed Business Information, Ltd, UK. Reprinted by permission via Tribune Media Services.

Nutrition for Optimum Athletic Performance—The Right Fuel Can Be the Difference

ELLEN COLEMAN, MA, MPH, RD, CSSD

Three primary factors influence athletic performance: genetics, training, and nutrition. Athletes have no influence over their heredity, but they can control their training and diet.

Athletes are constantly looking for a competitive edge. Though the appropriate diet won't guarantee athletic success, a poor diet can undermine training efforts. In many events, especially among elite athletes, the margin between victory and defeat is very small. Attention to nutrition can make that critical difference.

The foods an athlete chooses will influence performance in both training and competition. Diet may actually have its biggest impact on training. A healthful diet supports regular, intensive training and decreases the risk of illness and/or injury. Appropriate food choices can also enhance adaptations to the training stimulus.

Several prestigious organizations have recently issued guidelines on nutrition and athletic performance after meticulously reviewing the literature. This article will provide sports nutrition recommendations and highlight key points from these documents:

- the new International Olympic Committee Medical Commission consensus statement on sports nutrition, released in October 2010[1]; and
- the American Dietetic Association, American College of Sports Medicine, and Dietitians of Canada's 2009 update on their position statement on nutrition and athletic performance.[2]

These documents emphasize that diet has a significant influence on athletic performance. Athletes should adopt specific nutritional strategies before, during, and after training and competition to optimize their physical and mental performance and promote health. The proper amount of food, the composition of the meal, and the timing of food intake can help athletes train and perform more effectively and reduce the risk of illness and injury.[1,2]

Energy Intake

Energy requirements depend on an athlete's periodized training load and competition program and vary from day to day and with the competition schedule. An appropriate diet will help athletes reach an optimum body size and composition to achieve greater success in their sport.[1,2]

Excessive energy intake relative to expenditure increases body fat, which may hinder performance. Inadequate energy intake relative to energy expenditure impairs performance and adaptations to training.[1,2] Insufficient energy consumption causes the body to use both fat and lean tissue for fuel. Loss of lean tissue decreases strength and endurance and may compromise immune, endocrine, and musculoskeletal function.[2]

Energy availability is defined as "dietary energy intake minus exercise energy expenditure." Low energy availability should be avoided as it may be harmful to brain, reproductive, metabolic, and immune function and bone health.[1,2] The well-documented "Female Athlete Triad," consisting of low energy availability (with or without disordered eating), amenorrhea, and osteoporosis (alone or in combination), is a major concern and poses significant health risks to young and adult female athletes.

When energy intake is restricted to reduce body weight and/or fat mass, it is important to select nutrient-rich foods to reduce the risk of developing nutrient deficiencies that will impair health and performance.[1]

Dieting in young athletes should be discouraged as this may hinder their growth and development.[1] Athletes at risk of disordered eating patterns and reproductive disorders should be promptly referred to a qualified health professional for evaluation and treatment.[1]

Although exercise performance is influenced by body weight and composition, these physical measures should not be seen as criteria for sports performance. Athletes may be pressured to lose weight and body fat to improve their power-to-weight ratio (eg, running, distance cycling, triathlon), achieve a desirable body composition for aesthetic sports (eg, gymnastics, figure skating, diving), or compete in a specific weight class (eg, wrestling, lightweight rowing, boxing) in spite of having an appropriate weight for health and performance. Scholastic athletic governing bodies have instituted weight-loss procedure guidelines that limit the rate of loss for collegiate and high school wrestlers, but the potential for abuse still exists in other sports. Losses of both muscle and fat mass due to extreme energy restriction may adversely influence an athlete's performance and health.[2]

Body fat percentages of athletes vary depending on an athlete's gender and sport. The estimated minimal level of body fat compatible with health is 5 percent for males and 12 percent for females. However, optimal body fat percentages for an athlete may be much higher than these minimum levels and should be established on an individual basis. An athlete's optimal competitive body weight and relative body fatness should be determined when an athlete is healthy and performs at his or her best.[2]

A diet that provides adequate energy from a wide range of regularly available foods can meet the carbohydrate, protein, and fat requirements of training and competition.[1] Athletes do not need a diet substantially different than that recommended in the 2010 Dietary Guidelines for Americans.[2]

Carbohydrate

During high-intensity training, particularly prolonged exercise, an athlete should consume enough carbohydrate to meet the energy needs of the training program as well as replenish carbohydrate stores (muscle and liver glycogen stores) during recovery between training sessions and competitive events. For competitions lasting one hour or longer, the athlete should emphasize carbohydrate-rich foods in the hours and days before the event.[1]

Carbohydrate recommendations for athletes range from 5 to 12 g/kg/day, as shown in Table 1. These are general recommendations and should be adjusted with consideration of an athlete's total energy needs, specific training needs, and feedback from his or her training performance.[3]

Guidelines for carbohydrate intake should not be provided in terms of percentage contributions to total dietary energy intake. These recommendations are neither user friendly nor strongly related to the muscle's absolute need for fuel.[3]

Protein

Protein metabolism is influenced by exercise type (endurance vs. strength), exercise intensity, carbohydrate availability, training state, energy balance, gender, and age.[1]

Table 1   Daily Carbohydrate Recommendations for Athletes

- 5 to 7 g of carbohydrate/kg/day: athletes engaging in moderate-intensity exercise for 60 to 90 minutes per day
- 7 to 12 g of carbohydrate/kg/day: athletes engaging in moderate- to high-intensity endurance exercise for one to three hours
- 10 to 12 g of carbohydrate/kg/day: athletes participating in extreme endurance exercise for four to six hours per day (eg, Tour de France)

Athletes should take in more protein than the 0.8 g/kg/day recommended for the general population. Endurance athletes should consume 1.2 to 1.4 g/kg/day and strength athletes about 1.2 to 1.7 g/kg/day. The increase in contractile proteins allows a weightlifter to achieve a greater absolute power output, whereas an increased mitochondrial volume allows the endurance athlete to exercise for hours. However, consuming a varied diet that meets energy needs generally provides more protein than required, including any increases that may arise from high-level training.[1,2]

Athletes who severely restrict their energy intakes are at risk of failing to meet their protein needs. These include athletes in weight-restriction sports or aesthetically judged sports as well as athletes with disordered eating patterns. Inadequate protein intake can cause loss of muscle mass and compromise training adaptations and immune function.[2]

Athletes should consume high-quality protein regularly throughout the day to meet their protein requirements.[1] Consuming protein immediately after exercise may help increase net muscle protein balance, promote muscle tissue repair, and enhance adaptations involving synthesis of new proteins.[1-3]

Protein and amino acid supplements offer no advantages over protein-rich foods other than convenience. Although protein powders and amino acid supplements are widely used, they are a potential source for illegal substances such as anabolic steroids, which may not be listed on the ingredient label.[2]

Fat

Fat intake should be sufficient to provide essential fatty acids and fat-soluble vitamins as well as contribute energy for weight maintenance. The Acceptable Macronutrient Distribution range for fat (as established by the Food and Nutrition Board of the Institute of Medicine) of 20 percent to 35 percent of energy intake is appropriate for athletes.[2] Short-term fat adaptation ("fat loading") does not improve prolonged endurance exercise and may impair an athlete's ability to work at high intensities.[2]

Micronutrients

Vitamins and minerals play an important role in energy production, hemoglobin synthesis, maintenance of bone health, adequate immune function, and the protection of body tissues from oxidative damage. Micronutrients are also required to help build and repair muscle tissue following exercise.[2]

Consuming a varied diet that contains adequate micronutrients and energy, getting enough sleep, and reducing life stressors help enhance immunity and reduce the risk of infection.[1]

Athletes at greatest risk of poor micronutrient status usually restrict energy intake (especially over long periods), have severe weight-loss practices, eliminate one or more food groups from their diet, or rely on foods with a low nutrient density.[2]

Athletes should be particularly aware of their needs for calcium, vitamin D, and iron.[1,2] Inadequate dietary calcium and vitamin D increase the risk of low bone mineral density and stress fractures. Low energy availability, insufficient intake of dairy products (and other calcium-rich foods), and menstrual dysfunction greatly increase a female athlete's risk of having low bone mineral density.[1]

Athletes who live at northern latitudes or who train primarily indoors throughout the year, such as gymnasts and figure skaters, are at risk of poor vitamin D status, especially if they do not consume vitamin D-fortified foods. These athletes may benefit from vitamin D supplementation.[1,2]

Iron is required for the formation of hemoglobin, myoglobin, and enzymes involved in energy production. Iron depletion (low iron stores as measured by serum ferritin) is one of the most prevalent nutrient deficiencies observed among athletes, especially females. Iron deficiency, with or without anemia, can impair muscle function and limit work capacity. Athletes should consume a diet with high availability of iron.[2]

Female athletes, long-distance runners, adolescents, and vegetarians should be screened periodically to assess and monitor iron status. The decision to use iron supplements in athletes with depleted iron stores is usually made on an individual basis. Supplements are discontinued when the serum ferritin measurement returns to normal for an individual athlete.[2]

Hydration

Dehydration (loss of more than 2 percent of body mass) can impair performance in most events, particularly in warm and high-altitude environments. Dehydration also increases the risk of heat exhaustion and is a risk factor for heat stroke. Athletes should be well hydrated before exercise and drink sufficiently during exercise to limit dehydration to less than 2 percent of body mass.[1,2]

The amount and rate of fluid replacement depends on an individual's sweating rate, exercise duration, and opportunities to drink. It is not possible to propose a one-size-fits-all fluid and electrolyte replacement schedule due to the multiple factors that influence sweating rate and sweat electrolyte concentrations.[2]

Sports beverages containing carbohydrates and electrolytes may be consumed before, during, and after exercise to help maintain blood glucose concentration, provide fuel for muscles, and decrease the risk of dehydration and hyponatremia.[2] Guidelines for hydration management are as follows:

- **Before exercise:** Athletes should drink about 5 to 7 mL/kg of body weight (2 to 3 mg/lb) four hours before activity.
- **During exercise:** Athletes should monitor changes in body weight during training and competition to establish sweating rates for specific exercise and environmental conditions.[2] Consuming an appropriate amount of fluid during training sessions improves the quality of an athlete's workout and so enhances training adaptations. Athletes should not drink so much that they gain weight during exercise, as this increases the risk of developing hyponatremia.[1,2]

Sodium should be included when sweat losses are high, especially when exercise lasts more than about two hours. The average concentration of sodium in sweat is about 35 mmol/L, or about 800 mg/L. Chilled fluids may benefit performance in hot conditions.[1]

- **After exercise:** Athletes should drink 24 oz for each pound lost (1.5 L of fluid for each kilogram lost). To recover from exercise, athletes should replace the water and salt that is lost in sweat. When athletes must compete in several events in a short time period strategies to enhance recovery of fluid are important.[1,2]

Training Diet

Compared with the general population, athletes need additional energy to fuel physical activity and additional fluid to replace sweat losses. As energy requirements increase, athletes should first strive to consume the maximum number of servings appropriate for their energy needs from carbohydrate-rich foods: bread, cereals and grains, legumes, milk/milk alternatives, vegetables, and fruits.[2]

Athletes who are small or have lower energy requirements should focus on making nutrient-dense food choices to obtain adequate carbohydrate, protein, essential fats, and micronutrients.[2]

The food and fluid intake consumed around workouts should be individually determined and based on an athlete's gastrointestinal tolerance as well as the intensity and the duration of a workout.[2]

Preexercise Meal

Eating before exercise improves performance compared with exercising in a fasted state. The size and the timing of the preexercise meal are interrelated; smaller meals should be consumed closer to the event to allow for gastric emptying, whereas larger meals can be consumed when more time is available before exercise or competition. A carbohydrate feeding of 1 g/kg is appropriate one hour before exercise, whereas 4.5 g/kg can be consumed four hours before exercise as shown in Table 2.[2,3]

The preexercise meal should be high in carbohydrate (to maintain blood glucose and maximize glycogen stores), relatively low in fat and fiber (to facilitate gastric emptying and minimize gastrointestinal distress), moderate in protein, contain familiar foods, and provide sufficient fluid to contribute to hydration.[2]

If an athlete is unable to eat breakfast prior to early morning exercise, consuming about 30 g of easily digested carbohydrate five minutes before exercise may improve performance.

Table 2 Carbohydrate Recommendations for the Preexercise Meal

- Consume 1 g of carbohydrate/kg one hour before exercise.
- Consume 2 g of carbohydrate/kg two hours before exercise.
- Consume 3 g of carbohydrate/kg three hours before exercise.
- Consume 4 to 4.5 g of carbohydrate/kg four hours before exercise.

Table 3 Carbohydrate Content of Selected Foods

- 1 qt of Gatorade Thirst Quencher = 56 g
- 1 PowerBar Harvest = 43 g
- 2 Vanilla Bean GU gels = 50 g
- 28 Sport Beans = 50 g
- 6 Clif Shot Bloks = 48 g
- 3 large graham crackers = 66 g
- 4 Fig Newtons = 42 g
- 1 banana = 30 g

Fueling During Exercise

Consuming carbohydrate (30 to 60 g/hour) during endurance exercise or stop-and-go sports lasting one hour or more can enhance physical and cognitive performance by maintaining blood glucose levels and carbohydrate oxidation in the latter stages of exercise.[1,2] As the duration of the event increases, so does the amount of carbohydrate needed to optimize performance. Relatively high rates of intake (up to 90 g/hour) are needed to optimize performance in events lasting three hours or more.[2]

The maximum amount of carbohydrate that can be oxidized during exercise from a single carbohydrate source (eg, glucose) is about 1 g/minute or 60 g/hour because the transporter responsible for carbohydrate absorption in the intestine becomes saturated. A series of studies conducted by researchers at the University of Birmingham has shown that consuming between 1.8 to 2.4 g of carbohydrate per minute (108 to 144 g/hour) from a mixture of carbohydrates increases carbohydrate oxidation up to 75 to 104 g of carbohydrate per hour.[4]

Athletes should experiment with different sports drinks and sports foods during training to develop effective fueling strategies for competition. Consuming carbohydrate during training sessions also improves the quality of an athlete's workout and so enhances training adaptations. Choosing sports foods and drinks that contain a mixture of carbohydrates will maximize absorption from the gut and minimize gastrointestinal disturbances.[1] The carbohydrate content of selected foods is listed in Table 3.

Recovery Following Exercise

The restoration of muscle and liver glycogen stores is important for recovery following strenuous training. Athletes commonly engage in prolonged high-intensity workouts once or twice per day with a limited amount of time (six to 24 hours) to recover before the next exercise session. Utilizing successful refueling strategies following daily training sessions helps to optimize recovery and promote the desired adaptations to training.[1,2]

During the early period of recovery (up to four hours) after glycogen-depleting exercise, an athlete should consume about 1 g of carbohydrate/kg/hour.[3] When there are less than eight hours between exercise sessions, start consuming carbohydrate immediately after exercise to maximize recovery time. Recovery meals and snacks contribute to an athlete's daily carbohydrate requirements of 5 to 12 g of carbohydrate/kg/day.[3]

Table 4 Recovery Nutrition Strategies

- During the early period of recovery after glycogen-depleting exercise, consume 1 g of carbohydrate/kg/hour.
- When there are less than eight hours between exercise sessions, start consuming carbohydrate immediately after exercise to maximize recovery time.
- Consume 15 to 25 g of high-quality protein after each training session to stimulate muscle protein synthesis/repair.

Consuming foods or drinks providing 15 to 25 g of high-quality protein after each training session enhances muscle protein synthesis, promotes maintenance of lean tissue, and aids muscle repair.[1] Recovery meals and snacks contribute to an athlete's daily protein requirements of 1.2 to 1.7 g of protein/kg/day.[2] Table 4 provides recovery nutrition strategies.

Supplements and Ergogenic Aids

Vitamin and mineral supplements are not needed if adequate energy to maintain body weight is consumed from a variety of foods.[2] The use of supplements does not compensate for poor food choices and an inadequate diet.[1] Supplements that provide essential nutrients may be a short-term option when food intake or food choices are restricted due to travel or other factors.[1] The consumption of large amounts of some micronutrients via supplements may be harmful. Vitamin D may be needed in supplemental form when sun exposure is inadequate, particularly for those living in extreme northern latitudes.

Athletes seek that "secret ingredient" that will enhance their workout and give them the edge over their competitors. They want to believe in something magical that can improve performance more than hard training or a prudent diet. In many events, the difference between winning and losing is in divisions of seconds, so it is not surprising that athletes are susceptible to miraculous claims for sports supplements.

An enormous array of nutritional ergogenic aids are available to athletes. The desire for that elusive "magic bullet' may cause athletes to abandon sound nutrition practices and become victims of nutrition quackery. A few nutritional ergogenic aids (eg, creatine, caffeine, sodium bicarbonate) perform as claimed and may enhance athletic performance when used properly. Most, however, do not perform as claimed or give athletes the results they want. Some sports supplements may contain banned substances or be detrimental when taken in high doses for prolonged periods.[1,2]

Dietary supplements do not undergo evaluation for safety and effectiveness by the FDA prior to being marketed. Thus, nutritional ergogenic aids should be used with caution and only after careful product evaluation for safety, efficacy, potency, and legality (doping). Some supplements contain ingredients (anabolic steroids and stimulants) not declared on the label that are prohibited by national and international sports governing bodies. Innocent ingestion of prohibited substances is not an acceptable excuse; athletes are ultimately responsible for the product they ingest and any consequences.[1,2]

The use of supplements by young athletes should be discouraged. The focus should be on consuming a nutrient-dense diet to promote growth as well as a healthy body composition.[1]

Vegetarian Athletes

Vegetarian athletes may be at risk of low intakes of energy, protein, fat, and key micronutrients such as iron, calcium, vitamin D, riboflavin, zinc, and vitamin B12. Women in particular are vulnerable for nonanemic iron deficiency, which may limit endurance performance. Consultation with a sports dietitian is recommended to avoid these nutrition problems.[2]

Sports Dietitians

All athletes can benefit from the guidance of qualified sports nutrition professionals regarding their individual energy, nutrient, and fluid needs and developing sport-specific nutritional strategies for training, competition, and recovery.[1,2] In 2005, the Commission on Dietetic Registration created a specialty credential for food and nutrition professionals who specialize in sports dietetic practice. The board certified specialist in sports dietetics (CSSD) credential is designed as the premier professional sports nutrition credential in the United States. Specialists in sports dietetics provide evidence-based nutrition assessment, guidance, and counseling for health and performance for athletes, sport organizations, and physically active individuals and groups. The credential requires current RD status, maintenance of RD status for a minimum of two years, and documentation of 1,500 sports specialty practice hours as an RD within the past five years.[2]

Final Thoughts

Athletes should adopt nutrition strategies that optimize physical and mental performance and support good health. The proper amount of food, the composition of the meal, and the timing of food intake can help athletes train and perform more effectively and reduce the risk of illness and injury.

Athletes should consume adequate energy and macronutrients (especially carbohydrate and protein) during times of heavy physical activity to maintain body weight, replenish glycogen stores, and provide adequate protein to build and repair tissue. Athletes should also ingest adequate food and fluid before, during, and after exercise to maintain blood glucose concentration during exercise, maximize exercise performance, and optimize recovery. Athletes should be well hydrated before exercise and drink enough fluid during exercise (based on individual sweat rates) and after exercise to replace their fluid losses.

Vitamin and mineral supplements are not needed if an athlete consumes adequate energy to maintain body weight from a variety of foods. Nutritional ergogenic aids should be used cautiously and only after meticulous product evaluation for safety, effectiveness, potency, and legality.

A qualified sports dietitian (in the United States, a CSSD) should provide individualized nutrition guidance and counseling following a comprehensive nutrition assessment.[2]

References

1. International Olympic Committee Consensus Statement on Sports Nutrition. October 27, 2010. Available at: www.olympic.org/Documents/Reports/EN/CONSENSUS-FINAL-v8-en.pdf.
2. Rodriguez NR, Di Marco NM, Langley S, et al. Position of the American Dietetic Association, Dietitians of Canada, and the American College of Sports Medicine: Nutrition and athletic performance. *J Am Diet Assoc.* 2009;109(3):509–527.
3. Nutrition Working Group of the Medical Commission of the International Olympic Committee. Nutrition for athletes. June 2003. Available at: www.olympic.org/Documents/Reports/EN/en-report-1251.pdf.
4. Currell K, Jeukendrup AE. Superior endurance performance with ingestion of multiple transportable carbohydrates. *Med Sci Sports Exerc.* 2008;40:275–281.

Critical Thinking

1. Contrast carbohydrate and protein needs in athletes compared to a person with low physical activity.
2. Describe the benefit of consuming carbohydrates and protein after exercise.
3. Identify the micronutrients that should be of utmost importance among athletes.
4. Summarize the recommendations for hydration before, during, and after exercise.

Iron Nutrition and the Female Athlete: Countermeasures for the Prevention of Poor Iron Status

Laura J. Bass, MS, RD[1] and James P. McClung, PhD[1]

Iron is a trace element essential for many critical biological processes, including those involved in cognition and physical activity. Iron confers function through incorporation into proteins and enzymes. Many of these proteins and enzymes, such as myoglobin, cytochrome *c,* and hemoglobin are critical for the maintenance of human performance.[1] Poor iron status remains a worldwide public health concern and affects billions of people; in fact, iron deficiency is the most prevalent micro-nutrient deficiency disease in the world.[2] In the United States, iron deficiency and iron deficiency anemia, respectively, occur in up to 12% and 4% of women between the ages of 20 and 49 years.[3] Iron deficiency is defined clinically using cutoff values for a series of iron status indicators such as transferrin saturation and serum ferritin level. Iron deficiency anemia is clinically defined when individuals present with iron deficiency as well as hemoglobin values below a cutoff value.

Diminished iron status in athletes, sometimes referred to as "sports anemia," was first reported more than 40 years ago.[4] Although the first studies reporting reductions in iron status in athletes were conducted using male volunteers,[5,6] more recent work has described declines in indicators of iron status in female athletes following periods of physical training.[7] Similarly, research from our laboratory has detailed reductions in iron status in female military personnel during basic combat training, an 8- to 10-week course that includes a series of aerobic and muscle strength training activities.[8–10]

Poor iron status is of particular concern for female athletes. First, the prevalence of iron deficiency and iron deficiency anemia is greater in female athletes when compared to other demographic groups,[11] as they have difficulty maintaining iron balance because of insufficient dietary iron intake coupled with increased iron losses through mechanisms associated with heavy physical activity.[8] Second, iron deficiency and iron deficiency anemia are known to affect cognitive and physical function, which are paramount to athletic performance.[9] Iron supplementation and the consumption of iron-fortified foods could be useful for health professionals when recommending countermeasures for preventing poor iron status in female athletes. This review will detail recent studies of iron supplementation and fortification in physically active women, and compare and contrast the efficacy of these methods for maintaining iron balance.

Iron Balance in Female Athletes

Total body iron has been estimated at approximately 3.8 g in males and 2.3 g in females, although these estimates can shift based on body weight.[12] Although consuming adequate levels of iron through the diet is most important for maintaining positive balance, factors affecting iron loss also have a major impact on iron status (Figure 1). Athletes can have increased iron losses from gastrointestinal bleeding, which can occur following physical activity. In one report, median fecal hemoglobin concentrations increased by nearly 40 percent following marathon running; reported peak losses were 1.5 mg/g of feces.[13] Although the finite cause of increased gastrointestinal bleeding following physical activity remains unknown, contributors could include gut ischemia or aggravation of preexisting gut lesions. Sweat loss, a marginal, yet consistent factor for athletes, can affect iron status; estimates of iron loss from sweat range from 22 μg/L of sweat up to 6 mg/L but vary widely based on sweat collection techniques.[14] Furthermore, menstrual blood loss

[1]United States Army Research Institute of Environmental Medicine (USARIEM), Natick, MA, USA

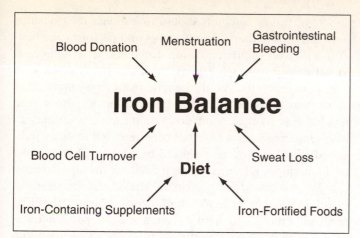

Figure 1   Factors contributing to iron balance

has been demonstrated to be a strong predictor of iron status, and female athletes prone to large menstrual losses can be at greater risk of iron deficiency or iron deficiency anemia. Although estimates of iron loss through menstruation vary and are largely driven by total menstrual blood loss, one recent report indicates mean daily iron losses ranging from 0.23 to 0.4 mg/d in a population of young women.[15]

Hepcidin, a recently discovered hormone regulator of iron homeostasis, can provide another mechanism affecting iron balance in athletes. Hepcidin regulates iron balance by degrading ferroportin, a protein responsible for iron transfer from the enterocyte and other cell types, thereby reducing the biologically available iron supply.[16] Although the expression of hepcidin is affected by iron status, the synthesis of this protein is also affected by the presence of proinflammatory cytokines, such as interleukin-6. As interleukin-6 can rise following acute bouts of physical activity,[17] it is possible that heavy bouts of exercise could stimulate hepcidin synthesis, with subsequent effects on iron balance in athletes. The observation that both male and female athletes exhibit an elevation in inflammatory markers, including interleukin-6, and that urinary hepcidin levels rise following exercise supports the link between physical activity, inflammation, and diminished iron status.[17–19]

Current recommendations for dietary iron intake are 15 mg/d for girls between the ages of 14 and 18 years and 18 mg/d for women 19 to 50 years old.[20] The recommendation for pregnant women is higher, 27 mg/d, because of gestational needs of the fetus and blood losses that occur during delivery. The bioavailability of dietary iron is largely dependent on the composition of the diet. Heme iron, predominantly found in animal protein, is better absorbed at 10 percent to 35 percent than nonheme iron, found mainly in plant foods. Nonheme iron is generally more abundant than heme iron in the diet; however, less than 10 percent of nonheme iron is absorbed.[21] A number of dietary factors affect nonheme iron absorption. Ascorbic acid, fermented foods, and factors in meat, poultry, and fish all enhance absorption,[22] whereas phytate, polyphenols, and other minerals inhibit iron absorption.[23] A strong predictor of both heme and nonheme iron absorption is iron status. Both heme and nonheme iron absorption are tightly regulated at the enterocyte[23] resulting in the efficient recycling of body iron. Iron bioavailability affects an individual's ability to obtain required levels of iron and could ultimately place certain populations, such as vegetarians, at higher risk for iron deficiency and iron deficiency anemia because of a lack of heme iron in the diet.

Supplementation for the Prevention of Iron Deficiency and Iron Deficiency Anemia in Female Athletes

Providing additional iron in the form of a dietary supplement is one method for achieving and maintaining optimal iron status in female athletes at risk for iron deficiency and iron deficiency anemia, and many studies have investigated this approach for preventing poor iron status. McClung et al[10] recently studied the effects of daily 100 mg ferrous sulfate supplementation on iron status and performance in female soldiers during basic combat training. In this randomized, placebo-controlled trial, those women who began basic combat training with iron deficiency anemia and who received the iron supplement exhibited a mean increase in hemoglobin concentration of 1.2 g/dL, which raised the group mean to 12.2 g/dL, a value above most clinical definitions of anemia.[10] These women also demonstrated significantly faster 2-mile run times when compared with the women with iron deficiency anemia who consumed the placebo. A 2-mile run has been demonstrated to correlate well with maximal oxygen uptake as a measure of endurance capacity.[24] Therefore, in this study, iron supplementation effectively increased hemoglobin concentrations above an anemic value, and presumably facilitated systemic oxygen transport, thereby contributing to improved performance in women who began the study with iron deficiency anemia.[10] In women who began basic combat training with normal iron status at baseline, decrements in serum ferritin and soluble transferrin receptor were observed during basic combat training, but these decrements were attenuated for those receiving the iron treatment, although running performance was not affected.[10] Attenuating declines in serum ferritin (an iron storage protein) and decreasing soluble transferrin receptor (an indicator of functional iron status) indicates improved maintenance of body iron stores.[25] Thus, iron supplementation provided a clear advantage for iron status and performance for females with iron deficiency anemia and although it prevented declines in iron status in females with normal iron status, a clear performance benefit was not apparent.

Although benefits of iron supplementation for female athletes with iron deficiency anemia have been well documented,[1,26] advantages are less clear in nonanemic women with iron deficiency. Some studies have demonstrated that supplementation of the iron deficient population can affect iron status and improve maximal oxygen uptake[27]; however, in female athletes with iron deficiency, iron supplementation has not always been demonstrated to improve physical performance. Recent studies have aimed to determine clinically relevant iron status biomarkers, other than hemoglobin concentration, that can provide a biochemical definition for the degree of iron deficiency that could affect performance in female athletes. For example, Brownlie et al[28,29] demonstrated that soluble transferrin receptor can be a useful biomarker to assess female athletes with iron deficiency who would benefit from iron supplementation for improved performance. In one supplementation trial, 100 mg of ferrous sulfate or placebo was provided daily for six weeks along with a prescribed exercise regimen. When supplemented, women with initial soluble transferrin receptor values greater than eight mg/L, indicating tissue iron deficiency, were able to improve time to finish during a 15-km cycling trial. However, supplementation was not associated with performance changes in women with baseline soluble transferrin receptor values less than eight mg/L.[28,29] Similarly, another recent study demonstrated that longitudinal increases in soluble transferrin receptor were associated with decreased performance on a two-mile run.[9] Together these findings suggest that soluble transferrin receptor is a useful biomarker for identifying iron deficient, nonanemic, female athletes whose diminished tissue iron stores could be affecting performance.

Serum ferritin is another iron status biomarker that could distinguish iron deficient females who would benefit from iron supplementation. Murray-Kolb and Beard[30] conducted a randomized, placebo-controlled trial, and studied the effects of 160 mg ferrous sulfate daily for 16 weeks on iron status and cognitive function in a group of women (n = 113), aged 18 to 35 years. This study documented diminished performance on cognitive tests in women with poor iron status at the beginning of the study, when compared with women with normal iron stores at baseline. Longitudinal comparisons demonstrated that women with a significant increase in serum ferritin, following the treatment period, also exhibited improved scores on cognitive tests, when compared with those women with no change in serum ferritin, suggesting that improving iron stores could prove beneficial for maintaining or improving cognitive performance.[30] However, caution is warranted when using serum ferritin as a biomarker to determine iron status since other factors, such as inflammation, can confound this measure.

Although clear benefits of providing supplemental iron to the female athlete with iron deficiency are not always apparent, future research should investigate relationships between bio-markers of iron status and performance benefits with iron supplementation. It would be advantageous to define a profile to identify those female athletes with iron deficiency that could benefit from iron supplementation and to avoid iron supplementation for those who would most likely obtain no benefit. Adverse effects of iron supplementation have not been reported in many published trials, however, it should be noted that the intake of high doses of iron, often provided in supplements, can be associated with oxidant stress and free radical cellular damage.[31] Clearly, high doses of iron should be avoided in those with hemochromatosis or other iron overload disorders. Iron is not readily excreted by men and post-menopausal women, thereby increasing the chance for overload if excess iron is consumed.[32] Women of childbearing age with regular menses are less at risk, yet it is not uncommon for female athletes to suffer menstrual cycle disruptions. Iron supplements should be provided with caution in an effort to prevent negative outcomes associated with iron overload.

Fortification for the Prevention of Iron Deficiency and Iron Deficiency Anemia in Female Athletes

As compared with supplementation, fortification of foods with iron can provide a tolerable and more sustainable method of delivery to the female athlete. Many successful public health initiatives using food fortification efforts have improved micronutrient status, including iron status in various populations. For example, iron-fortified fish sauce significantly reduced iron deficiency and iron deficiency anemia among Vietnamese people, and in South Africa, the fortification of curry powder reduced iron deficiency anemia in women from 22 percent to five percent.[33] It is hypothesized that the prevalence of iron deficiency and iron deficiency anemia in the United States is lower than other nations in part because of the fortification of wheat flour with iron, which started in the 1940s.[34] Consistent with that observation, when Sweden stopped fortifying wheat flour with iron in 1994, there was a decline in iron intake, and consequently an increase in the prevalence of iron deficiency was observed.[21] These data suggest that fortification is an effective long-term approach for improving and maintaining optimal iron status in large populations. In addition, obtaining nutrients from food sources provides enjoyment for many people,[35] which can enhance compliance, compared with nutrient consumption from supplements. For example, compliance with consumption of iron-fortified food bars was more than 90 percent, compared with less than 60 percent for iron supplements in a group of female soldiers during basic combat training (J. P. McClung, unpublished data, 2010), suggesting a preference for the fortified food. Increasing iron intake could be required for the duration of a female athletic career because of dietary habits and repeated exposure to the physiologic stressors associated with exercise. As such, iron fortification of food products could be an effective solution to assure sustained adequate intake.

Recently, the provision of iron through an iron-fortified sports bar was studied in a randomized, placebo-controlled study. In the study,[36] female soldiers consumed the bar throughout basic combat training, and performance and biological outcomes were assessed. Bars were consumed twice daily and each contained 100 mg ferrous sulfate in an encapsulated form. Consumption of fortified bars improved iron status in females with iron deficiency anemia, significantly increasing hemoglobin concentration and mitigating the increase in soluble transferrin receptor observed in the placebo group.[36] Whereas females with iron deficiency anemia experienced improvements in iron status, declines in iron status were not prevented in women with normal iron status or iron deficiency when consuming the iron-fortified bar. Previous studies have demonstrated that consumption of 100 mg of ferrous sulfate daily in supplement form was able to attenuate declines in iron status during military training in females with normal iron status,[10] which could indicate that iron bioavailability might not have been optimal in the iron-fortified bars, especially as the amount of elemental iron provided in the bars was more than double that provided in supplement form in a similar study.[10,36] Although ferrous sulfate is less bioavailable in food products than in capsule form, this source of iron is more bioavailable when compared with other iron fortification compounds,[37] making ferrous sulfate the form of iron preferred for both supplement and fortification use. It is often used in iron supplements but poses difficulties when incorporating it into food items as it decreases the shelf life of foods and can create flavors and color changes undesirable to the consumer.[37] Food scientists should strive to determine methods for including highly bioavailable iron during fortification while maintaining the integrity of the food product.

Consuming a well-balanced diet to include enhancers of iron absorption (ie, meat, poultry, fish, and foods high in ascorbic acid) increases the bioavailability of iron and improves absorption of iron from fortified foods.[33] Lyle et al[38] found that consumption of four to six ounces of meat per day with other foods high in iron was more successful in protecting iron stores when compared with daily supplementation with two levels of ferrous sulfate coupled with a diet low in iron. In this study,[38] groups were composed of women participating in a 12-week exercise program with normal iron status, iron deficiency, and iron deficiency anemia. Hemoglobin concentration increased significantly after 12 weeks in the group consuming meat and high iron foods, but not in the iron supplemented groups, suggesting

the quality of iron ingested in foods was superior and better absorbed despite a lower quantity of total iron consumed.[38] A daily intake of four to six ounces of lean muscle foods (considered part of a healthy and balanced diet as stated by the food guide pyramid)[39] effectively maintained and even improved some indicators of iron status in females participating in moderate exercise in this study, demonstrating that iron balance can be achieved for those who are physically active through the consumption of highly bioavailable iron food sources.

Best Practices for Obtaining Recommended Iron Intakes

Athletes who are known to be at risk for iron deficiency and iron deficiency anemia should be educated regarding which foods they should consume for high iron bioavailability. These include lean meats, poultry, and fish. Although beans contain nonheme iron and phytate, an iron absorption inhibitor, they are a source of iron for vegetarians. Enhancers of iron absorption, such as tomatoes and citrus fruit, which contain high amounts of ascorbic acid, should be encouraged with these foods as part of a complete meal, whereas inhibitors, such as products high in phytate, should be limited and consumed at other times. Incorporation of iron-fortified foods, such as fortified cereal products, into a diet can be a safe and cost-effective method of increasing dietary iron intake. These foods can be of particular benefit for female athletes who abstain from eating meat. Although iron-fortified foods have been successful for the general population for improving iron status, further studies should aim to determine if this is a viable approach for reducing iron deficiency and iron deficiency anemia in female athletes.

Female athletes and military personnel with iron deficiency anemia have shown physical performance and cognitive decrements, both of which were ameliorated with the provision of iron supplements.[10,30] For female athletes with iron deficiency anemia, supplementation can swiftly replete hemoglobin concentration, normalize iron status biomarkers, improve Vo_{2max}, increase energy efficiency, and result in cognitive improvements.[10,30] However, the efficacy of long-term iron supplementation for maintaining adequate iron levels, throughout the duration of an athlete's career, has not been studied. Long-duration iron supplementation might not be the optimal approach for maintaining iron status as high doses of iron, such as those often found in supplements, can produce gastrointestinal distress and lead to iron overload.[31] Although supplement use in female athletes with iron deficiency has resulted in some reported benefits, the iron-deficient, nonanemic population requires further study as benefits have not been consistently reported. Iron status biomarkers such as soluble transferrin receptor and serum ferritin can help to define a profile of iron deficient female athletes who are most likely to demonstrate performance benefits with improved iron intake. Given demonstrated compliance with iron-fortified food products, these products can provide an effective and sustainable method of increasing iron intake for those at risk of iron deficiency and iron deficiency anemia, especially when consumed as a part of a healthy diet containing foods with bioavailable iron.

References

1. Davies KJ, Maguire JJ, Brooks GA, Dallman PR, Packer L. Muscle mitochondria bioenergetics, oxygen supply, and work capacity during dietary iron deficiency and repletion. *Am J Physiol.* 1982;242:E418–E427.

2. DeMaeyer E, Adiels-Tegman M. The prevalence of anemia in the world. *World Health Stat Q.* 1985;38:306–316.

3. Looker AC, Cogswell ME, Gunter MT. Iron deficiency—United States, 1999–2000. *MMWR Morb Mortal Wkly Rep.* 2002;51:897–899.

4. Yoshimura H. Anemia during physical training (sports anemia). *Nutr Rev.* 1970;28:251–253.

5. de Wijn JF, de Jongste JC, Mosterd W, Willebrand D. Hemoglobin, packed cell volume, serum iron, and iron binding capacity of selected athletes during training. *J Sports Med.* 1971;11:42–51.

6. Radomski MW, Sabiston BH, Isoard P. Development of "sports anemia" in physically fit men after daily sustained submaximal exercise. *Aviat Space Environ Med.* 1980;51:41–45.

7. Magazanik A, Weinstein Y, Dlin RA, Derin M, Schwartzman S, Allalouf D. Iron deficiency caused by 7 weeks of intensive physical exercise. *Eur J Appl Physiol Occup Physiol.* 1988;57:198–202.

8. McClung JP, Marchitelli LJ, Friedl KE, Young AJ. Prevalence of iron deficiency and iron deficiency anemia among three populations of female military personnel in the US Army. *J Am Coll Nutr.* 2006;25:64–69.

9. McClung JP, Karl JP, Cable SJ, Williams KW, Young AJ, Lieberman HR. Longitudinal decrements in iron status during military training in female soldiers. *Br J Nutr.* 2009;102:605–609.

10. McClung JP, Karl JP, Cable SJ, et al. Randomized, double-blind, placebo-controlled trial of iron supplementation in female soldiers during military training: effects on iron status, physical performance, and mood. *Am J Clin Nutr.* 2009;90:124–131.

11. Hinton PS, Sinclair LM. Iron supplementation maintains ventilatory threshold and improves energetic efficiency in iron-deficient nonanemic athletes. *Eur J Clin Nutr.* 2007;61:30–39.

12. Yip R, Dallman PR. Iron. In: Ziegler EE, Filer LJ, eds. *Present Knowledge in Nutrition.* 7th ed. Washington, DC: ILSI Press; 1996:277–292.

13. Robertson JD, Maughan RJ, Davidson RJL. Faecal blood loss in response to exercise. *BMJ.* 1987;295:303–305.

14. Brune M, Magnussun B, Persson H, Hallberg L. Iron losses in sweat. *Am J Clin Nutr.* 1986;43:438–443.

15. Harvey LJ, Armah CN, Dainty JR, et al. Impact of menstrual blood loss and diet on iron deficiency among women in the UK. *BrJNutr.* 2005;94:557–564.

16. Ganz T, Nemeth E. Iron imports. IV. Hepcidin and regulation of body iron metabolism. *Am J Physiol Gastrointest Liver Physiol.* 2006;290:G199–G203.

17. Peeling P, Dawson B, Goodman C, et al. Training surface and intensity: inflammation, hemolysis, and hepcidin expression. *Med Sci Sports Exerc.* 2009;41:1138–1145.

18. Peeling P, Dawson B, Goodman C, et al. Cumulative effects of consecutive running sessions on hemolysis, inflammation and hepcidin activity. *Eur J Appl Physiol.* 2009;106:51–59.

19. Peeling P, Dawson B, Goodman C, et al. Effects of exercise on hepcidin response and iron metabolism during recovery. *Int J Sport Nutr Exerc Metab.* 2009;19:583–587.

20. Institute of Medicine. Iron In: *Dietary Reference Intakes.* Washington, DC: National Academies Press; 2001:290–393.

21. Zimmermann M, Hurrell R. Nutritional iron deficiency. *Lancet.* 2007;370:511–520.

22. Hallberg L, Rossander L, Brune M. Prevention of iron deficiency by diet. In: SJ Fomon, S Zlotkin, eds. *Nutritional Anemias.* New York, NY: Raven Press; 1992:169–181.

23. Hurrell R, Egli I. Iron bioavailability and dietary reference values. *Am J Clin Nutr.* 2010;91(suppl):S1461–S1467.

24. Mello RP, Murphy MM, Vogel JA. Relationship between a two mile run for time and maximal oxygen uptake. *J Appl Sport Sci Res.* 1988;2:9–12.

25. Cook JD, Skikne BS, Baynes RD. Screening strategies for nutritional iron deficiency. In: Fomon SJ, Zlotkin S, eds. *Nutritional Anemias.* New York, NY: Raven Press; 1992:159–168.

26. Gardner GW, Edgerton VR, Senewiratne B, Barnard RJ, Ohira Y. Physical work capacity and metabolic stress in subjects with iron deficiency anemia. *Am J Clin Nutr.* 1977;30:910–917.

27. LaManca JJ, Haymes EM. Effects of iron repletion on Vo2max, endurance, and blood lactate in women. *Med Sci Sports Exerc.* 1993;25:1386–1392.

28. Brownlie T IV, Utermohlen V, Hinton PS, Giordano C, Haas JD. Marginal iron deficiency without anemia impairs aerobic adaptation among previously untrained women. *Am J Clin Nutr.* 2002; 75:734–742.

29. Brownlie T IV, Utermohlen V, Hinton PS, Haas JD. Tissue iron deficiency without anemia impairs adaptation in endurance capacity after aerobic training in previously untrained women. *Am J Clin Nutr.* 2004;79:437–443.

30. Murray-Kolb LE, Beard JL. Iron treatment normalizes cognitive functioning in young women. *Am J Clin Nutr.* 2007;85:778–787.

31. Beard J, Tobin B. Iron status and exercise. *Am J Clin Nutr.* 2000; 72(suppl):S594–S597.

32. Muñoz M, Villar I, García-Erce JA. An update on iron physiology. *World J Gastroenterol.* 2009;15:4617–4626.

33. Allen L, de Benoist B, Dary O, Hurrell R, eds. *Guidelines on Food Fortification With Micronutrients.* Geneva, Switzerland: World Health Organization, Food and Agriculture Organization; 2006.

34. Hertrampf E. Iron fortification in the Americas. *Nutr Rev.* 2002; 60(7 pt 2):S22–S25.

35. Neary MT, Batterham RL. Gaining insights into food reward with functional neuroimaging. *Forum Nutr.* 2009;63: 152–163.

36. Karl JP, Lieberman HR, Cable SJ, Williams KW, Young AJ, McClung JP. Randomized, double-blind, placebo-controlled trial of an iron-fortified food product in female soldiers during military training: relations between iron status, serum hepcidin, and inflammation. *Am J Clin Nutr.* 2010;92:93–100.

37. Zimmermann MB, Winichagoon P, Gowachirapant S, et al. Comparison of the efficacy of wheat-based snacks fortified with ferrous sulfate, electrolytic iron, or hydrogen-reduced elemental iron: randomized, double-blind, controlled trial in Thai women. *Am J Clin Nutr.* 2005;82:1276–1282.

38. Lyle RM, Weaver CM, Sedlock DA, Rajaram S, Martin B, Melby CL. et al. Iron status in exercising women: the effect of oral iron therapy vs. increased consumption of muscle foods. *Am J Clin Nutr.* 1992;56:1049–1055.

39. United States Department of Agriculture. Food guide pyramid. www.mypyramid.gov. Accessed December 2, 2010.

Critical Thinking

1. Explain why female athletes are at higher risk of developing iron deficiency.

2. Discuss the efficacy of iron supplementation and fortification of food to improve iron status in iron-deficient female athletes and military personnel.

3. Describe the action of inflammation on iron status.

JAMES P. McCLUNG, United States Army Research Institute of Environmental Medicine (USARIEM), Kansas Street, Building 42, Natick, MA 01760, USA Email: james.mcclung@amedd.army.mil

Acknowledgments—The authors acknowledge Holly L. McClung for her editorial review of this article.

Authors' Note—The opinions or assertions contained herein are the private views of the authors and are not to be construed as official or as reflecting the views of the United States Army or the Department of Defense. Any citations of commercial organizations and trade names in this report do not constitute an official Department of the Army endorsement of approval of the products or services of these organizations.

Author Contributions—Laura J. Bass and James P. McClung contributed to the conception and design of this article.

Declaration of Conflicting Interests—The authors declared no potential conflicts of interests with respect to the authorship and/or publication of this article.

Funding—The authors disclosed receipt of the following financial support for the research and/or authorship of this article: Financial support for the production of this manuscript was provided by the United States Army Medical Research and Materiel Command (USAMRMC).

UNIT 4
Diet and Disease

Unit Selections

Learning Outcomes
After reading this unit, you will be able to:

- Discuss why it is more challenging for older adults to lose or maintain their body weight.

- Compare and contrast the physiological actions of glucose vs. fructose in the body.

- Illustrate the link between the consumption of high-fructose corn sweeteners and increased risk for heart disease, metabolic syndrome, type 2 diabetes, gout, and accumulation of visceral fat.

- Differentiate between type 1 and type 2 diabetes.

- Identify nutrients needed to maintain a strong immune system.

- Explain the physiology of the mental decline that occurs in Alzheimer's disease.

- List the foods and lifestyle behaviors that may slow the progression of dementia.

- Summarize the physiology of heartburn and identify the foods and lifestyle behaviors that increase the risk of heartburn.

- Define non-alcoholic steatohepatitis.

- Summarize the relationship of type 2 diabetes, obesity, insulin resistance, and fatty liver disease.

Student Website
www.mhhe.com/cls

Internet References
American Cancer Society
www.cancer.org
American Diabetes Association
www.diabetes.org
American Heart Association (AHA)
www.americanheart.org
Medline Plus
www.nlm.nih.gov/medlineplus
National Eating Disorders Association
www.nationaleatingdisorders.org

Research that focuses on the connection between diet and disease has unraveled the role of many nutrients in the delay of onset of certain diseases, prevention of diseases, and in some instances disease reversal. The challenging aspect of releasing results from nutrition research is communicating this information in a manner that is not controversial or contradictory to previously released messages. With the increasing interest in health and disease prevention among Americans, media outlets publish scientific findings prematurely and without the physiological context in which the message should be conveyed. Scientific research takes time to answer the questions about health, nutrition, disease, and medicine, whereas consumers want answers to these questions much quicker than scientifically possible.

Medical and nutrition research has changed since the mapping of the human genome. We have come to better understand the role of genetics in the expression of disease and its role in how we respond to dietary change. In addition, research about diet and disease has enabled us to understand the importance and uniqueness of the individual (age, gender, ethnicity, and genetics) and his or her particular response to dietary interventions. Individualizing one's diet to prevent disease and promote health is a concept that we will see developing in the future.

The prevalence of diet and lifestyle related diseases in the United States is astronomical. Heart disease, type 2 diabetes, obesity, stroke, high blood pressure, osteoporosis, and certain cancers are diet- and lifestyle-related conditions that affect millions of Americans. Proper nutrition plays a vital role in these diseases. Components of foods such as saturated fats, trans fats, sodium, and added sugars continue to be highlighted as the premier culprits of these diseases.

A recent area of nutrition research focus is the degree of added sugars that are consumed by Americans. The average American consumes 350 to 475 grams of added sugars each day. The most commonly consumed form of added sugars is high-fructose corn syrup, but other forms of sugar such as table sugar, honey, and cane juice are considered to be "added sugar" too. As more research explores the negative effects of high-fructose corn syrup on human health, food companies are developing products using other forms of sugar. These "natural sugars" still provide empty calories in the diet that may lead to weight gain if consumed in excess and not balanced by physical activity. Discretionary calories (calories consumed after nutrient needs are met from healthy food and beverage sources) are an effective way to think about the calories that are consumed in relation to the calories needed to provide adequate nutrient intakes. The USDA recommends discretionary calories of approximately 100 calories for women and 150 calories for men. Individual recommendations for discretionary calorie allowances can be calculated using myplate.gov.

High-fructose sweeteners have been linked to greater risk for heart disease, metabolic syndrome, type 2 diabetes, gout, and accumulation of visceral fat. The link may be caused by increased triglycerides and uric acid in the bloodstream secondary to the way fructose is metabolized.

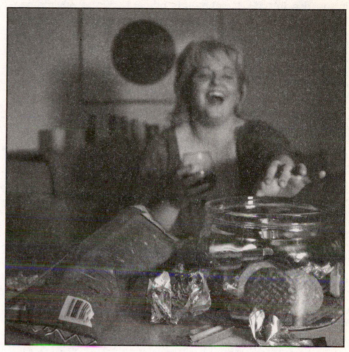

© BananaStock/PunchStock

Research supports the link between consumption of sugar-sweetened beverages and risk of type 2 diabetes, heart disease, hypertension, hypertriglyceridemia, gout, and weight gain. Added fructose has been tied to increased levels of triglycerides in the blood, decreased fat oxidation, increased LDL cholesterol, increased uric acid in the blood, and an increase in visceral fat. Epidemiological data supports a relationship between fructose sweeteners and heart attacks. Liquid calories from sugar-sweetened beverages are not only empty calories, but also promote increased calorie intake at meals, possibly through suppression of leptin, a hormone that triggers you to stop eating.

The number one concern of the health of the United States is the prevalence of overweight and obesity. Although much of the attention is centered on childhood obesity and tactics to prevent or curtail it, there is also an ongoing problem with overweight or obesity as our population ages. On average, Americans in their sixties are 10 pounds heavier than they were just a decade ago. A typical woman in her 40s weighs 168 pounds, compared to 143 pounds in the 1960s. People used to start midlife at a lower weight and lose weight when they reached their 50s. Humans need fewer calories as they age because of slower metabolism and the tendency to lose muscle mass and gain fat, especially abdominal fat. Since muscle burns more calories than fat, it is challenging to lose weight in older years and maintain weight while eating the usual intake. Staying lean and eating right can delay onset or prevent certain diseases that plague older Americans, such as osteoporosis, heart disease, hypertension, insulin resistance, memory loss, arthritis, and some cancers.

Approximately 25 million people in the United States have type 2 diabetes and 1 million have type 1 diabetes. The incidence of type 1 diabetes has been increasing at rates of 3–5 percent per year. The reason for the increase in incidence of type 1 diabetes is unclear. The Division of Diabetes Translation at the Centers for Disease Control speculates that the etiology in the rise in type 1 diabetes is primarily due to environmental factors. The article by Maryn McKenna reviews competing hypotheses that attempt to explain the rise in type 1 diabetes: the hygiene hypothesis and overload hypothesis.

The immune system is commonly taken for granted; however, it is a fascinating system of defense that is essential to our existence and optimal health. Proper nutrition and balanced nutrient intake is required for our immune system to function optimally. The article by Susan Percival describes the complex immune response and how nutrient deficiencies impair our immune system.

The articles in Unit 4 will be useful as a supplement to diet and chronic disease sections of general nutrition courses. The article topics add a slightly different view of the commonly known diet-related diseases and other diseases that are not publicized as often.

We Will Be What We Eat

When it comes to staving off the problems of aging, from bone and muscle loss to high blood pressure and heart disease, your diet is your friend—or enemy.

MERYL DAVIDS LANDAU

If your mental image of an older person is someone frail and thin, it may be time for an update. For the generation currently moving through middle age and beyond, a new concern is, well, growing: obesity. "We're already seeing a large number of obese elderly, and if we don't do something, that figure is sure to rise," laments David Kessler, former commissioner of the Food and Drug Administration and author of *The End of Overeating*. Government figures show that Americans in their 60s today are about 10 pounds heavier than their counterparts of just a decade ago. And an even more worrisome bulge is coming: A typical woman in her 40s now weighs 168 pounds, versus 143 pounds in the 1960s. "People used to start midlife [at a lower weight] and then lose weight when they got into their 50s, but that doesn't happen as much anymore," Kessler says.

People used to start midlife at a lower weight than they do now and then lose weight in their 50s, but not anymore.

If you're entering that danger zone now, be aware that it's not going to get any easier to lose weight, because people need fewer calories as they age. Blame slowing metabolism and the body's tendency starting in midlife to lose muscle mass—a process known as sarcopenia—and gain fat, especially around the abdomen. (Fat burns fewer calories than does muscle.) "All that conspires to make it harder for people to maintain the same body weight when they eat their usual diets," says Alice Lichtenstein, director of the Cardiovascular Nutrition Laboratory at Tufts University. "People have fewer discretionary calories to play with, so they need to make better food choices."

Why do those choices matter? First, carrying an extra 20 or 30 pounds with you into old age doesn't bode well for attempts to head off the myriad diseases that strike in midlife and later and are linked to weight—including diabetes, arthritis, heart disease, and some forms of cancer. (It's probably not a coincidence that one recent study finds that people in their 60s have more disabilities than in years past.)

But paying attention to what you eat isn't only about controlling weight; the need for certain vitamins and minerals increases with age. One is calcium, necessary to protect bones. Another is B_{12}, since some older adults make less of the stomach acid required to absorb the vitamin. More vitamin D also is required. "The skin gets less efficient at converting sunlight into this vitamin, so more is needed from other sources," Lichtenstein says. Fewer than 7 percent of Americans between 50 and 70 get enough vitamin D from the foods they eat, and fewer than 26 percent get enough calcium.

Staying lean and eating right are both crucial for maintaining health through the years. (Kessler recalls a fellow researcher at Yale who, upon realizing the panoply of diseases linked to body weight, promptly lost 30 pounds.) If weight is a problem, it is especially important to cut back on the processed foods that combine sugar and fat. Studies with rats indicate that when the two are added to chow, animals can't easily stop eating, says Kessler. This happens in humans, too, he says, and food manufacturers have taken note and added sugar and fat to many products.

So what should people eat? A healthful diet at midlife is the same as for younger adults—it's just that the stakes may be higher. The focus should be on fruit, vegetables, whole grains, low- and nonfat dairy, legumes, lean meats, and fish. For someone whose current diet is far from this ideal, Lichtenstein suggests starting small: Swap dark-green lettuce for iceberg, load more veggies on the dinner plate, eat more skinless chicken or beans in place of hamburger. And exercise. Walking briskly for at least 30 minutes every day makes it easier to get away with the occasional cookie. With some further fine-tuning of that basic healthful eating plan, you can greatly improve your odds of staving off the major barriers to a vital old age.

Bone Loss

No nutrient can stop bones from losing mass over time, but consuming sufficient calcium and vitamin D can slow the deterioration, says Felicia Cosman, an osteoporosis specialist at Helen Hayes Hospital in West Haverstraw, N.Y., and clinical director of the National Osteoporosis Foundation. Once a person reaches age 50, calcium requirements jump from 1,000 mg to 1,200 mg per day. Cosman recommends adding up the number of servings consumed in a typical day of dairy products and foods that are highly calcium-fortified, such as orange juice and cereal, and multiplying that by the 300 mg each most likely supplies. Add 200 to 300 mg for the combined trace amounts in leafy green vegetables, nuts, and other sources. Then get the remainder in a supplement. By midlife, adults also need at least 800 to 1,000 IU of vitamin D to help the body absorb calcium and, possibly, prevent other diseases, according to the NOF. Sources include fatty fish such as salmon (also important for heart health), egg yolks, and fortified foods, but most people need to supplement.

Heart Disease

By now, every American surely knows the roll call of foods that affect your heart, for better and for worse. Good for the ticker: monounsaturated fats like olive oil and the omega-3 fatty acids found in such cold-water fish as salmon and herring and in flaxseed and walnuts. Harmful: too much red meat and full-fat dairy, because of their saturated fat content, and margarine and baked goods, because of the trans fats they contain.

But expunging troublesome foods from your daily fare can be surprisingly difficult. "Although many supermarket products have removed the trans fats, they're hardly history. Restaurants, especially, continue to use them," cautions Robert Eckel, former president of the American Heart Association and a professor at the University of Colorado-Denver. Some food manufacturers, moreover, have simply swapped out their trans fats for saturated fat, which is equally problematic, Eckel says. Saturated fat should total no more than 7 percent of daily energy intake—about 16 grams for the average 2,000-calorie diet.

Recent research points to another potential heart danger. It's not fat; it's high-fructose corn syrup, commonly found in soda. The decades-long, 88,000-woman Nurses' Health Study found that, even controlling for weight and other unhealthful habits, drinking one 12-ounce can of regular soda daily boosts a woman's risk of later having a heart attack by 24 percent; two or more servings raise the risk by 35 percent. "We don't know exactly why this is, but fructose does increase uric acid and triglycerides in the blood, which are known contributors to hypertension and heart disease," says study coauthor Teresa Fung, associate professor of nutrition at Simmons College in Boston.

Hypertension

Lowering high blood pressure before it contributes to the development of heart disease is vital for people in midlife. It can be accomplished with an eating plan known as the DASH (Dietary Approaches to Stop Hypertension) diet. "The DASH diet has the same effect as taking a blood-pressure-lowering medication," Eckel says. The DASH-Sodium version, which subtracts salt, works as well as up to two medications. The plan is rich in fruits and vegetables (eight to 10 servings a day for someone on a 2,000-calorie diet), grains (six to eight servings daily, with most being whole grains), and low-fat protein sources. And it's low in saturated fats and added sugars. The biggest difference from standard healthful eating advice is DASH's focus on lowering

sodium, which can damage artery walls in people sensitive to the nutrient. The diet limits sodium to 2,300 mg a day, while DASH-Sodium slashes it to 1,500 mg—just two thirds of a teaspoon. It's not enough to go easier on the salt shaker; the National Institutes of Health recommends looking for low- or no-salt labels, limiting high-sodium foods like bacon and sauerkraut, and rinsing canned foods. (A one-day sample menu of a DASH eating plan is available on the *U.S. News* website at www.usnews.com/dash.)

Insulin Resistance

Research has repeatedly demonstrated that type 2 diabetes and insulin resistance (a precursor to the disease in which the body begins to respond less well to the hormone that clears glucose from the blood stream) can often be prevented or postponed with a healthful diet, exercise, and weight loss. That three-part combination, in fact, actually has been shown to be more effective than medication. An eating plan aimed at minimizing the risk of insulin resistance does not have to be complex. "I coach people to mentally divide their lunch and dinner plate into thirds, with one third protein, one third nonstarchy vegetables, and the final third a starch like brown rice, whole-wheat pasta, potatoes, or corn," says Nora Saul, a dietitian and diabetes educator at Harvard's Joslin Diabetes Center in Boston. It's also a good idea to get serious about cutting back on sugar and white flour, both of which have a high glycemic index and can spike blood glucose levels.

Memory Problems

Alas, there's no magic bullet that will guarantee protection from dementia. But researchers are finding that a Mediterranean diet—similar to a conventional healthful diet but with an emphasis on fish and olive oil—seems to lower the odds of developing cognitive problems. Scientists at Columbia University followed more than 1,300 people for up to 16 years; those most closely adhering to this diet developed Alzheimer's at half the rate of those who didn't. One caveat: Alcohol (particularly in the form of wine), one element of the Mediterranean Diet that has been suggested to enhance memory function, has not been proved to do so, says Gary Kennedy, director of geriatric psychiatry at Montefiore Medical Center in New York.

Joint Disease

Although age is a risk factor for arthritis, the breakdown of cartilage in the joints is not inevitable. Minimizing weight gain goes a long way toward avoiding this problem, because every extra pound translates to 3 pounds of pressure on the knees while walking. It is also a good idea to limit foods that encourage inflammation in the body, particularly omega-6 fatty acids (found in corn and soybean oils and many snack and fried foods), the Arthritis Foundation says.

Cancer

Some 45 percent of colon cancers, 38 percent of breast cancers, and 69 percent of esophageal cancers would never occur if Americans ate better, weighed less, and exercised more, estimates the American Institute for Cancer Research. "It's not just cancers of the digestive tract. What you eat and what you weigh affect certain other cancer types as well," says Alice Bender, AICR's nutrition communications manager. The organization recommends limiting red meat to 18 (cooked) ounces per week and loading up on plant-based foods, which are high in the phytochemicals and antioxidants known to inhibit cancer cell growth in lab animals. Those with the deepest colors—like purple grapes, blueberries, and leafy green vegetables—tend to have the most beneficial compounds. One recent study, for example, showed that eating foods such as broccoli and kale that have lots of sulforaphane, an antioxidant, suppresses a bacterium linked to stomach cancer.

It looks as if food is the best source of healthful nutrients. "Numerous studies on supplements—of vitamin C, lycopene, beta carotene, and even fiber—have all proved disappointing," Bender says. Yet another reason to swap that cookie for a carrot.

Critical Thinking

1. Why is it more difficult for people over the age of 50 to lose or maintain their weight?

2. Which nutrients are needed in higher quantities by older adults?

3. What is the DASH diet? How many servings of fruits and vegetables and how much sodium is recommended per day on the DASH diet?

Article 25

Sugar Overload
Curbing America's Sweet Tooth

What led the American Heart Association to issue its new scientific statement on "Dietary Sugars Intake and Cardiovascular Health"?

The association cited the "worldwide pandemic of obesity and cardiovascular disease" in explaining its "heightened concerns about the adverse effects of excessive consumption of sugars."[1]

"Added sugars have become such a predominant feature of the American diet that we can't help but recognize their major contribution to excess calories," explains Van Horn. The average American swallows 350 to 475 calories' worth of added sugars each day (depending on the type of data used to estimate intakes).

Exactly what *are* added sugars? They include high-fructose corn syrup, ordinary table sugar, honey, agave syrup, and all other sweeteners with calories. (In this article, the word "sugars" refers to them all.)

To hear some critics talk, high-fructose corn syrup is the real villain. Table sugar gets a free pass. (See "Fear of Fructose".)

In fact, high-fructose corn syrup is roughly half fructose and half glucose, as is table sugar (sucrose) once it breaks down in the body. And although the fructose half may cause some problems, the glucose half causes others. So if there's a villain, it's *all* sugars.

"Added sugars are added sugars," says Rachel Johnson, a professor of nutrition at the University of Vermont who chaired the heart association panel that issued the new sugars advice.

Who can afford the roughly 400 calories' worth of added sugars that the typical American consumes each day?

"No adults, except those who are extremely physically active—we're talking about the Michael Phelpses of the world," says Linda Van Horn, a professor of preventive medicine at the Northwestern University Feinberg School of Medicine in Chicago. "The rest of us have no business consuming that many calories from sugars."

There's new evidence that added sugars—or sugar-sweetened beverages—may raise the risk of obesity, heart disease, diabetes, and gout.

What's wrong with sugars? For starters, they're not good for your teeth, especially if they come in sticky foods. Here are 10 reasons to cut back.

1. **You can't afford the empty calories.** The American Heart Association based its advice on what scientists call "discretionary calories"—that is, how much room you have for empty calories once you've eaten all the

vegetables, fruit, lean protein, low-fat dairy, whole grains, and other foods you need to stay healthy. (It's like discretionary income that people can spend on luxuries once they've paid their bills.)

"There's no question that sugars are a major culprit in obesity, because they're a source of empty calories that most Americans don't need," says Van Horn. "They have no nutritional benefit whatsoever."

The fact is that most people simply can't afford a 500-calorie scone or a 600-calorie Venti White Chocolate Mocha when they stop at Starbucks.

"Added sugars either crowd out healthy foods, or they make you fat if you eat them in addition to healthy foods," explains Frank Sacks, a professor of cardiovascular disease prevention at the Harvard School of Public Health in Boston.

So the heart association turned to the discretionary calorie allowances calculated by the U.S. Department of Agriculture. (To find yours, go to mypyramid.gov.)

A typical woman, who should shoot for 1,800 calories a day, for example, would need about 1,600 calories a day from vegetables, fruits, lean protein, dairy foods, and whole grains to get the nutrients she needs.

That leaves about 200 calories to spend (like discretionary income) on whatever she wants. "We said, okay, half of that discretionary calorie allowance can come from solid fats and half can come from added sugars," explains Johnson. That's about 100 calories each.

A typical man should shoot for 2,200 calories a day. He gets about 150 calories to spend on each.

"Solid fats" include not just butter or margarine, but the extra fat you get if you choose dairy foods (milk, cheese, yogurt, ice cream) that aren't fat-free, poultry with skin, and cakes, cookies, pies, and other sweets that aren't fat-free. So unless you eat mostly fat-free foods, your 100-calorie solid-fat allowance is going to disappear quickly.

Sucrose

Sucrose (table sugar) is broken down—in the body and (to some extent) in foods—to half fructose and half glucose. At that point it is essentially identical to high-fructose corn syrup.

Sugar by Any Other Name

Here's the scoop on some popular sugars. Sucrose (table sugar) breaks down into 50% fructose, 50% glucose in the body.

Agave syrup or nectar *(84% fructose, 8% glucose, 8% sucrose).* From the Mexican Agave cactus.

Apple juice concentrate *(60% fructose, 27% glucose, 13% sucrose).* Made by cooking down apple juice.

Brown sugar *(97% sucrose, 1% fructose, 1% glucose).* Granulated white sugar mixed with a small amount of molasses.

Corn syrup *(8% to 96% glucose, 0% fructose, 0% sucrose).* A liquid made from cornstarch.

Evaporated cane juice *(100% sucrose).* Crystals made by evaporating liquid that has been pressed from sugarcane.

Fructose *(100% fructose).* Found naturally in fruits and vegetables. We get most of our fructose from high-fructose corn syrup.

Glucose or Dextrose *(100% glucose).* Small amounts are found naturally in fruit and vegetables, but most is made from cornstarch. It's also found in honey and most other sugars.

Grape juice concentrate *(52% fructose, 48% glucose).* Made by cooking down grape juice.

High-fructose corn syrup (HFCS) *(typically 55% fructose, 45% glucose or 58% glucose, 42% fructose).* Corn syrup with some of its glucose converted into fructose.

Honey *(50% fructose, 44% glucose, 1% sucrose).* Made by honeybees from plant nectar.

Maple syrup *(95% sucrose, 4% glucose, 1% fructose).* Boiled down tree sap from the sugar maple tree.

Molasses *(53% sucrose, 23% fructose, 21% glucose).* By-product of sugarcane refining. Blackstrap molasses is a good source of iron and calcium.

Orange juice concentrate *(46% sucrose, 28% fructose, 26% glucose).* Made by cooking down orange juice.

Raw sugar *(100% sucrose).* Partially refined sugar with some molasses left.

Table sugar, Confectioner's sugar, Baker's sugar, Powdered sugar *(100% sucrose).* Most is refined from sugarcane or beets.

Note: If percentages don't add up to 100, other sugars account for the difference.

Sources: USDA Nutrient Database and company information.

And guess what happens to your added sugars allowance if you want a glass of wine or beer.

"It's been shocking to some people when I've said that we've been fairly conservative, because if you're consuming alcohol regularly, you should be having even less added sugar," notes Johnson.

If you want more sugar, you can always burn more calories.

"What I tell people who can't live with the added-sugars recommendation is that they need to move more," says Johnson. "Then you can have more sugar."

2. **Sugar-sweetened beverages promote obesity.** We're eating 20 percent more added sugars now than we did in 1970. What's largely responsible for the leap in sugars intake?

"Soft drinks, soft drinks, soft drinks," says Johnson. In 1965, Americans got an average of 12 percent of their calories from beverages. In 2001, beverages accounted for 21 percent.[1]

"Soft drinks are the number-one source of added sugars in Americans' diets," says Johnson. And sugary liquids may make us fatter because they don't curb our appetite for more food.[2]

"When you give people liquid calories before a meal, they don't compensate by eating less at the meal or later, in the same way they do for calories from solid food," notes Johnson.

In a classic study at Purdue University, researchers gave 15 young adults 450 calories of sugars each day as either a liquid (a soft drink) or a solid (jelly beans).[3] After one month on the jelly beans, the volunteers compensated by eating less of other foods, so they gained no weight. But on the soft drinks, they actually ate slightly *more* food than before. That plus the calories in the soft drinks led them to gain weight.

Where's the Added Sugar?

Coke. Pepsi. Sprite. Regular sodas add the most sugar to a typical American's diet. But don't forget about coffee drinks, teas, sports drinks, and fruit drinks that have a health halo.

And in a recent trial that lasted 1½ years, people who cut back on liquid calories lost more weight than those who cut the same number of solid calories.[4]

"I keep telling people, 'If you're trying to cut back on added sugars, look at what you're drinking,'" says Johnson.

What's more, in a study of 51,000 women, those who went from drinking regular soda no more than once a week to at least once a day gained the most weight over four years.[5]

It's not just soda pop.

"If you look at consumption data, soft drinks are leveling off, but other sugar-sweetened beverages—sports drinks, energy drinks, sweetened teas—are taking off," Johnson notes.

"Just walk down the supermarket aisles. An entire one is filled with soft drinks and another is filled with other sugar-sweetened beverages that have a health halo."

3. **Sugar-sweetened drinks may raise the risk of heart disease.** "Sugars have for many years been considered neutral in their impact on cardiovascular disease," says Northwestern University's Linda Van Horn. "But in an obese environment like ours, we can't turn a blind eye to added sugars that contribute to excess calorie intake."

Fear of Fructose

"Made with no high-fructose corn syrup," brags the label of Thomas' Original English Muffins and dozens of other foods. What's wrong with high-fructose corn syrup (HFCS)?

Here's what the popular website run by Dr. Joseph Mercola (mercola.com) claims: "Part of what makes HFCS such an unhealthy product is that it is metabolized to fat in your body far more rapidly than any other sugar, and, because most fructose is consumed in liquid form (soda), its negative metabolic effects are significantly magnified."

"Among them: diabetes, obesity, metabolic syndrome, an increase in triglycerides and LDL (bad) cholesterol levels, liver disease."

There's some truth to some of those claims, but Mercola makes a common mistake: he seems to confuse high-fructose corn syrup with fructose, as though high-fructose corn syrup were mostly fructose. It's not.

"High-fructose corn syrup is typically 55 percent fructose, explains Kimber Stanhope, who conducts research on sugars at the University of California, Davis." "But sucrose, or table sugar, is 50 percent fructose."

Glucose makes up the rest of both HFCS and sucrose. So it's not surprising that researchers find few differences—in blood sugar, insulin, ghrelin (which stimulates appetite), or leptin (which curbs appetite)—when they pit high-fructose corn syrup against table sugar.[1]

"We still have no comparative data showing that HFCS or sucrose is better or worse than the other," says Stanhope.

What's the harm in minimizing high-fructose corn syrup? Nothing. "But people become so conscious of avoiding high-fructose corn syrup that they forget about avoiding other sweeteners," says University of Vermont researcher Rachel Johnson.

"I ate a granola bar the other day that listed brown rice syrup on the ingredient list. Doesn't that sound healthy? It's just a sweetener. Added sugars all add empty calories."

[1]*Am. J. Clin. Nutr. 87*: 1194, 2008.

Clearly, excess weight isn't good for the heart. A big belly is one part of the metabolic syndrome, which raises the risk of heart disease (and diabetes). But sugar-sweetened beverages may promote heart disease whether or not they make you gain weight.

When Harvard researchers tracked more than 88,000 women for 24 years, they found that—regardless of weight—those who drank at least two sugar-sweetened beverages a day had a 20 percent higher risk of heart disease than those who drank less than one sugar-sweetened beverage a month.[6]

"Our data suggest that soft drinks increase the risk above and beyond their impact on weight," notes study coauthor JoAnn Manson, a professor of medicine at Harvard Medical School.

And when scientists tracked 4,000 men and women in the Framingham Heart Study for four years, those who drank at least one soft drink a day had a 44 percent higher risk of being diagnosed with the metabolic syndrome than those who drank less than one soft drink a day, regardless of how much they weighed.[7]

Why else would sugar-sweetened drinks raise the risk of heart attacks? One possibility: the fructose in added sugars (like high-fructose corn syrup and table sugar) raises levels of fats called triglycerides. Higher-than-normal triglycerides are another sign of the metabolic syndrome.

4. **Fructose raises triglycerides.** Cholesterol isn't the only thing in blood that's linked to heart attacks. People with higher-than-normal triglycerides (at least 150) are also at risk, especially if their triglycerides soar after a meal.[8]
   And fructose raises triglycerides after meals.

For example, researchers at the University of Minnesota fed 24 men and women a diet that got 17 percent of its calories from either glucose or fructose.[9]

(That's a high dose, since Americans average 16 percent of their calories from added sugars, roughly half of it from fructose and half of it from glucose.)

After six weeks, triglyceride levels throughout the day were 32 percent higher when the men (but not the women) ate the high-fructose diet.

Peter Havel and colleagues at the University of California, Davis, got similar results when they studied 32 over-weight or obese men and women over 40. Participants got a hefty 25 percent of their calories from beverages sweetened with either fructose or glucose for 10 weeks.[10]

Once again, blood levels of triglycerides after a meal were higher on fructose than on glucose. "It's a strong and consistent effect," says researcher Kimber Stanhope, who works with Havel.

Triglycerides rose more in men, but they also rose in women, notes Stanhope, "possibly because the women in our study were older and heavier" than those in the earlier study.

Why would people on a high-fructose diet have higher triglycerides than people on a high-glucose diet?

When you consume a large dose of glucose, the liver doesn't pull much of it in if you don't need the calories. In contrast, fructose ends up in the liver whether you need the calories or not.

"The liver will take up nearly the entire amount of fructose," says Stanhope. "Very little of the fructose stays in the bloodstream."

What does the liver do with all that fructose? "It starts converting some of the fructose into fat," Stanhope explains. "Much of this fat gets sent into the bloodstream, resulting in higher levels of triglycerides."

That would explain why large doses of fructose boost triglyceride levels in the bloodstream and possibly in the liver. Would smaller doses do the same?

"We're testing lower doses right now," says Stanhope. "We're studying over 200 younger people, so it will take a while."

5. **Sugar-sweetened beverages may promote diabetes.**
   When researchers tracked roughly 91,000 women for eight years, those who drank at least one sugar-sweetened soft drink a day had an 83 percent higher risk of type 2 diabetes than those who drank less than one a month.[5]

When the scientists took weight out of the equation, soda drinkers had a 40 percent higher risk.

Tout de Sweet

A typical woman should get no more than 100 calories (about 6½ teaspoons) a day from added sugars, says the American Heart Association. A typical man should get no more than 150 calories (about 9½ teaspoons)—roughly what's in a 12 oz. can of Coke.

Here's how much added sugars you'd get in a sampling of popular foods. (The numbers don't include the naturally occurring sugars in fruit or milk.) To convert teaspoons to grams of sugar, multiply by 4. To convert teaspoons to calories from sugar, multiply by 16.

Food	Added Sugars (teaspoons)
Dairy	
Ice cream, vanilla (½ cup)	3
Chocolate milk, reduced fat 2% (8 fl. oz.)	3½
Yogurt, low-fat vanilla (6 oz.)	3½
Yogurt, low-fat fruit (6 oz.)	4½
Silk Chocolate Soymilk (8 fl. oz.)	5
TCBY Old Fashioned Vanilla Frozen Yogurt (regular cup, 8.7 oz.)	6*
Baskin-Robbins Vanilla Ice Cream Cone (double scoop, 8.4 oz.)	11½*
Chocolate shake, fast food (16 fl. oz.)	13
Dairy Queen Heath Blizzard (medium, 14.5 oz.)	26*
Baskin-Robbins Oreo Outrageous Sundae (12.6 oz.)	27*
Coldstone Creamery Founders Favorite (Gotta Have It, 14.6 oz.)	30½*
Beverages	
Propel Lemon (24 fl. oz.)	1½
Starbucks Caffè Mocha (grande, 16 fl. oz.)	3*
Starbucks Caramel Macchiato (grande, 16 fl. oz.)	4*
Starbucks Vanilla Latte (grande, 16 fl. oz.)	4*
Hawaiian Punch Fruit Juicy Red (8 fl. oz.)	4½*
SunnyD Tangy Original (8 fl. oz.)	4½*
Starbucks Cinnamon Dolce Latte (grande, 16 fl. oz.)	5*
Starbucks Tazo Shaken Iced Tea, any flavor (grande, 16 fl. oz.)	5
Gatorade Lemon-Lime (20 fl. oz.)	8½
Glacéau Vitamin Water Revive (20 fl. oz.)	8½
Starbucks Tazo Passion Shaken Iced Tea Lemonade (grande, 16 fl. oz.)	8½
Coca-Cola (12 fl. oz. can)	10
Snapple Lemon Tea (16 fl. oz.)	10½
Nestea Iced Tea Sweetened Lemon (16.9 fl. oz.)	12
Schweppes Tonic Water (20 fl. oz.)	14
SoBe Green Tea (20 fl. oz.)	15½
Sprite (20 fl. oz.)	16
Arizona Southern Style Sweet Tea (23 fl. oz.)	16½
Coca-Cola (20 fl. oz.)	16½
Minute Maid Lemonade (20 fl. oz.)	17
Pepsi (20 fl. oz.)	17½
Sunkist Orange Soda (20 fl. oz.)	21

Candy, Chocolate, etc.	Added Sugars (teaspoons)
Werther's Original Hard Candies (3 pieces, 0.6 oz.)	2½
Lindt Excellence 70% Cocoa Dark Chocolate (4 squares, 1.4 oz.)	3
Dove Dark Chocolate Promises (5 pieces, 1.4 oz.)	5
Hershey's Milk Chocolate Bar (1.6 oz.)	5½*
York Peppermint Patties (1 patty, 1.4 oz.)	6½
Jelly Belly Jelly Beans (35 pieces, 1.4 oz.)	7
M&M's Milk Chocolate (56 pieces, 1.7 oz.)	8
Maple syrup (¼ cup, 2.9 oz.)	12

Sweets (1 item, unless otherwise noted)	
Pepperidge Farm Milano, original (3 cookies, 1.2 oz.)	3
Entenmann's Crumb Coffee Cake (1/10 cake, 2 oz.)	3½
Mrs. Fields semi-sweet Chocolate Chip Cookie (1.2 oz.)	3½
Nabisco Oreo (3 cookies, 1.2 oz.)	3½
Pepperidge Farm Double Chocolate Milano (3 cookies, 1.4 oz.)	4
Entenmann's Rich Frosted Donut (2.1 oz.)	4½
Jell-O Strawberry (1 snack cup, 3.5 oz.)	4½
Sara Lee All Butter Pound Cake (1 slice, 2.7 oz.)	5
Entenmann's Glazed Buttermilk Donut (2.1 oz.)	5½
Krispy Kreme Chocolate Iced Kreme Filled Doughnut (3.1 oz.)	6
Entenmann's Chocolate Fudge Cake (½ cake, 2.3 oz.)	7
Krispy Kreme Glazed Chocolate Doughnut (2.8 oz.)	7
Starbucks Chocolate Chunk Cookie (3 oz.)	8
Starbucks Marble Loaf (1 slice, 3.8 oz.)	8
Panera Chocolate Chipper Cookie (3.3 oz.)	8½
Panera Chocolate Fudge Brownie (3.5 oz.)	8½
Starbucks Classic Coffee Cake (4 oz.)	8½
Hostess Twinkies (2 cakes, 3 oz.)	9
Starbucks Pumpkin Scone (4.2 oz.)	11
Entenmann's Super Cinnamon Buns (6 oz.)	11½
Hostess Sno Balls (2 cakes, 3.5 oz.)	11½
Panera Pecan Roll (5.5 oz.)	12
Panera Pumpkin Muffin (6 oz.)	12
Cinnabon Classic Cinnamon Roll (7.8 oz.)	14
Denny's Hershey's Chocolate Cake (1 slice, 5 oz.)	14
Dunkin' Donuts Coffee Cake Muffin (5.8 oz.)	14½
Uno Chicago Grill Chocolate Chocolate Malt Layer Cake (1 slice, 9.5 oz.)	25

Cereals & Cereal Bars	
Kashi TLC Trail Mix Chewy Granola Bar (1 bar, 1.2 oz.)	1½
General Mills Cinnamon Toast Crunch (¾ cup, 1.1 oz.)	2½
General Mills Honey Nut Cheerios (¾ cup, 1 oz.)	2½
Kellogg's Bite Size Frosted Mini-Wheats (24 biscuits, 2.1 oz.)	3
Kashi GoLean Crunch! Original (1 cup, 1.9 oz.)	3½
Kellogg's Cracklin' Oat Bran (¾ cup, 1.8 oz.)	4
Kashi GoLean Cookies 'N Cream Chewy Bar (1 bar, 2.8 oz.)	9

Miscellaneous	
Bush's Homestyle Baked Beans (½ cup, 4.5 oz.)	3
Cracker Jack (½ cup, 1 oz.)	4
Häagen-Dazs Chocolate Sorbet (½ cup, 3.7 oz.)	5

*CSPI estimate. Note: Added sugars are rounded to the nearest half teaspoon.

Sources: Company information and U.S. Department of Agriculture Nutrient Database. Chart compiled by Amy Ramsay.

Sweet Nothings

When researchers gave people either regular or diet soft drinks for several weeks, the participants gained weight only on the regular sodas.[1,2] But all non-caloric sweeteners are not created equal. Here's our take on their safety:

- **Acesulfame-potassium.** Tests conducted in the 1970s were of mediocre quality. One suggested an increased cancer risk in female rats.
- **Aspartame (NutraSweet, Equal).** Judging by two recent rat studies, it may slightly increase cancer risk. At the very least, new studies should be conducted.
- **Saccharin (Sweet'N Low).** In animal studies, it has caused cancer of the urinary bladder, uterus, ovaries, skin, blood vessels, and other organs.
- **Stevia.** Coke and Pepsi have started to use it to sweeten some beverages. It appears to be safe, though there should be more independent testing.
- **Sucralose (Splenda).** It appears to be safe, though there hasn't been much independent testing. (Sucralose isn't as natural as ads have implied. It's made by chlorinating sugar molecules.)

[1]Am. J. Clin. Nutr. 76: 721, 2002.
[2]Am. J. Clin. Nutr. 51: 963, 1990.

"Weight gain appears to account for half of the increased risk," says Manson.

What could explain the other half? "Sugar-sweetened soft drinks might also increase the risk of type 2 diabetes because they're high in rapidly absorbable carbohydrates," she suggests.

High-fructose corn syrup is roughly half fructose, which goes largely to the liver, so it doesn't raise blood sugar. But the glucose half of high-fructose corn syrup heads straight to the bloodstream.

"Consumption of sugar-sweetened soft drinks causes a fast and dramatic increase in blood sugar levels," says Manson. "In our studies, people who eat foods that raise blood sugar levels have a higher risk of diabetes."

6. **Fructose may boost visceral fat.** In the University of California, Davis, study, the 32 men and women gained about the same weight (roughly three pounds) after 10 weeks whether they drank beverages sweetened with fructose or glucose.[10] But there were differences.

The fructose eaters (especially the men) gained more deep abdominal—or visceral—fat than the glucose eaters. That's critical because visceral fat is linked to a higher risk of heart disease and diabetes.

In contrast, the glucose eaters gained more subcutaneous fat, which is just below the skin and is less likely to raise the risk of diabetes and heart disease.

Since this study was the first to see fructose's effect on visceral fat, Stanhope notes, "it would be good to see the result confirmed in other studies."

Another new finding: the fructose drinkers had a drop in insulin sensitivity. Reduced sensitivity to insulin is linked to a higher risk of heart disease and diabetes. But it's too early to know if Stanhope's results will hold up in future studies.

If fructose makes insulin less efficient, no one knows how. "It may be due to an increase in the amount of triglyceride stored in the liver," speculates Stanhope, "which could then lead to a chain of events that causes insulin receptors to perform less effectively."

7. **Fructose may raise the risk of gout.** Gout hurts. If your blood has too much uric acid, the excess ends up in joints (especially those of the big toe), where it can cause excruciating pain.

"Obesity is the major risk factor for gout because it's so common and it substantially increases the risk," says Gary Curhan, an associate professor of medicine at the Harvard Medical School.

But fructose is also a culprit. "We know that fructose increases uric acid, and that uric acid causes gout," says Curhan.

In a study of roughly 46,000 men, those who got at least 12 percent of their calories from fructose were nearly twice as likely to be diagnosed with gout over the next 12 years as those who got less than 7 percent of their calories from fructose.[11]

"After we adjusted for weight and all the other risk factors for gout that we know about, people with higher intakes of fructose had a substantially higher risk of gout," Curhan explains.

At least that's true in men, who are far more likely to get the disease. "We're just starting to look at women," says Curhan.

8. **Fructose may promote over-eating.** Leptin is a hormone made by fat cells. It's supposed to make you stop eating.

"Leptin tells your brain that you've got enough calories on board," says Robert Lustig, a professor of clinical pediatrics at the University of California, San Francisco, who served on the heart association sugar panel. "When you don't get that signal, you're still hungry."

When researchers fed rats a huge dose of fructose (60 percent of their diet) for six months, the animals became resistant to leptin—that is, leptin injections failed to curb their appetite.[12]

(Obese people can also be leptin-resistant. "They have lots of leptin, but it doesn't work," explains Lustig.)

Over time, a high-fructose diet blocks the leptin signal in the brain, notes Lustig. "So leptin can't extinguish hunger and can't extinguish reward." The result: you keep eating.

In fact, when the rats were allowed to eat as much palatable food as they wanted, they gained nearly twice as much weight as rats that got no fructose.

But so far, it's not clear what happens when people eat fructose in less-excessive amounts.

The Bottom Line

- Shoot for 100 calories (6½ teaspoons, or 25 grams) a day of added sugars if you're a woman and 150 calories (9½ teaspoons, or 38 grams) a day if you're a man. Even less may be better for your heart (see "What Should I Eat?" *Nutrition Action,* Oct. 2009).
- Don't drink sugar-sweetened beverages. Limit fruit juices to no more than 1 cup a day.
- Limit *all* added sugars, including high-fructose corn syrup, cane or beet sugar, evaporated cane juice, brown rice syrup, agave syrup, and honey.
- Don't worry about the naturally occurring sugar in fruit, milk, and plain yogurt.
- To estimate your calorie needs and get a more precise added-sugars limit, go to mypyramid.gov and click on "Get a personalized plan" in the "I Want To . . ." box.
- If a food contains little or no milk or fruit (which have natural sugars), the "Sugars" number on the package's Nutrition Facts panel will tell you how much added sugars are in each serving.

In two preliminary studies, 17 obese men and women and 12 normal-weight women had higher leptin levels over a 24-hour period when they consumed 30 percent of their calories from glucose-sweetened beverages with meals than when they consumed the same amount of fructose-sweetened beverages with meals.[13,14] Few other studies have been done.

Does that mean we should be eating foods sweetened with glucose, which is what's in ordinary corn syrup?

"Why do we need corn syrup anyway?" asks Lustig. "We're better off getting carbs from foods that are packaged naturally with their own fiber. If we got carbs from whole grains, vegetables, fruit, and beans, we wouldn't overeat."

Fruit contains fructose (as well as sucrose and glucose). Do we need to limit apples and oranges? "I'm not concerned about fructose from fruit," says Lustig. "How many oranges can you eat in one sitting?"

9. **Minimizing added sugars keeps a lid on blood pressure.** "There's a possibility that sugar raises blood pressure," says Frank Sacks of the Harvard School of Public Health. "But it's far from definitive."

However, what *is* clear is that there's little place for sugar in a diet that's designed to lower blood pressure (see *Nutrition Action,* Oct. 2009, cover story).

The OmniHeart Study tested three diets on people with hypertension (blood pressure at least 140 over 90) or pre-hyper-tension (blood pressure at least 120 over 80).[15] Each diet was rich in fruits, vegetables, low-fat dairy foods, beans, nuts, and other foods that supply potassium, magnesium, and other key nutrients.

"The higher-carb OmniHeart diet did a great job of lowering blood pressure," says Sacks. It had just five teaspoons (80 calories) of added sugars a day. In people with hypertension, it trimmed systolic blood pressure (the top number) by an impressive 13 points.

But, adds Sacks, "the other two Omni-Heart diets—which were higher in either protein or unsaturated fat—did better." Those diets, which contained only two or three teaspoons (30 to 50 calories) of added sugars a day, cut systolic blood pressure by 16 points in people with hypertension.

"There's not much room for added sugars in most people's diets," concludes Sacks. "And certainly not if you're trying to optimize your diet to lower blood pressure."

His advice: "I never drink liquid calories, and I keep sweets and snacks out of the house. It's okay to indulge once in a while, but if I get hungry at night and there are no sweets around, I eat nuts or an apple."

10. **Most sugary foods are junk.** Coca-Cola, Pepsi, Cinnabon, Krispy Kreme, Dunkin' Donuts, Snapple, Entenmann's, Hostess, Sara Lee, Little Debbie.

Just about any sweets made by those and similar companies are high in sugars and low in nutrients. Many are also packed with virtually worthless white flour. And many are now supersized. Do you need a Cinnabon that's the size of a boxed lunch?

To stick to the heart association's new recommendations, you'll need to use your added sugars calorie allowance wisely. (To find out how much added sugar is in popular foods, see "Tout de Sweet").

"Be discriminating," suggests the University of Vermont's Rachel Johnson. "People enjoy sweet taste, and if you're discriminating, it has a role in a healthy diet. We're not all going to eat non-fat plain yogurt."

But "they're called discretionary calories for a reason," she adds. "Use them to enhance the palatability of already nutritious foods."

"I'd rather see someone consume added sugars in a flavored yogurt or a whole-grain breakfast cereal or by putting maple syrup on oatmeal than consume them in a doughnut or soft drink."

Notes

1. *Circulation 120:* 1011, 2009.
2. *Physiol. Behav. 59:* 179, 1996.
3. *Int. J. Obesity 24:* 794, 2000.
4. *Am. J. Clin. Nutr. 89:* 1299, 2009.
5. *JAMA 292:* 927, 2004.
6. *Am. J. Clin. Nutr. 89:* 1037, 2009.
7. *Circulation 116:* 480, 2007.
8. *JAMA 298:* 309, 2007.
9. *Am. J. Clin. Nutr. 72:* 1128, 2000.
10. *J. Clin. Invest. 119:* 1322, 2009.
11. *BMJ 336:* 309, 2008.
12. *Am. J. Physiol. Regul. Integr. Comp. Physiol. 295:* 1370, 2008.
13. *J. Clin. Endocrinol. Metab. 89:* 2963, 2004.
14. *J. Clin. Endocrinol. Metab. 94:* 1562, 2009.
15. *JAMA 294:* 2455, 2005.

Critical Thinking

1. Describe the concept of discretionary calories. What are the recommended amount of discretionary calories for an average male and female?

2. Explain why consuming high-fructose corn sweeteners increases the risk for heart disease, metabolic syndrome, type 2 diabetes, gout, and accumulation of visceral (abdominal) fat.

3. Why do fructose sweeteners promote overeating? Identify the hormone that is involved.

Role of Sugar Intake in Beverages on Overweight and Health

Max Lafontan, PhD

The present overview will be limited to the analysis of the putative impact of sugar inclusion in beverages on health, obesity, and diabetes risk. Mechanisms of action and physiological end points will be highlighted to clarify the differences existing in the health impact of various kinds of sugars.

Sugars, Heterogeneity, Basic Biology, Major Metabolic Impacts and Health-Related Questions

The term *sugars* (carbohydrates) includes a large family of monosaccharides and disaccharides, which are naturally present in (or added to) food or beverages. Sugar is the most common word for saccharose (sucrose); it represents 75 percent of added sugars, whereas glucose syrup represents only 25 percent in France. The most commonly used sweetener in the United States is high-fructose corn syrup (55 percent fructose and 45 percent glucose). The mean sugar content of sugar-sweetened beverages (SSBs) commonly used in the United States is 10 g/100 g (ranging from 4.5 to 16 g/100 g). Sugar-sweetened beverages represent the major source of dietary fructose, as provided in various forms including carbonated soft drinks, juice-based beverages, 100 percent juices, flavored milk, gourmet coffees, and liquid meal replacement mixtures for weight loss. Fructose is also included in solid foods (pastries, desserts, and a number of processed foods). The introduction of high-fructose corn syrup in the 1970s in the United States has resulted in a 30 percent increase in total fructose intake in the last 20 years. It is associated with a remarkable increase in the rates of obesity and diabetes.[1–3]

Glycemic Index, Glycemic Load, and Feeding

The glycemic index (GI) is the method of indexing the glycemic response to a fixed amount of available carbohydrate from a test food, to the same amount of available carbohydrate from a standard food consumed by the same subject. Initially, the standard "food" was glucose, now it is white bread. The glycemic load (GL) is a ranking system integrating sugar content and portion size; it is the product of the GI and total carbohydrates in the food portion. Detailed data on GI and GL are reported by Foster-Powell et al.[4] Foods with high GI are suspected to be the dietary factor that promotes repeated insulin release and contributes to the settlement of chronic diseases in patients at risk. Drinking SSBs when eating food contributes to a high GI of the overall diet.

Glucose and Fructose Possess Strikingly Different Metabolic Fates

Main alimentary polysaccharide hydrolysis generates glucose, fructose, and galactose, which are absorbed by the intestinal cells and delivered into circulation. Glucose and fructose have different metabolic fates in terms of absorptive processes, metabolic effects, and actions on leptin, ghrelin, and insulin secretion. Growing evidence suggests direct and opposite actions of glucose and fructose on hypothalamic neurons and food intake.

The site, rate, and extent of carbohydrate digestion and absorption from the gut are keys to understanding the many roles of carbohydrates. Glucose and galactose are absorbed via a Na^+/glucose cotransporter (SGLT1), whereas fructose is absorbed further down the duodenum by a non–Na^+-dependent process (Glut 5 transporter). The gastrointestinal system plays an important role in the neuroendocrine regulation of food intake. Recent mechanisms governing sugars and other nutrient sensing and peptide secretion by enteroendocrine cells have been discovered. Novel taste-like pathways exist in the enteroendocrine cells, which express several G protein–coupled receptors identified as taste receptors similar to those previously found in the taste buds on the tongue.[5] Several enteroendocrine cell types throughout the gut express T1R2/3 sweet taste G protein—coupled receptors, T2R-family bitter receptors, and/or the taste-specific G protein $G\alpha_{gustducin}$.[6] The combination of T1R2+3 recognizes natural sugars such as sucrose and glucose and also artificial sweeteners such as saccharin and acesulfame K.[7]

Glucose is an energy-providing substrate; glucose consumption by muscle considerably increases during physical exercise. Glucose oxidized during physical activity comes from glycogen stores in the liver and muscles and from ingested carbohydrates. Oxidation of other hexoses (eg, fructose and galactose) is lower than that of glucose. They must be transformed into glucose by the liver before utilization by skeletal muscle. Glucose need depends on the type of exercise, its intensity and duration, age, sex, and the level of physical training of the subjects. Nutrition recommendations for men and women performing exercise must be adapted to their individual needs according to the exercise performed.

Outside its role as an energy-providing substrate in numerous tissues, glucose is also an important signaling molecule. Glucose is involved in the regulation of the expression of genes regulating glycolysis and lipogenesis via a pathway involving a new transcription factor (ie, carbohydrate regulatory element binding protein).[8] Fructose metabolism has unique characteristics; it is largely metabolized in the liver (50 percent–70 percent), with the rest being metabolized by the kidneys and adipocytes. Fructose possesses beneficial effects at low concentrations (hepatic glucose uptake) while exerting a number of deleterious effects when chronically consumed in excess (hepatic steatosis, insulin resistance, inflammation, and hyperuricemia).[9]

Glucose sensing is an important function of the brain.[10] Two populations of glucose-sensing neurons have been identified in hypothalamic areas: those that are excited (ie, increased electrical activity) and those that are inhibited (ie, decreased activity). They are triggered at different glucose concentrations. Unlike glucose, which suppresses food intake, fructose increases food intake when metabolized by the central nervous system. Fructose has the opposite effect of glucose on the AMP activated kinase/malonyl–CoA signaling system and thereby feeding behavior. Thus, increased fructose metabolism within the brain increases food intake and obesity risk.[11]

Sugars and Sweetness Are Important in Establishing Lifelong Food Habits

It is important to understand the early factors that determine choice and ingestion, when designing strategies to enhance the health of infants, children, and adults. Early experiences set the stage for later food choices, and they are important in establishing lifelong food habits.[12] Different brain regions are responsive to sweetness intensity and pleasantness perceptions in humans.[13] Psychological and behavioral components of sweetness are very complex. Full development of this question is considered to be outside the present review.

Glucose, Insulin Secretion, and Glucotoxicity

High dietary GI and GL have been associated with an increased risk of developing type 2 diabetes mellitus in large prospective studies.[14] The foods that were the most consistently associated with increased risk of type 2 diabetes are white rice, white bread, potatoes, and SSBs. Type 2 diabetes is a complex syndrome of polygenic nature; the genetic susceptibility of the pancreas β cells determines the risk of developing the disease. Increased plasma glucose and free fatty acids may exert, in the long term, toxic influences on β-cell function. When glucose is in excess, instead of flowing uniquely and normally through oxidative phosphorylation, metabolites overflow into alternative pathways causing oxidative stress and leading to β-cell dysfunction.[15]

Comments on the Obesity Epidemic

Adipocyte number is settled early in life during childhood and adolescence. An increasing number of nations face childhood obesity problems. Obese children are at a high risk of becoming irreversibly obese adults. Most obese adults have been obese since childhood, with less than 10 percent of children with normal weight going on to develop adult obesity. By contrast, more than three-fourths of obese children go on to become obese adults. Obesity has its genesis in childhood. Interventional focus should be placed in early life.[16] Risk factors and causes of obesity in children include a number of parameters (ie, genetic, antenatal life, auxologic parameters at birth, early postnatal development, socioeconomic conditions of the parents, physical activity, dieting, etc).

Increased lipid storage in already developed fat cells (adipocytes) is thought to be the most important event of fat mass expansion. Adipocyte number is a major determinant for the fat mass in adults. As previously suspected in the 1970s, a recent study has confirmed that the number of adipocytes existing in adulthood is set during childhood and adolescence. The number of fat cells stays constant in adulthood in lean and obese individuals, even after marked weight loss. Approximately 10 percent of fat cells are renewed annually at all adult ages and levels of body mass index. A tight regulation of fat cell numbers occurs during adulthood.[17] Thus, it is clear that an excess number of fat cells represent an important element of the future of fat mass status. The number of adipocytes for lean and obese individuals is set before the age of 20 years. Adipocyte number is subject to little variation during adulthood; changes are limited to variations in cell size. Even after significant weight loss in adulthood and reduced adipocyte volume, the adipocyte number remains the same.

Glucose uptake is essential for triacylglycerol synthesis in human fat cells. Glucose uptake by fat cells operates under the control of the Glut 4 glucose transporter. Insulin stimulates fatty acids and glucose uptake and activates lipoprotein lipase activity and triglyceride synthesis.[18] It is easily understandable that whenever insulin release is potently stimulated by high GI food or SSB intake, a potent signal for fat storage will be provided to the fat cell by insulin. Erratic and/or frequent intake of SSBs could represent a risk of fat storage in patients at risk of developing obesity, depending on their activity level. Cumulative daily imbalances in energy intake affect body fat mass.[19] If intake exceeds expenditure by 2 percent daily (ie, <1 can of SSBs) for a year, the result would be an increase of 75 312 kJ, or approximately 2.3 kg. A major program to control childhood obesity must be established at all the levels of health care delivery. The necessary measures include education of the public regarding the risk factors for childhood obesity: (1) limit consumption of sucrose- and fructose-containing drinks and foods with high carbohydrate and fat contents, (2) assume correct hydration by water drinking, and (3) promote exercise programs at home and at school.

What Do Epidemiological Studies Tell Us: Interest and Limits of Cross-sectional, Longitudinal, and Intervention Studies?

Overweight among children has increased dramatically during the past 2 decades and is reaching epidemic proportions. The obesity epidemic is a crisis that requires action before all the scientific evidence is settled. A number of questions have been raised concerning the putative impact of SSBs on health and obesity epidemics. Energy intake is positively associated with consumption of soft drinks.[20] For example, mean adjusted energy intake was 7656 kJ/d for school-aged children who were not consumers of SSBs, compared with 8443 kJ/d for children who consumed an average of 250 mL of soda per day.[21]

Influential global reports have asserted that SSBs play a key role in the etiology of overweight and obesity.[22,23] Cross-sectional studies are the most common. A number of comprehensive scientific reviews of the evidence have tended to be cautious, less straightforward, and with a number of controversies that cannot be detailed here. A recent systematic review and meta-analysis have concluded that the strength of the relationship was near zero and contested some previous positive results.[24] However, this meta-analysis was open to criticisms. Concerning longitudinal studies, half of a group of 18 showed a significant positive result between SSB intake and body mass index; the effect appears to be rather small. The effects of potential confounding factors from other components of the diet, physical activity, and other lifestyle factors are not sufficiently assessed in the majority of such studies, as recently discussed.[25]

Intervention trials represent the best level of evidence to test a hypothesis. Avoidance of SSBs may help to prevent further weight gain in overweight children or obese subjects.[26, 27] The relative effects of dietary sugars (glucose vs fructose) were compared during a 10-week consumption period. Overweight and obese subjects consumed glucose- or fructose-sweetened beverages providing 25 percent of energy requirements for 10 weeks. It was demonstrated that dietary fructose specifically increases hepatic de novo lipogenesis, promotes dyslipidemia, decreases insulin sensitivity, and increases visceral adiposity in overweight/obese adults.[28] Results of intervention trials are promising, although they remain quite rare, difficult to settle, and expensive.

Conclusions and Future Trends

Despite the large number of studies on the role of sugar intake in beverages on overweight and health, definitive conclusions are not easily drawn from studies. Publication biases have been highlighted recently.[25] Industry-funded studies tend to reveal smaller effects than other studies. Cross-sectional studies are the most abundant types of studies but they cannot establish cause-effect relationships and are rarely conclusive. The effects observed in longitudinal studies are often seen in the studies of smaller size, but could be affected by modification of other aspects of diet and lifestyle. It is necessary to be careful with industry-funded studies, which have a tendency to reveal smaller effects.

The recent results of an intervention study provide the best arguments to infer causality. It is expected that this kind of intervention approach will be expanded in the future in the different populations of the planet because nutritional habits and sugar composition of SSBs could differ noticeably. Intervention trials must be developed to delineate the doses of SSBs promoting adverse changes of plasma lipids and a decrease in insulin sensitivity in different populations at risk for health problems. More studies of adequate duration must also be performed among children and in overweight consumers of SSBs. When considering weight changes and obesity-related questions related to SSB consumption, it is important to take into account population differences and genetic parameters. Lifestyle influences (eg, other components of the diet and physical activity) must also be considered in the studies.

References

1. Bray GA, Nielsen SJ, Popkin BM. Consumption of high-fructose corn syrup in beverages may play a role in the epidemic of obesity. *Am J Clin Nutr.* 2004;79:537–543.
2. Havel PJ. Dietary fructose: implications for dysregulation of energy homeostasis and lipid/carbohydrate metabolism. *Nutr Rev.* 2005;63:133–157.
3. Johnson RJ, Segal MS, Sautin Y, et al. Potential role of sugar (fructose) in the epidemic of hypertension, obesity and the metabolic syndrome, diabetes, kidney disease, and cardiovascular disease. *Am J Clin Nutr.* 2007;86:899–906.
4. Foster-Powell K, Holt SH, Brand-Miller JC. International table of glycemic index and glycemic load values: 2002. *Am J Clin Nutr.* 2002;76:5–56.
5. Cummings DE, Overduin J. Gastrointestinal regulation of food intake. *J Clin Invest.* 2007;117:13–23.
6. Rozengurt E. Taste receptors in the gastrointestinal tract. I. Bitter taste receptors and alpha-gustducin in the mammalian gut. *Am J Physiol Gastrointest Liver Physiol.* 2006;291:G171–G177.
7. Li X, Staszewski L, Xu H, et al. Human receptors for sweet and umami taste. *Proc Natl Acad Sci USA.* 2002;99:4692–4696.
8. Postic C, Dentin R, Denechaud PD, et al. ChREBP, a transcriptional regulator of glucose and lipid metabolism. *Annu Rev Nutr.* 2007;27:179–192.
9. Johnson RJ, Perez-Pozo SE, Sautin YY, et al. Hypothesis: could excessive fructose intake and uric acid cause type 2 diabetes? *Endocr Rev.* 2009;30:96–116.
10. Gonzalez JA, Reimann F, Burdakov D. Dissociation between sensing and metabolism of glucose in sugar sensing neurones. *J Physiol.* 2009;587:41–48.
11. Lane MD, Cha SH. Effect of glucose and fructose on food intake via malonyl-CoA signaling in the brain. *Biochem Biophys Res Commun.* 2009;382:1–5.
12. Beauchamp GK, Mennella JA. Early flavor learning and its impact on later feeding behavior. *J Pediatr Gastroenterol Nutr.* 2009;48(1 suppl):S25–S30.

13. Small DM, Gregory MD, Mak YE, et al. Dissociation of neural representation of intensity and affective valuation in human gustation. *Neuron*. 2003;39:701–711.

14. Willett W, Manson J, Liu S. Glycemic index, glycemic load, and risk of type 2 diabetes. *Am J Clin Nutr*. 2002;76:274S–280S.

15. Poitout V, Robertson RP. Glucolipotoxicity: fuel excess and beta-cell dysfunction. *Endocr Rev*. 2008;29:351–366.

16. August GP, Caprio S, Fennoy I, et al. Prevention and treatment of pediatric obesity: an endocrine society clinical practice guideline based on expert opinion. *J Clin Endocrinol Metab*. 2008;93:4576–4599.

17. Spalding KL, Arner E, Westermark PO, et al. Dynamics of fat cell turnover in humans. *Nature*. 2008;453:783–787.

18. Lafontan M. Advances in adipose tissue metabolism. *Int J Obes (Lond)*. 2008;32(suppl 7):S39–S51.

19. Rosenbaum M, Leibel RL, Hirsch J. Obesity. *N Engl J Med*. 1997;337:396–407.

20. Ludwig DS, Peterson KE, Gortmaker SL. Relation between consumption of sugar-sweetened drinks and childhood obesity: a prospective, observational analysis. *Lancet*. 2001;357:505–508.

21. Harnack L, Stang J, Story M. Soft drink consumption among US children and adolescents: nutritional consequences. *J Am Diet Assoc*. 1999;99:436–441.

22. World Health Organization and Food and Agriculture Organization. *Diet, Nutrition and the Prevention of Chronic Diseases*. Geneva, Switzerland: WHO; 2003.

23. World Cancer Fund Food. *Nutrition, Physical activity and the Prevention of Cancer*. Washington, DC: American Institute for Cancer Research; 2007.

24. Forshee RA, Anderson PA, Storey ML. Sugar-sweetened beverages and body mass index in children and adolescents: a meta-analysis. *Am J Clin Nutr*. 2008;87:1662–1671.

25. Gibson S. Sugar-sweetened soft drinks and obesity: a systematic review of the evidence from observational studies and interventions. *Nutr Res Rev*. 2008;21:134–147.

26. Ebbeling CB, Feldman HA, Osganian SK, et al. Effects of decreasing sugar-sweetened beverage consumption on body weight in adolescents: a randomized, controlled pilot study. *Pediatrics*. 2006;117:673–680.

27. Sichieri R, Paula Trotte A, de Souza RA, et al. School randomised trial on prevention of excessive weight gain by discouraging students from drinking sodas. *Public Health Nutr*. 2009;12:197–202.

28. Stanhope KL, Schwarz JM, Keim NL, et al. Consuming fructose-sweetened, not glucose-sweetened, beverages increases visceral adiposity and lipids and decreases insulin sensitivity in overweight/obese humans. *J Clin Invest*. 2009;119:1322–1334.

Critical Thinking

1. Compare and contrast the physiological actions of glucose vs fructose in the body.

2. List the diseases caused by excess intake of fructose, particularly from high-fructose sweeteners.

3. Explain why fructose is implicated in the increased prevalence of type 2 diabetes and obesity.

4. Evaluate why the results from the majority of research on fructose, diabetes, and obesity are rarely conclusive. What type of research needs to be conducted to provide more conclusive evidence?

MAX LAFONTAN, PHD, is director of research, Unité Inserm 858, Institut de Médecine Moléculaire de Rangueil, and Université Paul Sabatier, Toulouse, France. The author is not receiving any funding for research investigations from Danone Waters but has received consulting fees from a paid advisory board for the review. Dr Lafontan has received speaker and consultancy honorarium from Danone Waters R&D.

Sugar Belly

How Much Is Too Much Sugar?

Soft drinks, sports drinks, fruit drinks, energy drinks, coffee drinks, cupcakes, cookies, muffins, doughnuts, granola bars, chocolate, ice cream, sweetened yogurt, cereal, candy. The list of sweet temptations is endless.

The average American now consumes 22 to 28 teaspoons of *added sugars* a day—mostly high-fructose corn syrup and ordinary table sugar (sucrose). That's 350 to 440 empty calories that few of us can afford.

How much added sugar is too much? Cutting back to 100 calories (6½ teaspoons) a day for women and 150 calories (9½ teaspoons) a day for men might mean slimmer waistlines and a lower risk of disease.

BONNIE LIEBMAN

Obesity

Do sugary foods and drinks deserve more blame for America's obesity epidemic than other foods?

"There is strong evidence linking sugar-sweetened beverages to weight," says Vasanti Malik, a research fellow at the Harvard School of Public Health.

For example, when she and her colleagues tracked more than 50,000 women for four years, they found that weight gain was greatest (about 10 pounds) among women who went from drinking no more than one sugar-sweetened drink a week to at least one a day.[1]

"But most industry-funded studies have reported no association," she notes. "This back-and-forth with industry has been muddying the waters."

For example, a 2009 meta-analysis by scientists with industry ties found no link between soft drinks and weight in children.[2]

"But there were some errors in the way they scaled the data," Malik explains.

What's more, some studies in the industry-funded analysis only compared soda drinkers to non-soda drinkers *who consumed the same number of calories.*

"It doesn't make sense to adjust for total calories because extra calories may explain how sugar-sweetened beverages lead to obesity," says Malik.

"When we re-analyzed the data correctly, there was an association between weight and sugar-sweetened beverages."[3]

What about the added sugars in solid foods? "There's not as much evidence for them," says Malik. "We haven't looked at that carefully yet."

"We focused on sugar-sweetened beverages because they're the largest contributor of added sugar intake," she adds, "and because of the lack of compensation for liquid calories."

Studies find that people may "compensate" for the calories they get from solid foods by eating less later in the day. But that doesn't seem to happen when people drink liquid calories.[4]

"In one study, people given jelly beans consumed less at subsequent meals than those who were given the same calories as liquid sugary beverages," says Malik.

More evidence that sugary beverages can plaster on the pounds: In three studies, scientists randomly assigned people to consume either sugary beverages (made with sugar or high-fructose corn syrup) versus diet beverages (usually made with aspartame) for three to 10 weeks.[5-7] Sure enough, only those who consumed sugar or high-fructose corn syrup gained weight.

But now researchers are hot on the trail of a new lead: Is the fructose that makes up roughly half of most added sugars more likely to migrate to your belly than elsewhere?

A Beeline to the Belly

Clearly, too many calories from anything—sugary beverages, beer, burgers, fries, pizza, ice cream, or dozens of other foods—explains why many American waists have been replaced by a spare tire.

Sugars 101

Sucrose (table sugar) is broken down—in the body and (to some extent) in foods—to half fructose and half glucose. At that point it is almost identical to most high-fructose corn syrup. Fruit contains a mixture of fructose, sucrose, and glucose.

And studies haven't found that you'd gain more pounds from, say, 100 calories of added sugars than from 100 calories of other foods. But calories from fructose (which is found only in added sugars and fruit) may be more likely than other calories to aim for your waist.

To find out if fructose is destined to end up around your midsection, researchers compare fructose to glucose (which is found in added sugars but is also the building block of starches).

The first solid evidence came in 2009. Researchers gave 32 overweight or obese middle-aged men and women 25 percent of their calories from beverages sweetened with either fructose or glucose for 10 weeks.[8]

Both groups gained the same weight (about three pounds). But their new fat didn't all go to the same place.

"We saw an increase in visceral fat in people fed fructose," says study author Kimber Stanhope of the University of California, Davis.

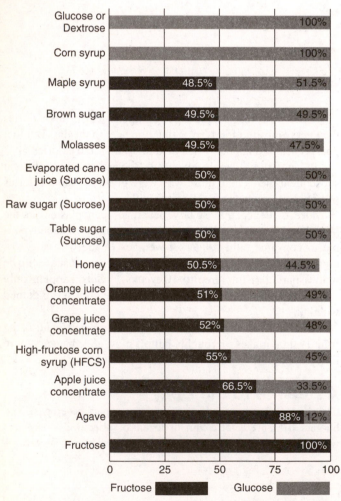

Glucose or Dextrose 100%
Corn syrup 100%
Maple syrup 48.5% / 51.5%
Brown sugar 49.5% / 49.5%
Molasses 49.5% / 47.5%
Evaporated cane juice (Sucrose) 50% / 50%
Raw sugar (Sucrose) 50% / 50%
Table sugar (Sucrose) 50% / 50%
Honey 50.5% / 44.5%
Orange juice concentrate 51% / 49%
Grape juice concentrate 52% / 48%
High-fructose corn syrup (HFCS) 55% / 45%
Apple juice concentrate 66.5% / 33.5%
Agave 88% / 12%
Fructose 100%

Scale: 0 25 50 75 100

Fructose ■   Glucose ■

* Sucrose is shown as its component sugars (fructose and glucose). Note: If percentages don't add up to 100, other sugars account for the difference.

Sugar by Any Other Name   With a few exceptions (like agave and corn syrup), most sweeteners and the naturally occurring sugars in fruit break down into roughly half fructose and half glucose in the body.* The natural sugar in milk (lactose) breaks down into half glucose and half galactose.

Sources: USDA Nutrient Database and company information.

Visceral (deep belly) fat is more closely linked to a higher risk of heart disease and diabetes than subcutaneous (just below the skin) fat. (See "Where's the Fat?")

"The high-fructose corn syrup industry's scientific consultants criticized our study," says Stanhope. "They said, 'This is meaningless. No one consumes foods sweetened with pure fructose so no one consumes that much fructose.'"

Now two new studies have reported similar results with less fructose:

• **Danish scientists** assigned 47 overweight men and women to drink a liter (not quite three 12 oz. cans) a day of one of four drinks: regular cola (sweetened with sucrose), reduced-fat milk, diet cola (sweetened with aspartame), or water.[9] (Sucrose is half glucose and half fructose.)

  After six months, visceral fat went up only in those drinking regular cola. "The increase in visceral fat was quite impressive," says Stanhope.

  And a liter isn't much. Roughly half the population doesn't drink sugary beverages, but among the drinkers, 50 percent swallow at least half a liter a day and 5 percent gulp down at least $1^1/_3$ liters.[10]

• **Swiss researchers** assigned 29 healthy, normal-weight men to drink beverages with one of the following: 10 teaspoons of fructose, 20 teaspoons of fructose, 10 teaspoons of glucose, 20 teaspoons of glucose, or 20 teaspoons of sucrose each day.[11]

  "Those aren't large amounts," notes Stanhope. A 12 oz. can of soda has about 10 teaspoons of sugars (roughly half fructose and half glucose). The 10-teaspoon dose was only about 7 percent of the men's calories.

  After just three weeks, waist-to-hip ratio rose slightly only in the men who got fructose (alone or in sucrose), but not glucose. (Measuring waist-to-hip ratio isn't as accurate as measuring visceral fat, but when your waist expands, it's often because visceral fat expands.)

"With three studies now, these data suggest that added sugars cause an increase in visceral fat," says Stanhope.

And links between visceral fat and sugary foods or drinks are now showing up elsewhere. When University of Minnesota researchers studied nearly 800 men and women, those who drank the most sugar-sweetened beverages had more visceral fat and larger waists.[12]

"We observed greater overall abdominal fat with increasing sugar-sweetened beverage consumption, and the increase in visceral fat was driving it," says Andrew Odegaard, a research associate at the University of Minnesota School of Public Health.

Where's The Fat?

The fructose in most added sugars appears to boost liver, muscle, and visceral fat. Excess fat anywhere in the body increases the risk of insulin resistance and diabetes. But a fatty liver and visceral fat may increase your risk the most.

And among roughly 560 teenagers, those who consumed the most fructose (from beverages and food) had the most visceral fat, as well as the most insulin resistance, higher blood pressure, and higher blood sugar levels.[13]

"We took into account a lot of variables that could make this relationship spurious—fiber, calorie intake, fat and lean mass, socioeconomic status, physical activity," says author Norman Pollock, an assistant professor of pediatrics at the Georgia Health Sciences University in Augusta. "But the relationship with visceral fat was still there."

It's not as though added sugars are the only cause of a ballooning belly. Most of our expanding waistlines is due to eating too many calories, period.

But each notch on that belt could have serious consequences for your health.

"From what we understand, visceral fat may be what really drives insulin resistance and cardiometabolic disorders like type 2 diabetes and heart disease," says Odegaard.

Diabetes & Heart Disease

The link between diabetes and sugars is clearest when researchers look at sugary drinks.

"We summarized the results from eight studies," explains Harvard's Vasanti Malik. All told, the meta-analysis pooled data on more than 300,000 people.[14] The results: "For each 12 oz. serving of a sugar-sweetened beverage you drink per day, you're getting about a 15 percent increased risk for diabetes," says Malik. "So it really doesn't take much to increase your risk."

"Fewer studies have looked at cardiovascular disease," she observes. "But we found an increased risk."

When Malik and colleagues tracked 88,000 nurses for 24 years, those who consumed at least two sugar-sweetened beverages a day had a 35 percent higher risk of heart attack than those who drank less than one a month.[15]

Sugar-sweetened-beverage drinkers also have a higher risk of the metabolic syndrome, which can lead to type 2 diabetes or heart disease.[14,16] (You have the metabolic syndrome if you have at least three of the following: elevated blood sugar, blood triglycerides, blood pressure, or waist circumference, or low HDL cholesterol.)

"In our meta-analysis, people who drank two or more sugar-sweetened beverages a day had about a 20 percent increased risk of the metabolic syndrome compared to those who drank none or less than one per month," says Malik.

And it's not just that can of Coke. In 2010, researchers at Emory University reported that among a nationally representative sample of more than 6,000 adults, those who got more sugars from drinks and foods had lower HDL ("good") cholesterol and higher triglyceride levels in their blood.[17]

"Elevated triglycerides, together with elevated LDL ("bad") cholesterol, contributes to changes in our blood vessels that increase the risk of heart disease," explains Emory's Jean Welsh.

"The job of HDL is to carry away the triglycerides and the bad cholesterol so that they don't cause damage."

But none of those studies can prove cause-and-effect. "To find out if fructose is causing adverse effects, you have to give people fructose or glucose drinks for months," says Pollock.

That's just what the latest studies did.

Look to the Liver

In the Danish study, the people who drank a liter a day of sucrose-sweetened cola didn't just have more visceral fat. Their liver and muscle fat more than doubled.[9]

"That's a substantial increase," notes Stanhope. "We had suggested that consuming high amounts of fructose-containing sugars could lead to an increase in liver fat. This is the first well-controlled study to show it."

Why does liver fat matter? When the body stores fat anywhere but in fat cells, it's called "ectopic" fat. And ectopic fat, especially in the liver, means trouble.

"When liver fat levels go up, that may trigger the sequence of events that leads to insulin resistance," says Stanhope. That's

---

Sugar vs. Sugar

"No High Fructose LOW Corn Syrup," says the Kashi GoLean label.

Is high-fructose corn syrup worse than table sugar (sucrose), even though both are roughly half fructose and half glucose?

"Added sugars—whether they come from sucrose, high-fructose corn syrup, or fruit juice concentrates—all have equal adverse effects metabolically," says Harvard University's Vasanti Malik. "This obsession with high-fructose corn syrup is a little misguided."

In January, researchers at the University of Florida reported that people who were given 24 ounces of Dr Pepper sweetened with high-fructose corn syrup had higher blood sugar levels over the next six hours than those who got sucrose-sweetened Dr Pepper.[1] But other short-term studies have found no difference.[2]

"If you're getting a lot of fructose, it doesn't matter where it's coming from," says the Georgia Health Sciences University's Norman Pollock. "Even 100 percent fruit juice could be bad if you're consuming large quantities."

In fact, in some studies, people who drank more fruit juice had a greater risk of type 2 diabetes or weight gain.[3,4]

"The sugars in juices are natural, but it's still a large amount of sugar," explains Malik. "We saw an increased risk of diabetes with juices but not whole fruit, which suggests that the fiber in fruit—which isn't in the juice —might ameliorate the risk of diabetes."

Her advice: "Drink water, tea, or coffee, keeping the sweeteners and creamers minimal in the coffees and teas. If you want a little flavor, try sparkling waters with a twist of lime or orange. You can cut a little lime or lemon rind or orange peel and add them yourself."

[1] *Metabolism (2011),* DOI:l 10.1016/j.metabol.2011.09.013.
[2] *Am. J. Clin. Nutr 87:* 1194, 2008.
[3] *Diabetes Care 31:* 1311, 2008.
[4] *JAMA 292:* 927, 2004.

Sweet Somethings

Here's how much added sugars you'd get in a sampling of popular foods. (The numbers don't include the naturally occurring sugars in fruit or milk ingredients.)

Most women should get no more than 100 calories (6½ teaspoons) a day from added sugars. Most men should get no more than 150 calories (9½ teaspoons). To convert teaspoons to grams of sugar, multiply by 4. To convert teaspoons to calories from sugar, multiply by 16.

Sweets (1 cookie, piece of cake, etc., unless noted)	Calories	Added Sugar (tsp.)
Kashi TLC Oatmeal Dark Chocolate Cookies (1 oz.)	130	2
Pepperidge Farm Nantucket Dark Chocolate Soft Baked Cookies (1.1 oz.)	140	2.5
Krispy Kreme Original Glazed Doughnut (1.7 oz.)	190	2.5
Nabisco Chips Ahoy! Original (3 cookies, 1.2 oz.)	160	3
Pepperidge Farm Milano Cookies (3 cookies, 1.2 oz.)	180	3
Nabisco Oreo (3 cookies, 1.2 oz.)	160	3.5
Newman's Own Organics Original Newman-O's (3 cookies, 1.3 oz.)	170	3.5
Entenmann's Ultimate Crumb Cake (1/10 cake, 2 oz.)	250	4
Entenmann's Rich Frosted Donut (2.1 oz.)	300	4.5
Sara Lee All Butter Pound Cake (¼ cake, 2.7 oz.)	300	5
Pepperidge Farm Golden 3-Layer Cake (1/8 cake, 2.5 oz.)	230	6.5
Krispy Kreme Glazed Chocolate Cake Doughnut (2.8 oz.)	300	6.5
Au Bon Pain Chocolate Mocha Whoopie Pie (3 oz.)	330	6.5
Marie Calender's Southern Pecan Pie (1/8 pie, 4 oz.)	490	6.5
Marie Calender's Lemon Meringue Pie (1/9 pie, 4.3 oz.)	320	8.5
Starbucks Marble Pound Cake (3.8 oz.)	350	8.5
Panera Chocolate Chipper cookie (3.3 oz.)	440	8.5
Entenmann's Cinnamon Danish (4 oz.)	460	8.5
Starbucks Cinnamon Chip Scone (4.2 oz.)	480	8.5
Entenmann's Jumbo Iced Honey Bun (5 oz.)	660	8.5
Au Bon Pain Red Velvet Cupcake (3.1 oz.)	400	9
Starbucks Reduced-Fat Cinnamon Swirl Coffee Cake (4 oz.)	340	10
Au Bon Pain Hazelnut Mocha Brownie (4 oz.)	450	10.5
Dunkin' Donuts Chocolate Chip Muffin	610	14
Panera Chocolate Fudge Brownie with icing (4.3 oz.)	470	14.5
Cinnabon Classic Roll	880	15
Cinnabon Caramel Pecanbon	1,080	19
IHOP CINN-A-STACK Pancakes (4) with Old Fashioned Syrup (¼ cup)	1,110	23.5
The Cheesecake Factory Black-Out Cake	1,330	38
Candy, Chocolate, etc. (1 bar, box, etc., unless noted)		
Lindt Excellence 70 percent Cocoa Smooth Dark (4 squares, 1.4 oz.)	250	3
Planters Sweet 'N Crunchy Peanuts (1 oz.)	140	3.5
Dove Dark Chocolate Silky Smooth Promises (5 pieces, 1.4 oz.)	210	5
Hershey's Milk Chocolate Kisses (9 pieces, 1.4 oz.)	200	6
Hershey's Milk Chocolate bar (1.5 oz.)	210	6
Ghirardelli Chocolate Dark & Mint Squares (3 squares, 1.6 oz.)	210	6.5
M&M's Milk Chocolate (1.7 oz.)	230	8
Junior Mints, theater size (4 oz.)	480	22.5
Cereals		
Quaker Lower Sugar Maple & Brown Sugar Instant Oatmeal (1 pkt., 1.2 oz.)	120	1
Kellogg's Original All-Bran (½ cup, 1.1 oz.)	80	1.5

	Calories	Added Sugar *(tsp.)*
Post Honey Roasted Honey Bunches of Oats *(¾ cup, 1 oz.)*	120	1.5
General Mills Honey Nut Cheerios *(¾ cup, 1 oz.)*	110	2.5
Kellogg's Vanilla Almond Special K *(¾ cup, 1 oz.)*	110	2.5
Quaker Maple & Brown Sugar Instant Oatmeal *(1 pkt, 1.5 oz.)*	160	2.5
Kellogg's Raisin Bran *(1 cup, 2.1 oz.)*	190	2.5
Bear Naked Maple Pecan Granola *(½ cup, 2.2 oz.)*	260	2.5
Kellogg's Frosted Mini-Wheats Bite Size *(21 biscuits, 1.9 oz.)*	190	3
Kashi GoLean Crunch! *(1 cup, 1.9 oz.)*	190	3.5
Post Just Bunches! Honey Roasted Honey Bunches of Oats *(²/₃ cup, 2 oz.)*	250	3.5
Cereal & Granola Bars *(1 bar)*		
Kashi TLC Honey Almond Flax Chewy Granola Bar *(1.2 oz.)*	140	1.5
Fiber One Oats & Chocolate Chewy Bar *(1.4 oz.)*	140	2.5
Nature Valley Vanilla Chewy Yogurt Bar *(1.2 oz.)*	140	3.5
Quaker Dark Chocolatey Chewy Dipps Granola Bar *(1.1 oz.)*	140	3.5
Kellogg's Special K Chocolate Caramel Protein Meal Bar *(1.6 oz.)*	170	4
Kashi GoLean Chocolate Malted Crisp Bar *(1.9 oz.)*	190	4.5
Clif Bar Maple Nut *(2.4 oz.)*	250	5.5
Beverages		
Silk Vanilla Soymilk, refrigerated *(8 fl oz.)*	100	2
Starbucks Caramel Macchiato *(grande, 16 fl oz.)*	240	4*
Starbucks Vanilla Latte *(grande, 16 fl oz.)*	250	4*
Silk Chocolate Soymilk, refrigerated *(8 fl oz.)*	140	5
Starbucks Tazo Black Shaken Iced Tea *(grande, 16 fl oz.)*	80	5.5
Ocean Spray Cranberry Juice Cocktail *(8 fl oz.)*	120	5.5*
Schweppes Tonic Water *(12 fl oz.)*	130	8
Gatorade Perform Lemon-Lime *(20 fl oz.)*	130	9
Starbucks White Chocolate Mocha *(grande, 16 fl oz.)*	470	9*
Coca-Cola *(12 fl oz.)*	140	10
AriZona Extra Sweet Green Tea *(23.5 fl oz.)*	260	17
McDonald's Sweet Tea *(large, 32 fl oz.)*	280	17.5
Starbucks Java Chip Frappuccino *(venti, 24 fl oz.)*	560	18.5*
Dairy		
Häagen-Dazs Chocolate Ice Cream *(3.7 oz.)*	260	3*
Dannon All Natural Vanilla Yogurt *(6 oz.)*	150	4*
Häagen-Dazs Zesty Lemon Sorbet *(4 oz.)*	120	7
Cold Stone Creamery Sweet Cream Ice Cream *(Love it, 8 oz.)*	530	8.5*
TCBY Golden Vanilla Yogurt *(large, 13.4 fl oz.)*	400	9.5*
Pinkberry Original Frozen Yogurt *(large, 13 oz.)*	370	14.5*
Cold Stone Creamery Very Vanilla Shake *(Gotta Have It, 24 fl oz.)*	1,550	32.5*
Other		
Wholesome Sweeteners Organic Raw Blue Agave *(1 Tbs.)*	60	4
Honey *(1 Tbs.)*	60	4.5
Betty Crocker Rich & Creamy Chocolate Frosting *(2 Tbs.)*	130	4.5
Nutella *(2 Tbs.)*	200	5*

*Estimate. Note: added sugars are rounded to the nearest half teaspoon.

Source: Company information.

when insulin loses its ability to admit blood sugar into cells. It's often the first step on the road to diabetes or heart disease.

The liver may also explain why fructose leads to higher levels of triglycerides.

"Fructose gets metabolized by the liver very quickly," says Welsh. "When there is more sugar than the liver can process, it converts the sugar to fat. Some of the fat goes into the bloodstream, and that's why we get elevated triglycerides."

What's more, in Stanhope's study, the fructose drinkers burned less fat (and more carbohydrate).[18] "The body doesn't make fat and burn fat at the same time," she explains.

"In our study, fat oxidation got blocked every time people drank the fructose drink because that fructose is getting turned into fat."

Also troubling: "We saw an increase in small, dense LDL when people drank fructose," says Stanhope. Those are cholesterol-carrying particles that are more damaging to arteries than fluffy, large LDL.

And Stanhope noticed something else. "LDL increased as much in the high-fructose corn syrup group as in the pure fructose group. That was surprising because the high-fructose corn syrup group got less fructose."[19]

"Do fructose and glucose together exacerbate the problems?" she asks. "We can't say at this point. But it's possible that because fructose is activating the pathways by which sugar gets turned into fat, more of the glucose is getting turned into fat, too."

As if that weren't enough, fructose may also lead to gout, a painful inflammation due to a buildup of uric acid in joints.

"Fructose has been shown to increase uric acid," says Malik. "And gout has also been associated with sugar-sweetened beverages."[20]

The problem isn't just that fructose boosts several risk factors for diabetes and cardiovascular disease.

"It's that those risk factors—abdominal obesity, high triglycerides, and insulin resistance—all exacerbate each other," says Stanhope. "You get a vicious circle going."

A case in point: "Some researchers argue that if you increase visceral fat, it sends out more inflammatory factors, which go back to the liver, where they promote more insulin resistance," she explains.

Another example: "Fructose-containing sugars increase fat-making in the liver, which causes insulin resistance," says Stanhope. "But insulin resistance also increases fat-making in the liver, so all the processes get revved up."

Healthier? A slice of Starbucks Reduced-Fat Cinnamon Swirl Coffee Cake has 10 teaspoons of added sugars.

"That's why the metabolic syndrome is so difficult to treat with one medication," she adds. "Everything is feeding on everything else."

Empty Calories

How much is too much added sugar? In 2009, the American Heart Association suggested a limit: no more than 100 calories a day for women and no more than 150 calories a day for men.[21]

The heart association wasn't just concerned about "the worldwide pandemic of obesity and cardiovascular disease," but also about the healthy foods that added sugar replaces.

"To follow recommendations to lower the risk of heart disease, diabetes, osteoporosis, hypertension, you name it, you have to use most of your calories for fruits, vegetables, grains, milk, meat, fish, poultry, and oils," explains Susan Krebs-Smith of the National Cancer Institute. "Very few calories are left over for empty calories."

In her recent analysis of a nationally representative survey of more than 16,000 people, roughly 78 percent of women and 67 percent of men ate too much added sugar.[22]

"For example, for someone who eats 2,000 calories a day, 'too much' was more than 130 calories' worth of added sugar," she says.

Not surprisingly, more than 90 percent of the people also came up short on green and orange vegetables, beans, dairy, and whole grains. "Most calories need to count for something nutritionally," adds Krebs-Smith.

But growing evidence suggests that added sugars aren't just empty calories. They're harmful calories.

"We saw huge metabolic differences between people who consumed fructose instead of glucose, despite the same weight gain," says Stanhope.

"Many people believe that excess calories are the problem, and it doesn't matter where they come from. But now we know that that's not true."

The Bottom Line

- Shoot for 100 calories (6½ teaspoons) a day of added sugars if you're a woman and 150 calories (9½ teaspoons) a day if you're a man. Even less may be better for your heart. (See "What Should I Eat?" Oct. 2009, p. 1.)
- Don't drink sugar-sweetened beverages. Limit fruit juices to no more than I cup a day.
- Limit all added sugars, including high-fructose corn syrup, cane or beet sugar, evaporated cane juice, brown rice syrup, agave syrup, and honey.
- Don't worry about the naturally occurring sugar in fruit, milk, and plain yogurt.
- If a food has little or no milk or fruit (which contain natural sugars), the "Sugars" number on the package's Nutrition Facts panel will tell you how many grams of added sugars are in each serving. Multiply the grams by 4 to get calories from sugar. Divide the grams by 4 to get teaspoons of sugar.

Notes

1. *JAMA 292:* 927, 2004.
2. *Am. J. Clin. Nutn 87:* 1662, 2008.
3. *Am. J. Clin. Nutr. 89:* 438, 2009.
4. *Int. J. Obes. 24:* 794, 2000.
5. *Am. J. Clin. Nutn 51:* 963, 1990.
6. *Am. J. Clin. Nutr. 76:* 721, 2002.
7. *Br. J. Nutr. 97:* 193, 2002.
8. *J. Clin. Invest. 119:* 1322, 2009.
9. *Am. J. Clin. Nutr 95:* 283, 2012.
10. cdc.gov/nchs/data/databriefs/db71.htm.
11. *Am. J. Clin. Nutr. 94:* 479, 2011.
12. *Obesity 20:* 689, 2011.
13. *J. Nutr. 142:* 251, 2012.
14. *Diabetes Care 33:* 2477, 2010.
15. *Am. J. Clin. Nutn 89:* 1037, 2009.
16. *Circulation 116:* 480, 2007.
17. *JAMA 303:* 1490, 2010.
18. *Eur. J. Clin. Nutr. 66:* 201, 2012.
19. *J. Clin. Endocrinol. Metab. 96:* E1596, 2011.
20. *BMJ 336:* 309, 2008.
21. *Circulation 120:* 1011, 2009.
22. *J. Nutr. 140:* 1832, 2010.

Critical Thinking

1. Describe the conclusions from the research studies conducted in Denmark and Switzerland on the effect of soda on visceral fat.
2. Identify the organs that are impacted by the increased fat accumulation linked to drinking soda.
3. Explain why drinking soda leads to higher levels of fat in the blood and stored in the body.

A Diabetes Cliffhanger

Researchers are baffled by the worldwide increase in type 1 diabetes, the less common form of the disease

MARYN MCKENNA

When public health officials fret about the soaring incidence of diabetes in the U.S. and worldwide, they are generally referring to type 2 diabetes. About 90 percent of the nearly 350 million people around the world who have diabetes suffer from the type 2 form of the illness, which mostly starts causing problems in the 40s and 50s and is tied to the stress that extra pounds place on the body's ability to regulate blood glucose. About 25 million people in the U.S. have type 2 diabetes, and another million have type 1 diabetes, which typically strikes in childhood and can be controlled only with daily doses of insulin.

For reasons that are completely mysterious, however, the incidence of type 1 diabetes has been increasing throughout the globe at rates that range from 3 to 5 percent a year. Although the second trend is less well publicized, it is still deeply troubling, because this form of the illness has the potential to disable or kill people so much earlier in their lives.

No one knows exactly why type 1 diabetes is rising. Solving that mystery—and, if possible, reducing or reversing the trend—has become an urgent problem for public health researchers everywhere. So far they feel they have only one solid clue.

"Increases such as the ones that have been reported cannot be explained by a change in genes in such a short period," says Giuseppina Imperatore, who leads a team of epidemiologists in the Division of Diabetes Translation at the U.S. Centers for Disease Control and Prevention. "So environmental factors are probably major players in this increase."

A Challenge of Counting

Type 1 and type 2 diabetes share the same underlying defect—an inability to deploy insulin in a manner that keeps blood sugar from rising too high—but they arise out of almost opposite processes. Type 1, which once was known as juvenile diabetes, is an autoimmune disease in which the body attacks its own cells—namely, the beta cells of the pancreas—destroying their ability to make insulin. In type 2, formerly known as adult-onset diabetes, tissues that need insulin to take up glucose (such as the liver, muscles and fat) become resistant to insulin's

presence. The insulin-producing cells respond by going into overdrive, first making more of the hormone than normal and then losing the ability to keep up with the excess glucose in the blood. Some people end up unable to make insulin at all.

The first strong signal that the incidence of type 1 diabetes was on the rise came in 2006, from a World Health Organization project known as DIAMOND (a combination of words in several languages for worldwide diabetes). That survey, which looked at 10 years of records from 112 diabetes research centers in 57 countries, found that type 1 had risen an average of 5.3 percent a year in North America, 4 percent in Asia and 3.2 percent in Europe.

Statistics from Europe—where the single-payer health care systems that care for residents throughout their lives generate rich stores of data—back up that first finding. In 2009 researchers from a second project called EURODIAB compared diabetes incidence across 17 countries and found not only that type 1 was rising—by 3.9 percent a year on average—but also that it was increasing most quickly among children younger than five. By 2020, they predicted, new cases of type 1 diabetes in that age group will nearly double, from 3,600 children to an estimated 7,076 children.

Most assessments of diabetes in the U.S. have been more partial and local. There is one comprehensive national surveillance project, the federally funded SEARCH for Diabetes in Youth study, which published data in 2007. Because that was an initial report, however, researchers could not compare it with earlier years. Still, when looked at against the findings of other studies, it suggests a rising tide. For example, the 2007 study found higher rates of type 1 in the U.S. than did the WHO's worldwide study of the year before. In addition, the SEARCH study results were sharply higher than regional studies from the 1990s in Alabama, Colorado and Pennsylvania.

Competing Hypotheses

The challenge for explaining the rising trend in type 1 diabetes is that if the increases are occurring worldwide, the causes must also be. So investigators have had to look for influences

Annual Percent Change in Type 1 Diabetes Incidence by Region and Age Group (1990–1999)

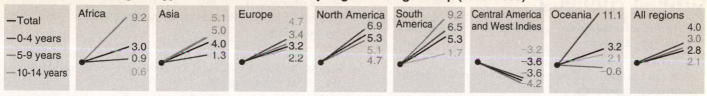

Global mystery: Although some regions (Africa, Asia) are starting from a lower base than others (North America, Europe), the incidence of type 1 diabetes is growing everywhere except the West Indies (where the decline can be traced to one country—Cuba).

that stretch globally and consider the possibility that different factors may be more important in some regions than in others.

The list of possible culprits is long. Researchers have, for example, suggested that gluten, the protein in wheat, may play a role because type 1 patients seem to be at higher risk for celiac disease and the amount of gluten most people consume (in highly processed foods) has grown over the decades. Scientists have also inquired into how soon infants are fed root vegetables. Stored tubers can be contaminated with microscopic fungi that seem to promote the development of diabetes in mice.

None of those lines of research, though, have returned results that are solid enough to motivate other scientists to stake their careers on studying them. So far, in fact, the search for a culprit resembles the next-to-last scene in an Agatha Christie mystery—the one in which the detective explains which of the many suspects could not possibly have committed the crime.

The last scene in the drama, unfortunately, still has not been written. Currently the suspects getting the closest scrutiny are infections with bacteria, viruses or parasites. The presumptive etiology: a version of the "hygiene hypothesis" that links clean modern lifestyles and allergies.

The hygiene hypothesis proposes that early exposure to infections or soil organisms teaches the developing immune system how to maintain itself in balance and so keeps it from reacting in an uncontrolled way later in life when it encounters allergens such as dust and ragweed. Living hygienically, it goes on to say, has deprived children of those early exposures, fueling an epidemic of allergies. The diabetes version of the hygiene hypothesis proposes that when the immune system learns not to overreact to allergens, it also learns to tolerate compounds from the body's own tissues—and therefore prevents the autoimmune attack that destroys the ability to make insulin.

Some circumstantial evidence supports that proposal. Children with multiple siblings—who might bring infections home from day care or school—are less likely to be hospitalized for type 1 diabetes (a proxy measure for incidence). The disease is also less common in children who attend day care themselves, and it is more common in specially bred mice that do not encounter infections because they are raised in a sterile environment.

By themselves, however, those findings do not make the case. Christopher Cardwell, a lecturer in medical statistics at Queen's University Belfast, has conducted meta-analyses of associations between type 1 and birth order, maternal age at birth, and birth by cesarean section, all of which affect the organisms to which young children are exposed. "All of these seemed to be associated," he says, "but they all were in my opinion fairly weak associations. None were of a magnitude that could explain the increasing incidence over time."

Back to Fat

Recently the search for a cause behind the rise of type 1 diabetes has taken an unexpected turn. Some investigators are reconsidering the role of an old adversary: being overweight or obese.

That suspicion might seem counterintuitive given that diabetes dogma holds that being overweight tugs the body toward producing large amounts of insulin (as in type 2), not too little insulin. But some contend that the stress of producing all that extra insulin can burn out the insulin-producing beta cells of the pancreas and push a child whose beta cells are already under attack into developing type 1 diabetes. This idea, called the accelerator or overload hypothesis, proposes that "if you have a kid who is chubby, that extra adiposity is going to challenge the pancreatic beta cells," says Rebecca Lipton, an emeritus professor at the University of Chicago. "In a child who has already started the autoimmune process, those beta cells are just going to fail more quickly, because they are being forced to put out more insulin than in a thin child."

Overweight makes a logical perpetrator. People are packing on the pounds in rich countries and poor ones. Of course, investigators want to do more than just to explain the rise of type 1 diabetes; they want to prevent it. Unfortunately, if excess weight is a major contributor to the problem, that task will not be easy. No one, so far, has been able to slow the global obesity epidemic. (By 2048, according to researchers from Johns Hopkins University, all American adults will be at least overweight if present trends continue.) Until societies can ensure that most children (not to mention adults) are more physically active, eat healthfully and maintain a normal weight, diabetes researchers will be in the position of detectives who, having solved a murder, realize they can do nothing to prevent the next one.

Critical Thinking

1. Differentiate the physiological differences between type 1 and type 2 diabetes.

2. Contrast the competing hypotheses that attempt to explain the rise in type 1 diabetes: the hygiene hypothesis and the overload hypothesis.

3. Explain why type 1 is considered an autoimmune disease.

Maryn McKenna is a journalist, a blogger and author of two books about public health. She writes about infectious diseases, global health and food policy.

Source: "Incidence and Trends of Childhood Type 1 Diabetes Worldwide 1990–1999," by Diamond Project Group, *In Diabetic Medicine,* Vol. 23, No. 8: August 2006

Nutrition and Immunity

Balancing Diet and Immune Function

Susan S. Percival, PhD

This article briefly reviews the components of the immune system with emphasis on a particular leukocyte, the gamma delta ($\gamma\delta$) T cell. The importance of nutrition in this large and complex system cannot be underestimated. All nutrients, macro and micro, are required in an optimum balance for the proper function of immunity. The issue is that an optimum balance specifically for the role of immunity in humans is not well understood. This article describes some of the consequences of nutrient deficiencies, but more importantly discusses foods that help maintain or balance the immune response by the $\gamma\delta$ T cell. The consequences of an immune system that is out of balance are also discussed.

Functional Immunity
Parts and Location

Immune cells originate in the bone marrow. Some cells differentiate there, in the marrow (neutrophils, other granulocytes, and B cells), whereas others travel to the thymus (T cells) to differentiate. Some cells, for example, monocytes, travel through the blood and differentiate into macrophages in the tissues. Whereas the blood cells are the best studied because of their accessibility, many of our immune cells reside in the skin and the epithelial linings of the gut, lung, and reproductive system. The gut, because of its large surface area, is the largest immune organ in the body.

Three Modes of Operation

The first mode of operation is known as surveillance (Figure). To survey their environment, the immune cells migrate in and out of the lymph, blood, and tissues. Some maintain residence in tissues or lymph, whereas others never stop moving. Both static cells and migrating cells can be "samplers," testing their immediate surroundings for evidence of foreign invaders. Surveillance

destroys foreign invaders without any symptoms of illness. One particular cell involved in surveillance is the $\gamma\delta$ T cell, whose importance is a central focus of this report.

The second mode of operation is the activation or response. If surveillance is not enough to combat the foreign invader, the immune system goes into action, which is known as the response mode. First, signaling molecules such as cytokines (peptides), leukotrienes, and prostaglandins (lipids) are synthesized and secreted, resulting in a complex network of communication signals to other cells of the immune system. Cell numbers expand greatly, and eventually, the foreigner is destroyed by cytotoxic activity of the immune cells. Symptoms of illness, including inflammation and fever, accompany the response.

To understand the response capacity of immunity, the general organization will be covered first. In most of the literature, immunity is organized into 2 systems, the innate immune system and the adaptive (or acquired) immune system (Table). The cells of our innate immune system react within minutes to a foreign invasion. They kill pathogen using free radicals and other toxic chemicals, and they recognize foreign invaders by their nonspecific patterns. The innate cells express receptors on their cell surfaces that recognize nonspecific patterns known as pathogen-associated molecular patterns (PAMPs). Bacteria, for example, contain unique molecules such as lipopolysaccharide, not found in any other plant or animal. Other PAMPs are derived from viruses, protozoa, and fungi and include molecules such as peptidoglycans, lipoproteins, flagellin, double-stranded and single-stranded RNA from viruses, imidazoquinolines, CpG DNA motifs, and teichoic acids. Our innate immune system uses pattern recognition receptors to detect PAMP, and this recognition results in an immune response. Interaction of the PAMP with the pattern recognition receptors sets off a chain reaction of signaling molecules such as cytokines,

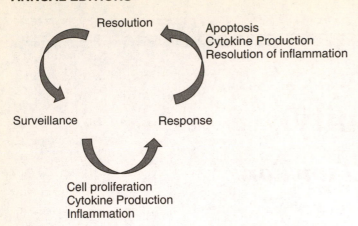

Figure. The cyclic nature of immunity. Surveillance is the nonsymptomatic mode of handling foreign invaders. When surveillance is not enough, activation of the immune response occurs, driven by cytokines and lipid mediators. Once the foreign invader has been disposed of, then an active process operates to resolve inflammation so that it returns to surveillance.

prostaglandins, and leukotrienes. These mediators, in turn, cause activation of the adaptive (or acquired) immune cells, the alpha beta ($\alpha\beta$) T cells and the B cells. The adaptive cells may take up to days to fully respond. They get their signals not only from the innate cells' signaling molecules but also from antigen-presenting cells. Each T or B cell of the adaptive immune system produces a unique receptor, and each cell responds to very specific antigens, not just a generalized pattern. Cells of the adaptive immune system have the ability to distinguish between self and nonself. Their mode of killing is by initiating apoptosis or programmed cell death. These cells are influenced by previous exposures to pathogens and thus are said to have memory.

Finally, the third mode is the return to normal surveillance. When the pathogen has been destroyed, the immune system returns to surveillance mode. This return to normal surveillance is an active process utilizing specific cells such as $\gamma\delta$ T cells, macrophages, natural killer cells, and CD8$^+$ T cells to destroy activated immune cells to end the response. The consequence of not ending the response is chronic inflammation and is discussed in the following section.

Nutritional Aspects
Nutrient Deficiencies
Many examples exist in the literature of specific nutrient deficiencies that result in impaired immunity and an impaired immune response. Protein-calorie malnutrition, essential lipid deficiency, and vitamin and mineral deficits all result in some aspect of impaired immunity. Nutrients are important for synthesis and secretion of signaling molecules, cell proliferation, free radical generation, and the active process of immune suppression at the end of the response. Lacking any nutrient would impair the response.

Nutrition for Surveillance and for the Response
A healthy, balanced diet provides all nutrients necessary for adequate operation of the surveillance mode because that is the normal condition under which nutrient requirements were determined. However, it is much more difficult to study the increased nutrient requirements during the immune response, but considering that cell proliferation is a major part of the response, all nutrients are required in greater quantity. To determine how much of an increased need occurs during the response, nutrient requirements would have to be studied at the onset of illness. Some of the nutrients for which information is available and that show a greater need in the context of the immune response include conditionally essential amino acids,[1,2] zinc,[3] and magnesium.[4] An exception to the generalized statement that all nutrients are needed in greater

Table. Origin and Function of Immune Cells

Branch	Cell	Differentiation Location	Specialized Function
Acquired	B cell	Bone marrow	Secret antibodies
	T cell	Thymus	Cytotoxic, helper, regulatory
Innate	Monocyte	Bone marrow	Further differentiates to macrophages
	Macrophage	Tissues (see monocyte)	Phagocytosis, respiratory burst
	Neutrophils	Bone marrow	Phagocytosis, respiratory burst
	Other granulocytes:	Bone marrow	Various: basophils, eosinophils, mast cells
Characteristics of both	$\gamma\delta$ T cell	Thymus	Cytotoxic, regulatory
	Natural killer cell	Bone marrow	Cytotoxic

amounts is iron, because it appears to be sequestered during an immune response.

Other indirect evidence that suggests initiating an immune response requires more nutrients is due to the nature of the response itself: in addition to the demands for cellular proliferation, the immune response must synthesize and secrete signaling molecules and antibodies. Although it is difficult to pinpoint exactly how much more of a specific nutrient is needed, some research suggests that greater doses of nutrients may reduce the severity of a cold or flu. A meta-analysis[5] suggests that gram quantities of vitamin C taken regularly had no effect on the incidence of common cold symptoms but were beneficial in that they reduced the duration of the cold. However, a subgroup exposed to extreme conditions (exercise and/or cold weather) did have a reduced incidence when supplemented with gram quantities of vitamin C. The mechanism by which vitamin C works to reduce severity of an illness is not clear.

Folic acid and other B vitamins that are involved in 1-carbon metabolism are also considered critical nutrients for the response mode. Because of the rapid proliferation of many immune cell types, the need to synthesize DNA, transcribe message, and translate proteins may require more of these vitamins.

Vitamins A and D, because of their role in cellular differentiation and transcription, are theoretically required in greater amount when mounting an immune response. The stores of nutrients may be enough to handle the increased need without requiring an increased intake, but nonetheless are used by the body to a greater extent for an immune response.

During the response, assessing nutrient requirements is more challenging. Nutrients are required in greater quantity when the immune system is responding, but what ones, and how much, is not known. Studying simple illness in humans is not easy, unless perhaps it is under controlled conditions, such as a viral challenge. Humans are genetically or environmentally dissimilar, but even more challenging is that humans have differences in vaccination histories as well as immunological memories. In other words, different people will respond in different ways to the same challenge.

Consequences of Not Ending an Immune Response

Inflammation is a necessary component of the immune response. What is inflammation, exactly? It is a collection of symptoms described more than 2000 years ago as swelling, due to increased permeability of the capillaries resulting in edema, redness, and heat due to increased blood flow, and pain due to stimulation of nerve endings.

Some of these symptoms occur because of the release of reactive oxygen species that are part of the killing mechanism of the innate immune system. Other symptoms are from the effect of the cytokines and lipid mediators that drive the inflammatory process and set the stage for both the eradication of the foreign invader and the repair of damaged tissues. Normally, mechanisms are in place to restore the immune response to its surveillance mode. However, in some circumstances, the immune system inappropriately stays "on" because it is chronically stimulated by some foreign invasion that cannot be eradicated, or the mechanism to turn inflammation off is impaired. Chronic inflammation is thought to be responsible for many diseases.

Conversely, the disease itself might be a cause of chronic inflammation. Heart disease, cancer, rheumatoid arthritis, inflammatory bowel disease, and some neurological disorders have symptoms that suggest chronic inflammation may be involved in the disease process. Reactive oxygen species that are generated during chronic inflammation may cause damage to host macromolecules if not contained or neutralized. For example, oxidized low-density lipoprotein molecules may be viewed as foreign by the immune system and are taken up by macrophages in the arterial vessel walls. Reactive oxygen species may damage cellular DNA, and this damage may have some relationship to cancer, although cancer is much more complex than simple DNA damage. Oxidation of proteins affects the elasticity of cell membranes and may impair function of enzymes. Some neurological disorders are associated with oxidized proteins in the brain. Damage to carbohydrate moieties, specifically those in the joint fluids such as hyaluronic acid, is thought to be associated with some forms of arthritis. To summarize, inflammation is important for an immune response, but there are circumstances where it may be dysregulated. Can diet help alleviate some of the repercussions of chronic inflammation? And, importantly, can dietary factors be helpful in helping to resolve the inflammation after it is no longer needed for the immune response?

Good evidence has been published that omega-3 fatty acids play a role in resolving inflammation when the response is no longer needed. The omega-3 fatty acids of importance are eicosapentaenoic acid and docosahexaenoic acid, 20:5n-3 and 20:6n-3, respectively. The synthesis of lipid mediators from these fatty acids produces inflammatory products of lower bioactivity compared with those derived from arachidonic acid, 20:4n-6. Moreover, eicosapentaenoic acid and docosahexaenoic acid can produce lipid mediators with anti-inflammatory activity. The potent anti-inflammatory mediators are known as the resolvins and protectins.[6]

Priming as a Means to Optimize Immune Response

The ability to prime our immune cells is poorly defined, mechanistically. B cells are primed as a result of vaccinations. In this sense, B cells are trained to recognize an attenuated foreign invader and forms memory cells that can respond faster and more effectively in the event that foreign invader is encountered again.

Certain molecules prime the immune cell without overtly activating the cell because they interact only weakly. Known as nonmicrobial priming, it is a fairly new concept in relation to dietary compounds and results in upregulation of mRNA transcripts but no translation of protein.[7] The immune cell is primed by certain food ingredients and is now able to respond quicker and more effectively to eradicate the real foreign invader because the building blocks are already present. Some of the molecules that can weakly interact with immune cells and prime them are found in foods of plant origin. The complex molecular structure of some phytochemicals may look similar to a PAMP, but not similar enough to result in activation.

Evidence That Some Food Ingredients Prime Immune Cells

This portion of the article discusses recent research showing evidence of priming of the $\gamma\delta$ T cell by food and food components. First, the $\gamma\delta$ T cell is briefly described, and then, the food components that prime this cell are briefly reviewed.

The $\gamma\delta$ T cell resides mainly in the skin and in the epithelial linings of the gut, lungs, and reproductive tract. There they act as a first line of defense against pathogens that are eaten or inhaled. About 5 percent to 8 percent of human T cells in the blood are the $\gamma\delta$ T cells, with the remainder circulating T cells the more common $\alpha\beta$ T cell. Although they are a T cell, carrying the T-cell receptor (TCR), they behave more like innate cells in that they recognize PAMPs and do not require recognition of the major histocompatibility complex as does the $\alpha\beta$ T cell.

Generally, the $\gamma\delta$ T cells are studied with those isolated from the blood because acquiring them from tissue, in humans, at least, is not feasible. Some of the $\gamma\delta$ T cells may be naive, meaning they have not interacted with pathogen. But some may have already surveyed their environment, have interacted with foreign objects, and are now migrating through the blood to other locations.[8] Thus, some of the $\gamma\delta$ T cells isolated from the blood have been exposed to food components in the gut, and the functional changes due to diet can be measured in $\gamma\delta$ T cells obtained from blood samples, regardless of whether the food components have been absorbed.

In addition to the ability of $\gamma\delta$ T cells to kill pathogen-infected cells and malignant cells, they are also necessary to turn off the immune response. In animal models where the $\gamma\delta$ TCR is knocked out, the animals are inflamed.[9,10] Adding another inflammatory stress to $\gamma\delta$-TCR knock-out mouse model is fatal. The researchers showed that $\gamma\delta$ cells physically interacted with activated macrophages, resulting in macrophage cell death, and were required to end the response. If dietary compounds can enhance the function of $\gamma\delta$ T cells, then diet may be instrumental in providing anti-inflammatory activity as well.

The relationship between diet and the $\gamma\delta$ T cell was first published in 1999.[11,12] These studies showed that drinking tea beverage compared with coffee resulted in an increased $\gamma\delta$ T-cell proliferation and interferon γ synthesis. The mechanism by which tea was thought to work was through a unique amino acid, L-theanine. After L-theanine is consumed, it is hydrolyzed to glutamic acid and ethylamine by the kidney.[13,14] Ethylamine is thought to be the nonmicrobial antigen that interacts with the $\gamma\delta$ T cell.

If a compound from tea interacts with the $\gamma\delta$ T cell, we asked if other fruits and/or vegetables also interact with this cell. In 2 studies, $\gamma\delta$ T-cell numbers were increased in the blood when subjects were fed a fruit and vegetable concentrate[15] or grape juice from Concord grapes (publication in review). The cellular proliferative capacity was not changed, but in 1 study,[15] a reduction in circulating interferon γ was observed, which suggests lower inflammatory activity.

A capsule containing a standardized mixture of tea components, L-theanine and catechins, showed an ability to functionally change $\gamma\delta$ T cells after consumption.[16,17] In these studies, people consumed a defined amount of L-theanine with tea catechins for 10 weeks. White blood cells from the subjects were then incubated ex vivo, with the compound responsible for priming them, ethylamine, and the results showed a greater activation and proliferation of $\gamma\delta$ T cells from subjects consuming L-theanine compared with those obtained from people consuming the placebo. A greater concentration of interferon γ was also produced by the cells from the L-theanine consumers. One of the inflammatory biomarkers that were measured was reduced, whereas a second one went unchanged.[16] The subjects taking the tea components experienced fewer cold and flu symptoms during the study.

Results of these studies led to the hypothesis that the phytochemicals found in plants can prime the $\gamma\delta$ T cell. Other in vitro research showed that $\gamma\delta$ T cells interact with proanthocyanidins and result in increased proliferation and activation.[18] Despite limitations to in vitro cell culture studies, we hypothesize that in vivo the $\gamma\delta$ T cells obtained from blood may have interacted with phytochemicals while residing in the gut. γδ T cells migrate out of the gut into the bloodstream where they are isolated and shown to have functional changes. The hypothesis of nonmicrobial priming suggests that the weak interaction of food phytochemicals with the cells does not activate the cell, but only primes it to respond better and faster to a secondary stimulus.[7] Although phytochemicals are not essential for life, as is a classic nutrient, they are beneficial to health.

Summary

All nutrients are important for maintaining immunity and providing appropriate amounts of protein, fat, carbohydrate, vitamins, and minerals for the surveillance mode of keeping us from getting sick. More nutrients are required during pathogen invasion, but it proves more difficult to study exactly what is the "right" balance of nutrients that are required to provide an optimal response when invaded by pathogen.

The food ingredients mentioned in relation to priming of the γδ T cells are plant-derived compounds. Thus, the best advice for a healthy immune system is to consume fruits and vegetables and includes tea. Vitamin C, folic acid and other B vitamins, vitamins A and D, phytochemicals, and food fiber all work to keep the immune system functioning without overresponsiveness (inflammation) or underresponsiveness (illness). These compounds do not appear to be stored in the body; therefore, to maintain a primed state requires daily consumption, to maximize exposure and thus benefits. Priming immune cells promotes a faster and stronger response. γδ T cells are unique cells that are important in surveillance, response, and ending the response. They appear to be supported by dietary compounds in a manner consistent with health benefits.

References

1. Furst P. Conditionally indispensable amino acids (glutamine, cyst(e)ine, tyrosine, arginine, ornithine, taurine) in enteral feeding and the dipeptide concept. *Nestle Nutr Workshop Ser Clin Perform Prog.* 2000;3:199–217; discussion 217–219, 199–217.
2. Manhart N, Stehle P. Nutritive amino acids—effective modulators of the immune response. *Forum Nutr.* 2003;56:151–154.
3. Raqib R, Roy SK, Rahman MJ, et al. Effect of zinc supplementation on immune and inflammatory responses in pediatric patients with shigellosis. *Am J Clin Nutr.* 2004;79:444–450.
4. Tam M, Gomez S, Gonzalez-Gross M, Marcos A. Possible roles of magnesium on the immune system. *Eur J Clin Nutr.* 2003;57:1193–1197.
5. Douglas RM, Hemila H, Chalker E, Treacy B. Vitamin C for preventing and treating the common cold. *Cochrane Database Syst Rev.* 2007:CD000980.c.
6. Galli C, Calder PC. Effects of fat and fatty acid intake on inflammatory and immune responses: a critical review. *Ann Nutr Metab.* 2009;55:123–139.
7. Jutila MA, Holderness J, Graff JC, Hedges JF. Antigen-independent priming: a transitional response of bovine gamma delta T-cells to infection. *Anim Health Res Rev.* 2008;17:1–11.
8. Brandes M, Willimann K, Lang AB, et al. Flexible migration program regulates gamma delta T-cell involvement in humoral immunity. *Blood.* 2003;102:3693–3701.
9. Carding SR, Egan PJ. Gamma delta T cells: functional plasticity and heterogeneity. *Nat Rev Immunol.* 2002;2:336–345.
10. Egan PJ, Carding SR. Downmodulation of the inflammatory response to bacterial infection by gamma delta T cells cytotoxic for activated macrophages. *J Exp Med.* 2000;191:2145–2158.
11. Bukowski JF, Morita CT, Brenner MB. Human γδ T cells recognize alkylamines derived from microbes, edible plants, and tea: implications for innate immunity. *Immunity.* 1999;11:57–65.
12. Kamath AB, Wang L, Das H, Li L, Reinhold VN, Bukowski JF. Antigens in tea-beverage prime human Vgamma 2Vdelta 2 T cells in vitro and in vivo for memory and nonmemory antibacterial cytokine responses. *Proc Natl Acad Sci U S A.* 2003;100:6009–6014.
13. Mitchell SC, Zhang AQ, Smith RL. Ethylamine in human urine. *Clin Chim Acta.* 2000;302:69–78.
14. Unno T, Suzuki Y, Kakuda T, Hayakawa T, Tsuge H. Metabolism of theanine, gamma-glutamylethylamide, in rats. *J Agric Food Chem.* 1999;47:1593–1596.
15. Nantz MP, Rowe CA, Nieves C Jr, Percival SS. Immunity and antioxidant capacity in humans is enhanced by consumption of a dried, encapsulated fruit and vegetable juice concentrate. *J Nutr.* 2006;136:2606–2610.
16. Nantz MP, Rowe CA, Bukowski JF, Percival SS. Standardized capsule of *Camellia sinensis* lowers cardiovascular risk factors in a randomized, double-blind, placebo-controlled study. *Nutrition.* 2009;25:147–154.
17. Rowe CA, Nantz MP, Bukowski JF, Percival SS. Specific formulation of *Camellia sinensis* prevents cold and flu symptoms and enhances γδ T cell function: a randomized, double-blind, placebo-controlled study. *J Am Coll Nutr.* 2007;26:445–452.
18. Holderness J, Jackiw L, Kimmel E, et al. Select plant tannins induce IL-2Ralpha up-regulation and augment cell division in gamma delta T cells. *J Immunol.* 2007;179:6468–6478.

Critical Thinking

1. List the nutrients that support the proper function of T cells.

2. Summarize the immune response to a pathogen and the type of nutrients involved in each phase.

3. Discuss the challenges of conducting research on the nutrient requirements of the immune response.

SUSAN S. PERCIVAL, PHD, is a professor of nutritional sciences in the Department of Food Science and Human Nutrition at the University of Florida, Gainesville. Her educational background includes a master's of science degree from the University of California, Davis, and a PhD from the University of Texas, Austin. She did her postdoctoral research in the Department of Biochemistry and Biophysics at Texas A&M University. From 1978 to 1981, she was tenure track faculty at the University of Rhode Island prior to an educational leave to pursue her doctorate. In 2004, she took an 8-month sabbatical leave at the National Institutes of Health with the Nutritional Sciences Research Group at the National Cancer Institute. She currently teaches courses on current issues in dietary supplements, research planning, and nutrition and immunity. Her current research deals with how dietary components influence immunity. Experimental models in cell culture, mice, and in humans reveal that certain dietary components including bioactive compounds from fruits and vegetables, herbs and spices, red wine, and green tea affect specific branches of immunity. These plant bioactive food components have benefits not only with their protective antioxidant capacity, but also through their ability to affect intracellular signaling pathways and prime immune cells to activate faster and to a greater extent when stimulated to do so. Funding acknowledgements: University of Florida Agriculture Experiment Station, IFAS.

Article 30

How to Save Your Brain

It's most people's biggest health fear. But whether you get dementia, scientists now believe, is mostly a matter of lifestyle; it hinges on what you eat every single day. Here's a guide to making the choices that will preserve a healthy mind—starting right now!

NIKHIL SWAMINATHAN

When it comes to aging, life can be cruel. There's plenty to . . . well . . . let's come right out and say it: think about. What will happen to my looks? What will happen to my body? Will I still be able to pursue my interests? What will happen to my mind?

That last question is now the second leading health concern (after cancer) among adults in at least four Western countries—France, Germany, and Spain, as well as the United States—according to a recent survey by the Harvard University School of Public Health and the Alzheimer Europe consortium. Fear of developing dementia would likely stir even more concern if Americans didn't mistakenly believe a cure for Alzheimer's disease exists (more than 45 percent of U.S. respondents think there is an effective treatment). Despite the lack of a cure, great progress has been made in the past three decades in understanding the disease.

The most common cause of dementia, or severe cognitive decline, and the sixth leading cause of death in the U. S., Alzheimer's disease is marked by difficulty storing new memories and recalling recent events, loss of ability to track day-to-day information, a disrupted sense of time and space, social withdrawal, irritability, and mood swings. The neurodegenerative condition typically manifests after age 60. Life expectancy in the U.S. is currently about 78 years and rising. The 5.4 million Americans who suffer from the illness include 13 percent of those over age 65.

Scientists attribute the debilitating disorder to the gradual accumulation between brain cells of a toxic protein, beta-amyloid, that blocks the transmission of information from cell to cell, wipes out synapses, and disrupts basic neuron function, leading to cell death. Inflammatory processes are also involved in memory loss.

The vast majority of Alzheimer's cases—over 99 percent —occur spontaneously; they are not linked to genetic factors. But they are linked to obesity. Researchers find that the same lifestyle choices that lead people to become obese or develop heart disease also increase the risk of developing dementia.

It comes down to this: Choices we make throughout life about what we put in our bodies may protect against Alzheimer's, or delay its onset. At the very least, says neuroscientist Gary Wenk, "We can slow down the time that it takes for someone to get symptoms." Professor of psychology, neuroscience, and molecular virology, immunology, and medical genetics at The Ohio State University, Wenk is author of the book *Your Brain on Food*.

Heading off dementia, he insists, starts with what we eat. Food should be thought of the same way as the drugs we put in our body. They're all made up of chemicals. Everything we consume prompts a reaction in the brain. Picking the right foods can minimize damage to neurons and preserve a healthy mind as you age.

Public Enemy Number One

It's oxygen—you know, the molecule without which you can't live. We have a complex relationship with the element: We desperately need it to breathe, and it is absolutely essential for metabolism, that is, converting the food we eat into energy. However, it causes us to age.

Proteins, fats, and carbohydrates are made up of chains of carbon atoms bonded together in a variety of ways. The body is built to break down the chains into the basic sugar glucose, which actually fuels our cells. Left over are carbon bonds that are cleared out by every breath we take—inhale oxygen, which binds with carbon to escort it out the body, exhale carbon dioxide. Biology 101.

Unfortunately, rogue, unbound oxygen molecules—free radicals—that invariably form during energy metabolism are toxic to body cells, essentially causing them to rust over time. Normally, the hemoglobin molecule in blood regulates oxygen levels throughout the body so that cells are not overexposed to it. Aging also weakens our natural defenses against free radicals, putting all our cells (including neurons) at risk.

Antioxidant molecules are abundant in nature; plants maintain elaborate systems of them, and they are found notably in colorful fruits and vegetables (compounds like vitamins A, C, and E, beta carotene, and capsaicin, the spice in chili peppers). A diet rich in antioxidants combats the oxidative stress we are constantly under.

In the brain, antioxidants slow neurodegeneration. "The chemicals that give fruits their color are exactly what we want to protect us from oxygen," says Wenk. In fact, by eating foods rich in antioxidants, we're taking advantage of the way another life-form has devised to defend itself against environmental harm. From their own sources of proteins and carbohydrates, plant cells synthesize the chemicals we recognize as antioxidants as shields against bacteria, viruses, and the oxidative stress resulting from exposure to ultraviolet light or the toxin ozone.

"EVERYDAY, YOUR BRAIN (AND BODY) AGES A LITTLE BIT, AND EVERYDAY THERE'S AN OPPORTUNITY TO HELP IT NOT TO."

Because of the basic similarities of evolved life processes, the plant protectors can also help human cells from showing the wear and tear of existence. Blueberries, broccoli, grapes, prunes, strawberries, spinach, artichokes, apples—all contain large amounts of antioxidants, as do herbs and spices like rosemary, turmeric, thyme, and oregano. Bright, yellow-orange turmeric is a classic ingredient in the curries that are a staple of Indian cooking. Please note: The incidence of Alzheimer's disease in India is one-sixth that of the U.S.

Adding antioxidant-rich foods to your diet is a fine hedge against dementia. But you need to add more than one. There are thousands of antioxidants—scientists haven't even come close to discovering them all, although they are now testing some of them, including turmeric, as therapeutic agents. Each has a unique combination of chemicals that fight oxidative damage in a distinctive manner.

Regularly consuming a battery of antioxidants through daily diet negates the need for vitamins and supplements, which, Wenk points out, offer little protection against Alzheimer's disease. "There's a parallel between our health and cancer, which, we've learned over the past 50 years, is something people get when they're exposed to low doses of something day after day," he says. "Every day, your brain (and body) ages a little bit, and every day there's an opportunity to help it not to."

What Your Brain Wants

First thing in the morning, after several hours of sleep, the brain is running low on glucose. Once awake, it's on the hunt for exactly the foods that deliver heaps of glucose. In short, it's jonesing for fries.

Fast carbohydrate sources prompt bursts of insulin, a peptide (or small protein) secreted by the pancreas in response glucose. Insulin's job is to get glucose into cells; in the brain, it ushers glucose into needy neurons. Exquisitely sensitive to glucose levels, insulin rushes into the bloodstream; rapid spikes in insulin levels in response to sugary foods are followed just as quickly by rapid declines in the hormone, as it pushes glucose into cells for energy. The result: You're hungry again a couple of hours later. So, you snack. (A bag of potato chips, perhaps?)

"THE PURPOSE OF EATING ANYTIME AFTER 5 P.M. IS TO GET ENOUGH NUTRIENTS TO GET YOU THROUGH THE NIGHT."

Eating big meals loaded with simple carbohydrates (high glycemic meals), a common practice in the U.S., can, over time, undermine the insulin system. So critical is this metabolic mechanism that the health of the insulin system predicts how well you're aging. When insulin signaling isn't working properly and glucose isn't getting into cells—insulin resistance—neurons are deprived of the

What About our Vices?

Don't assume that a brain-saving diet forbids goodies such as alcohol and chocolate. If consumed in moderation—of course—even daily, such indulgences can be beneficial.

Epidemiologists have evidence that alcohol protects against Alzheimer's disease. It's a powerful solute that helps dissolve fat in the body, offering cardiovascular protection that benefits the brain as well. The trick is not to consume so much that the liver becomes fatty. Red wine contains, in addition, the antioxidant resveratrol, effective against aging. Prefer beer? The hops that give beer its color also have antioxidant properties. Have a bite to eat first; it helps slow absorption of alcohol so you don't get drunk.

That bite could be a small bar of chocolate. "There's no better compound in nature in terms of flavonoids," says Wenk. Dark chocolate is best, due to its high cocoa content. Men who eat chocolate regularly, in fact, are known to live longer than men who do not.

As we age, our bodies don't harness the anti-inflammation powers of chocolate and other foods as well as they once did. There is, however, a substitute, shown to protect against Alzheimer's disease among people in their 60s and 70s. It's marijuana, studies in Wenk's lab show. Inhaled, the chemicals in marijuana travel easily into the brain, where they reduce inflammation and also stimulate neurogenesis, the birth of new neurons, another ability that attenuates with age. Wenk finds that a puff a day is sufficiently anti-inflammatory, although he doesn't encourage anyone to start smoking weed. Aside from the fact that it's not legal in most of the U.S., "it might cause the munchies," he says, "and that's not going to help."

fuel they need for cognition and self-control. Insulin resistance is correlated with increased formation of toxic beta-amyloid in the brain and with type 2 diabetes.

Eating several big meals a day compounds the risk. Instead, Wenk suggests eating only one big meal a day, and its timing is crucial: a varied breakfast. Edibles providing a variety of nutrients that are digested slowly yield sustained energy for the day in a way that minimizes wear and tear on the body. That way, you'll require only small refueling bites the rest of the time you're awake. Envision a breakfast that marries complex carbohydrates, such as oatmeal, a whole grain bagel, grapefruit, or low-fat yogurt; a burst of antioxidants, perhaps in the form of orange juice; and eggs or, say, turkey sausage for protein. You could even throw in a doughnut to give your brain the simple sugar punch it so desperately wants.

Don't forget to add coffee or tea. Your brain will also crave caffeine when you wake. Throughout the night, levels build up of the neurotransmitter adenosine, and that buildup blocks the function of neurons that make another neurotransmitter, acetylcholine, which is critical for paying attention and learning. Caffeine frees up acetylcholine neurons to make you more functional. Coffee and tea also contain antioxidant and anti-inflammatory compounds known as flavonoids.

Coffee protects your brain against aging in yet another way. People who drink five or more cups a day are 85 percent less likely to develop Parkinson's disease, which, in addition to its trademark tremors, can also cause dementia. The downside to a lot of caffeine is insomnia, jitteriness, and stomach problems. Good for the brain. Not so good for the body.

A Nibble Here or There

After breakfast, Wenk recommends, graze every hour or half hour, as needed, on fruit or nuts; due to their fiber (fruit) and fat (nuts) content, they release their payload at a stately pace and are metabolized slowly. There's no rush of chemicals to the brain. Lunch, Wenk says, should be low-fat and colorful. Think: chicken salad or fish and steamed vegetables. The afternoon should hold more nibbles followed by a small dinner.

Free yourself from the notion that dinner consists of appetizer, entrée, and dessert. Most calories should be consumed up front, to give the brain the energy it needs to get through the day. Dinner, Wenk explains, is an opportunity to load up on compounds not eaten earlier—foods with omega-3 fats, such as salmon, kiwi, or walnuts, which help neurons maintain their structural integrity. Says Wenk: "As far as the brain is concerned, the purpose of eating after 5 P.M. is to get enough nutrients to get you through the night without waking up."

All in Moderation

Even with the damage oxygen inflicts on the body, you can't not eat. That said, one very workable strategy for avoiding oxygen overexposure is simply to eat less. "Then you don't have to eat so many other things to protect you from the foods you did eat," Wenk observes.

What To Ditch From Your Diet Now

Obesity is the leading cause of preventable death in the world. According to actuarial charts, body mass index is the most accurate predictor of life span. The excess food it takes to make the normal person obese uses a lot of oxygen for processing. Says Wenk: "First fat ages you, then it kills you."

Once excess calories are turned into fat and stored, fat cells release cytokines, little proteins sent out by the immune system to destroy such interlopers as bacteria. They attack by causing inflammation, which eradicates the foreign bodies. Like much warfare, however, there's collateral damage; neighboring cells are caught in the cross fire. In the brain, inflammation abets dementia—so much so that arthritis sufferers, who typically down lots of anti-inflammatory drugs, tend to bypass dementia.

Taking megadoses of anti-inflammatory drugs has its own risks: gastrointestinal bleeding. Far safer to decrease the size of your belly. A recent report fingered the foods that most lead to long-term weight gain: French fries, potato chips, sugary drinks, red meat, and processed meats such as hot dogs, Eaten regularly, they cause obesity, upping the risk of high cholesterol levels, type 2 diabetes, and dementia.

Caloric-restriction diets (eliminating up to 40 percent of food intake per day) not only slow the aging process but offer cognitive benefits. The trade-off, however, is less energy, less activity, weak bone structure, and frailer musculature. To benefit from such a regimen takes a little experimentation. If you typically eat 2,000 calories a day, try cutting back to 1,600 and seeing whether you still have enough energy for some exercise. Since exercise requires energy—and, thus, oxygen—Wenk recommends two hours a week of aerobic exercise, or as little as three 20-minute walks per week.

When epidemiologists interview older people, those who maintain good mental and physical health often don't report being extremely active, which could cause long-term joint pain that also contributes to aging. "What people tell us is they were frequently active, did a little something everyday, and that seems to have biased them to live longer," Wenk explains. "They didn't tend to overeat, they didn't tend to overexercise. In fact, they didn't tend to live lives of extremes at all. It was always the moderation."

The Age Factor

Your age might also influence the zeal with which you consider adopting Wenk's brain-saving lifestyle. It is, he insists, like investing in the stock market: "If you start early, in your 30s, then you've got time to do the right things. In your 60s, there's less time to invest in your health."

Genetic makeup is a consideration in when to adopt a brain-saving diet. Heritability of Alzheimer's disease, though rare, appears to travel through the female line, Wenk points out. Anyone whose grandmother, mother, or aunt has developed dementia should consider the protective power of immediate lifestyle change.

Since metabolism slows with age, leading many to gain weight later in life, your best brain-saving regimen may be dropping the number of calories you're taking in. Taking weight off is a crucial step in saving one's brain. "The sooner you get started the better," advises Wenk.

In general though, thirtysomethings might begin to incorporate more colorful vegetables into their diet, or shift the bulk of their food intake to earlier in the day. By the time people hit 60, they might do well to remember the lyrics to the Rolling Stones' hit "Ruby Tuesday":

"There's no time to lose, I heard her say/Catch your dreams before they slip away/Dying all the time/Lose your dreams and you will lose your mind/Ain't life unkind?"

Critical Thinking

1. Describe the physiological events in the brain that lead to the decline in mental acuity associated with Alzheimer's disease.

2. Identify the antioxidant nutrients that may slow the progression of dementia.

3. Explain why coffee and tea may enhance attention, learning, and overall brain function.

NIKHIL SWAMINATHAN is an editor at *Archaeology Magazine* in New York.

Soothe the Fire in Your Belly

When to treat heartburn on your own and when to get help.

CONSUMER REPORTS ON HEALTH

Nearly everyone has experienced heartburn after eating a sumptuous or simply oversized meal. For many, the distress dies down within an hour or so—with or without the help of Rolaids or Tums—making it seem like nothing to worry about.

But the millions who suffer from frequent heartburn might actually have a chronic condition called gastroesophageal reflux disease, or GERD. Left untreated it can damage the esophagus and even lead to cancer.

Lifestyle changes and over-the-counter medication can provide relief for many people, but it's important to know if your symptoms are serious enough to warrant a trip to the doctor. And when should you turn to potent medications called proton pump inhibitors (PPIs) to extinguish the flames?

More than 50 million people in the United States experience heartburn every month, and about 15 million have daily flare-ups, according to the National Institute of Diabetes and Digestive and Kidney Diseases. The cost of treating the condition can quickly add up. The average person with GERD, a related ailment, spends an estimated $3,355 a year on medication and other treatments to help keep symptoms under control. Obese people, smokers, and pregnant women are more likely to suffer from GERD, but it can strike otherwise healthy men and women at any age.

How Heartburn Happens

When you swallow food, it travels down your throat to your esophagus into your stomach, which produces acid to help break it down so that it can be digested. Your lower esophageal sphincter, a muscle at the entrance to your stomach, is supposed to close after the food passes through to keep stomach acid from going into the esophagus. But if it doesn't, and acid reaches the esophagus (along with food), you'll feel a burning sensation. It usually starts just below your breastbone and can radiate into your throat. You might also notice a sour or bitter taste in your mouth or throat.

Occasional heartburn is generally not worrisome or dangerous, and can be relieved with diet and lifestyle changes and, if necessary, over-the-counter antacids or other medications. However, if you have heartburn twice a week or more, and it recurs for weeks or months, or if you frequently regurgitate food (with or without heartburn), consider seeing your doctor to be checked for GERD.

In contrast to occasional heartburn, GERD can be dangerous. Over time, the refluxed acid can inflame and erode the lining of the esophagus, resulting in esophagitis. You may feel a chronic soreness in your lower throat or chest.

Most cases of esophagitis are relatively mild, but when it is left untreated, bleeding, scarring, and narrowing of the esophagus can occur, making eating and swallowing painful and difficult. People who have uncontrolled GERD for years have a higher risk of developing cancer of the esophagus, though it's rare.

Fortunately, changes in your diet and lifestyle might be all you need to alleviate the problem. Those measures include eating smaller meals, not lying down for at least three hours after eating, losing weight if needed, and avoiding alcohol.

Certain food and beverages can trigger heartburn in some people, such as citrus fruit, chocolate, coffee or other caffeinated

Choosing the right remedy

Heartburn medication	When appropriate
Antacids (*Maalox, Mylanta, Rolaids, Tums,* and generics)	For occasional heartburn (less than twice a week). You should also make lifestyle changes, such as avoiding food that triggers heartburn and eating smaller meals.
H2 blockers (*Pepcid, Zantac,* and generics)	For occasional heartburn not relieved by antacids and lifestyle changes, or before eating a known heartburn trigger.
Proton pump inhibitors (*Prevacid, Prilosec,* and generics)	For frequent heartburn not relieved by lifestyle changes, antacids, or H2 blockers. After two weeks of use, check with your doctor to determine if you have GERD.

beverages, fried food, garlic, onions, spicy or fatty food, and tomato-rich food, such as marinara sauce, salsa, and pizza.

Drinking alcoholic beverages may increase GERD symptoms, which over time can cause damage to the lining of the esophagus. Symptoms may resolve after you stop drinking.

Smoking weakens the lower esophageal sphincter muscle and increases the risk of GERD (and other diseases), so if you smoke, you should quit. To help reduce heartburn flare-ups while you're asleep, try placing wood blocks beneath your bedposts to raise the head of your bed 6 to 8 inches. Avoid wearing tight clothing or belts that push on your abdomen, since compressing that area can contribute to reflux.

Medication

If diet and lifestyle changes don't help, it might be time to try an antacid, such as *Maalox, Mylanta, Rolaids,* or *Tums.* Some people might need something stronger to relieve their symptoms. In that case, try an acid-reducing H2 blocker such as famotidine (*Pepcid AC* and generic), nizatidine (*Axid AR*), or ranitidine (*Zantac 75, Zantac 150,* and generic). Those drugs help about half of sufferers and can be bought over-the-counter. You might also consider using an over-the-counter PPI, such as lansoprazole (*Prevacid 24HR*), for up to two weeks to see if it eases your symptoms.

If you've tried these options and still have heartburn at least twice a week for several weeks, it's time for a doctor to determine if you have GERD and if it has damaged your esophagus. If you have the condition, he or she will probably recommend that you have an upper endoscopy. This procedure, done under light anesthesia, involves the insertion of a lighted, flexible endoscope tube into your throat and down into the esophagus. The doctor can also use the endoscope to do a biopsy to test for cancer or Barrett's esophagus, which can lead to cancer.

If you have GERD your doctor will probably prescribe a PPI, such as esomeprazole (*Nexium*), lansoprazole (*Prevacid* and generic), or omeprazole (*Prilosec* and generic). Those popular drugs substantially reduce the amount of stomach acid produced, making the contents of your stomach less erosive. If there's already damage to your esophagus, reducing the amount of acid can help it heal.

But many doctors also think that PPIs are overused, a problem that is exacerbated by heavy advertising from pharmaceutical companies. The federal Agency for Healthcare Research and Quality (AHRQ) also noted a widespread overuse of PPIs (as well as other drugs used to treat GERD) in a September 2011 report. Ads have helped propel those drugs to top-selling slots among all prescription medication.

One PPI, *Nexium,* racked up $6.2 billion in sales in 2011, making it the third highest-selling prescription drug in the U.S. last year, according to IMS Health, an industry group that monitors drug sales. But studies have found that up to 70 percent of people who take a PPI may not have GERD and may not need such a potent, expensive medication.

PPIs can also cause serious side effects, including an increased risk of diarrhea associated with Clostridium difficile, an acute, sometimes chronic ailment that can lead to severe intestinal problems and, in rare cases, death. Long-term use can deplete magnesium levels, which can trigger muscle spasms, an irregular heartbeat, and convulsions. Other potential side effects include a higher risk of pneumonia and certain bone fractures, including breaks in the wrist, forearm, and spine.

PPIs can also interact with other medication, so before you take one, make sure it's compatible with other drugs you take. One of the most serious interactions occurs with omeprazole (*Prilosec* and generic) and clopidogrel (*Plavix*), a blood thinner used to reduce the risk of clots that could lead to a heart attack or stroke. According to the U.S. Food and Drug Administration, omeprazole can reduce the effectiveness of *Plavix* by about half, increasing the risk of a heart attack or stroke. *Nexium* and the H2 blocker cimetidine (*Tagamet* and generic) might also interact with *Plavix* in the same way as *Prilosec.*

Is it heartburn or a heart attack?

It's no surprise that people who have heartburn sometimes fear that they're having a heart attack because the symptoms can be very similar. But delaying treatment for a heart attack can be a matter of life and death. Some typical heart attack signs are listed below. Not all people experience the same ones. If you're in doubt, don't take a chance. Chew and swallow a 325-milligram aspirin tablet and call for emergency help.

	Heart attack	Heartburn
Sensation	Pressure, squeezing, tightness, or pain in the center of the chest. Might last for several minutes or go away and come back.	Burning in throat that generally occurs after eating. Can be accompanied by a bitter or sour taste at the back of throat.
Location	Pain or discomfort generally starts in the center of your chest ond spreads to one or both arms, your back, stomach, neck, or jaw.	Pain is usually felt below the breastbone or ribs. It usually doesn't radiate to your shoulders, arms, or neck, but can.
Quick tests	Pain often goes away quickly after taking nitroglycerin, but not everyone will have this medication readily available.	Sensation often goes away soon after taking an antacid, such as Rolaids or Tums.

Other clues	Breaking into a cold sweat, fainting, light-headedness, nausea, rapid heartbeat, shortness of breath.	Pain tends to increase when bending over, exercising, lifting heavy objects, or lying down.
Action	Call for emergency help if you suspect you're having a heart attack. Also chew and swallow a 325-milligram aspirin tablet.	Make lifestyle changes and, if necessary, take heartburn medication.

If you need a PPI, Consumer Reports' Best Buy Drugs report recommends first trying an over-the-counter option, such as generic omeprazole, *Prilosec OTC,* or *Prevacid 24HR.* At less than $1 a day, they cost almost one-tenth the price of several of the prescription alternatives. And for most people, they are as effective as the prescription drugs. But check with your insurance provider to see if over-the-counter PPIs are covered. If not, it may be less expensive to get a prescription PPI because it might only cost you a $5 to $10 drug co-payment.

There's no clear answer about when to consider stopping a PPI, because that decision varies. For some people with GERD, symptoms go away after drug treatment and lifestyle changes, or they recur only periodically. Others appear to have a lifelong battle with GERD, so they may need to continue taking a PPI daily to keep symptoms under control. Some people might even need to consider surgery.

If you are diagnosed with GERD and are given a PPI prescription, ask your doctor how long you should take the medicine. After a few weeks or months, you may be able to slowly taper off the drug and eventually stop taking it without issue. If your symptoms return, you can often resume taking the medicine.

Considering Surgery

If lifestyle changes and medication haven't helped, then surgery may be an option. The standard procedure for GERD is laparoscopic fundoplication, in which the upper part of the stomach is sewn around the lower part of the esophagus. This is intended to help strengthen the sphincter muscle. It often helps relieve reflux symptoms and decrease the use of heartburn medication, according to the 2011 report from the AHRQ.

But some people who have surgery may still need to take drugs. Also, serious side effects can arise from the surgery, including infections, a hernia, and difficulty swallowing. So laparoscopic fundoplication should be used only as a last resort.

Critical Thinking

1. Differentiate between heartburn and gastroesophageal reflux disease (GERD).
2. Identify the groups of individuals who are at higher risk of GERD.
3. Describe the physiology of heartburn and GERD.

When the Liver Gets Fatty

Havard Health Letter

As Americans have gotten fatter, so have their livers, and some hearts may suffer as a result.

There's a fair amount of guesswork to the estimates, but perhaps as many as 20 percent of American adults have some degree of fatty liver disease, a condition that used to occur almost exclusively in people who drink excessively. The epidemics of obesity and diabetes are to blame. Fatty liver affects between 70 percent and 90 percent of people with those conditions, so as obesity and diabetes have become more common, so has fatty liver disease.

Fatty liver disease isn't confined to any one group, and there don't seem to be pronounced gender differences, but studies suggest that Latinos are disproportionately affected. It's primarily a condition of middle age, although children may get it, too. Fatty liver disease is rapidly becoming more common in Asia, and some research suggests that men in India may be especially susceptible.

Plumped-up Liver Cells

The prevailing theory is that the condition gets started because of insulin resistance, which is, in turn, frequently a consequence of obesity and excess fat tissue in the abdomen. When people are insulin resistant, their muscle, fat, and liver cells don't respond normally to insulin, so levels of the hormone—and the blood sugar it ushers into cells—build up in the blood. As a result, the risk of developing diabetes and heart disease increases. But insulin resistance is a complicated metabolic state that also includes an increase in the amount of free fatty acids circulating in the blood.

Fatty liver disease occurs when some of those fat molecules accumulate inside liver cells. The presence of those fattened cells can then lead to inflammation in the liver and damage to surrounding liver tissue. Once that happens, if excess alcohol is not involved, the condition is called nonalcoholic steatohepatitis (*steato-* for fat and *–hepatitis* because the liver is inflamed). Fortunately, that unwieldy name boils down to a handier acronym, NASH. Estimates vary quite a bit, but it seems that 5 percent to 10 percent of people with fatty liver disease go on to develop NASH.

NASH is often a relatively stable, low-grade condition that people live with for years, with few if any symptoms. But it can also start a cascade of serious damage to the liver and attempts by the organ to regenerate itself that culminate in an abundance of scar tissue and impaired liver function—a condition called cirrhosis. Cirrhosis is irreversible and can lead to total failure of the liver. It also is associated with an increased risk for developing liver cancer.

Some studies have shown as few as 3 percent of people with NASH developing cirrhosis, while others have shown as many as 26 percent doing so. There's no test or risk factor that predicts who will develop cirrhosis and who won't, although one study did find that people who are older or whose initial liver biopsies showed more inflammation were at greater risk. It's clear, though, that the prognosis for NASH is far better than it is for steatohepatitis that's the result of heavy alcohol consumption. Perhaps as many as half of all those with alcoholic steatohepatitis (which lacks a handy acronym) go on to develop cirrhosis.

It's just a theory at this point, but people with fatty liver disease and NASH may need to be more worried about heart disease and stroke than about serious liver problems. An article published in *The New England Journal of Medicine* in late 2009 argued that the inflammatory and other factors pumped out by a fat-afflicted liver promote the atherosclerotic process that damages the insides of arteries and makes blood more likely to clot, a combination that can lead to heart attack or stroke. The evidence the authors cited is intriguing, if circumstantial. They pointed to a study showing that people with NASH are twice as likely to die from heart attack or stroke as people without it. And NASH seems to add to the risks that come with excess weight. Overweight men with NASH have higher levels of C-reactive protein, an inflammatory factor, and fibrinogen, a clotting factor, than overweight men without NASH. Moreover, the levels of those and other factors go up as NASH gets more severe.

Diagnosis Requires a Biopsy

Most people with fatty liver disease don't have symptoms, and that's true even if it has developed into NASH. Only occasionally do people feel run-down, or they have an achy feeling in the upper right side of the abdomen, where the liver is located. So, more often than not, fatty liver disease and NASH are discovered incidentally, starting with higher than normal levels of

The Fatty Liver

How It Starts and What It Can Lead to: Abdominal obesity and metabolic syndrome* cause insulin resistance. Insulin resistance increases fatty acid levels in the blood.

Fat accumulates in liver cells

- Up to 20 percent of Americans have fatty livers
- Usually there are no symptoms
- Weight loss can make the liver less fatty
- Excessive alcohol also make the liver fatty

Fat in liver cells causes inflammation and damage to liver tissue

- The medical term is *steatohepatitis* (*steato-* for fat and *-hepatitis* for liver inflammation)
- Steatohepatitis that's not related to alcohol is called nonalcoholic steatohepatitis, or NASH
- A liver biopsy is the only way to definitely diagnose NASH
- Weight loss is the main treatment; vitamin E has shown some promise

Further liver damage results in liver fibrosis and cirrhosis

- Fibrosis is a buildup of fibrous tissue; cirrhosis is a buildup of scar tissue
- Between 3 percent and 26 percent of NASH patients develop cirrhosis
- A small number of people with cirrhosis develop liver cancer

NASH has been linked to an increased risk of heart attack and stroke

- A liver affected by NASH may produce inflammatory factors that promote the atherosclerotic process that narrows blood vessels
- NASH may be just another aspect of metabolic syndrome
- The cause of NASH, not NASH itself, may increase heart attack and stroke risk

* Metabolic syndrome is abdominal obesity along with high triglycerides, high blood pressure, high blood sugar, and low HDL cholesterol.

liver enzymes on a routine blood test. Ultrasound imaging, the same technology used to get pictures of developing fetuses, can be informative: the liver looks bright because the fat shows up as white on the image. But neither an ultrasound nor a CT or MRI scan is completely reliable for making a diagnosis. The fat in the liver is visible, but not the NASH-related inflammation. Some researchers have developed formulas that use a simple blood test and measurements of various hormones, inflammatory factors, and liver enzymes to arrive at a diagnosis, but this work is at a preliminary stage.

Currently, a liver biopsy is the only way to make a definitive diagnosis of fatty liver or NASH. Liver biopsies involve inserting a long needle into the right side of the abdomen and extracting a small piece of liver tissue that can be examined under a microscope. Liver biopsies are an invasive procedure, so they aren't entirely free of risk and complications, but they're also fairly routine these days and can be done on an outpatient basis.

Whether a doctor will order a biopsy to nail down a diagnosis depends on many factors, including whether the person is obese or has diabetes or shows other signs of liver trouble.

Weight Loss is the Treatment

There's been a fair amount of research into using diabetes drugs to treat NASH, even in people who don't have diabetes. Rosiglitazone (sold as Avandia) and pioglitazone (sold as Actos) have been the leading candidates because they reduce insulin resistance, the root cause of fatty livers. They're not looking so promising these days. The FDA has moved to sharply curtail the use of Avandia because it seems to cause heart problems. The results of an important trial published in 2010 in *The New England Journal of Medicine* showed Actos to be no better than a placebo in improving NASH in people without diabetes.

Another diabetes drug, metformin (Glucophage), might prove to be an effective treatment, but there isn't enough evidence yet. Vitamin E is a possibility: the same trial that showed Actos wasn't effective showed some improvement in the livers of people who took large doses (800 IU daily) of the vitamin. But many doctors are wary about prescribing large doses of vitamin E because they've been associated with an increased risk of bleeding. Besides, the improvements in the liver were limited. Fish oil has produced some favorable results, and clinical trials are under way, but it can't be endorsed yet.

These setbacks and uncertainties have left weight loss (ideally from changes in diet and an increase in physical activity) as the only recommended treatment for most cases of fatty liver disease and NASH. In many cases, weight loss seems to have a very direct effect: as people lose weight, the fatty liver becomes less fatty. Crash dieting is a bad idea, though, because rapid weight loss (losing 4 pounds a week or more) can wind up damaging the liver. Of course, if sustained weight loss were easy, a lot of today's health problems would be solved, not just fatty liver disease and NASH.

In addition to encouraging people to lose weight, doctors will often advise people with diabetes who have fatty liver disease or NASH to be vigilant about controlling their blood sugar.

The Bottom Line

Many parts of the body come to grief once people become obese or develop diabetes. It's not surprising that our livers do too, given how central they are to a whole suite of metabolic processes. There's some evidence that a fatty liver may add to the already high risk of heart disease among people who are obese or have diabetes. Fatty livers can also develop into cirrhotic ones if the inflammatory processes take off.

But there are two bright spots in the take-home message about fatty livers. First, most cases stay relatively stable and don't result in serious liver disease. Second, the treatment is not an expensive drug with side effects, but losing weight—and that will benefit many other parts of the body besides the liver.

Critical Thinking

1. Define non-alcoholic steatohepatitis.

2. Explain the relationship of type 2 diabetes and obesity, insulin resistance, and fatty liver disease.

3. How does the prognosis of liver disease caused by excessive alcohol differ from NASH?

4. What is the most effective treatment currently available for NASH?

Excerpted from *Harvard Health Letter,* January 2011. Copyright © 2011 by the President and Fellow of Harvard College. Reprinted with permission via Copyright Clearance Center. www.health.harvard.edu/health.

UNIT 5

Obesity and Weight Control

Unit Selections

Learning Outcomes

After reading this unit, you will be able to:

- Identify the primary factors that have contributed to the obesity epidemic in the world.

- Describe the behavioral approach to weight loss and why it is so effective.

- Interpret the most recent obesity rate data from the National Health and Nutrition Examination Survey (NHANES).

- Evaluate the possible reasons for changes in taste preferences, food cravings, and mental functions that have been reported by individuals who have bariatric surgery.

- Summarize the history of Weight Watchers and the most recent changes in the Points Plus system.

- Compare the actions of the hormones that influence food intake.

- Define food deserts. Where are they more likely to occur?

- Summarize the "food environment" in the United States. Explain why many health professionals refer to our food environment as toxic.

- Develop recommendations of how families can effectively impact the nutrition and health of their children.

- Describe how the Federal Trade Commission, the Centers for Disease Control and Prevention, the Food and Drug Administration, and the Department of Agriculture together are tackling the way food is marketed to children.

- Discuss the health consequences associated with children being overweight or obese.

- Explain how negative stigmas and prevalence of negative messages regarding obesity can potentiate the development of eating disorders.

Student Website

www.mhhe.com/cls

Internet References

American Society of Exercise Physiologists (ASEP)
www.asep.org
Calorie Control Council
www.caloriecontrol.org
Overweight & Obesity
www.cdc.gov/obesity
Shape Up America!
www.shapeup.org

Overweight and obesity have become epidemic in the United States during the last century and are rising at a dangerous rate worldwide. According to the National Health and Nutrition Examination Survey, 35 percent of U.S. adults (78 million people) have a body mass index (BMI) over 30, which is the cut-off for a diagnosis of obesity. Another third of the U.S. population is considered overweight, with BMI of 25–29.9. Therefore, two-thirds of the U.S. population is overweight or obese. Reports suggest that by the year 2050, half of the U.S. population will be considered obese if current trends continue; however, recent analysis indicates that the rate of increase in overweight and obesity in the United States is nearing a plateau rather than the upward slope. The latest statistics from the Centers for Disease Control and Prevention suggest that there has been a slight increase in obesity rates since 2005 compared to the significant increase climb in obesity rates from 1980 to 2005.

Overweight and obesity is prevalent in males and females of all ages, races, and ethnic groups. Data from the National Health and Nutrition Examination Survey (NHANES) have shown that obesity rates among non-Hispanic black women and Mexican American women have increased since 2004. More adult men are now overweight or obese as compared to women. From this data, 74 percent of men and 64 percent of women are overweight or obese.

Prevention efforts are geared toward curtailing obese children from maturing into obese adults. Overweight and obesity burden our current healthcare system and government-supported healthcare reimbursement programs with exorbitant costs of obesity-related chronic diseases. The major health consequences of obesity are heart disease, diabetes, gallbladder disease, osteoarthritis, and some cancers. The cost for treating the degenerative diseases secondary to obesity is approximately $100 billion per year in the United States.

Even though health and nutrition professionals have tried to prevent and combat obesity with behavior modification, a healthy diet, and exercise, it seems that these traditional ways have not proven effective. Fast-food restaurants are the mainstay for many Americans because they offer quick, inexpensive food. Supersizing has become the norm because, in many instances, it's cheaper to order a biggie combo than smaller items individually. Americans are so accustomed to our fast food nation that many people become infuriated when asked to pull up and wait an extra minute for a 2,400-calorie meal. The problem is exacerbated by the food industry's historical plight to earn profi t and market share by providing U.S. consumers with the fatty, sugary, and salty foods that we demand.

Food companies spend millions of dollars in advertising foods loaded with simple sugars, fat, and salt. Their aggressive advertising, coupled with food accessibility and large portion sizes, has impacted the current obesity pandemic. Other obstacles to maintaining a healthy diet are low accessibility and the high cost of eating a healthy diet.

Scientists have reported that fat is a dynamically active endocrine organ that releases hormones and inflammatory proteins

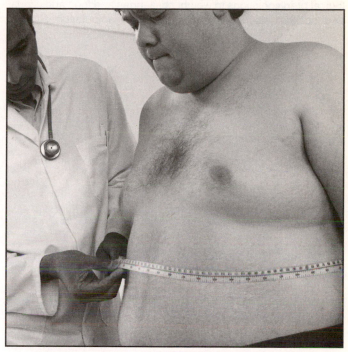

© Science Photo Library RF/Getty Images

that may predispose a person to chronic diseases such as heart disease. In addition, research has discovered the role of the "hunger hormone" and how individual differences affect our ability to lose weight. A positive association was recently found between obesity, especially central obesity, and different types of cancer. Thus, there is a great need for a multifaceted public health approach that would involve mobilization of private and public sectors and focus on building better coping skills and increasing activity.

Globalization is causing the rest of the world and especially developing third world countries to mimic the unhealthy Western diet that contributes to obesity. Obesity and its health consequences are now becoming a global epidemic. Sweetened beverages and the sedentary Western way of life that has been adopted by many developing countries are some of the major contributors of this epidemic.

Intervention and prevention should be the top priorities of policymakers. At the public sector, inclusion of health officials, researchers, educators, legislators, transportation experts, urban planners, and businesses to cooperate in formulating ways to combat obesity is crucial. A sound public health policy would require that weight-loss therapies have long-term maintenance and relapse-prevention measures built into them. Healthy People 2010 is the U.S. government's prevention agenda designed to ensure high quality of life and reduce health risks. One of the 28 areas it focuses on is overweight and obesity. Its main objectives are to reduce the proportion of overweight and obese children, teens, and adults by half and to increase the proportion of adults who are at a healthy weight.

Another perspective to consider about the obesogenic environment in the United States is the affect it is having on people who have or may develop disordered eating. An obesogenic environment is an environment that has norms of inadequate physical activity, consumption of too many calories, promotion of energy-dense foods, a large number of obese people with biological predispositions to weight challenges and food addictions, and societal discrimination and media manipulation of ideal body image. This environment may contribute to disordered eating behavior in people prone to the disease. Conflicting messages such as very thin is beautiful and eating energy-dense foods is attractive and desirable can lead to feelings of helplessness, psychological distress, and self-dislike.

The articles in this chapter may be used to supplement information presented in the energy balance section of general nutrition courses.

How to Fix the Obesity Crisis

Although science has revealed a lot about metabolic processes that influence our weight, the key to success may lie elsewhere.

DAVID H. FREEDMAN

Obesity is a national health crisis—that much we know. If current trends continue, it will soon surpass smoking in the U.S. as the biggest single factor in early death, reduced quality of life and added health care costs. A third of adults in the U.S. are obese, according to the Centers for Disease Control and Prevention, and another third are overweight, with Americans getting fatter every year. Obesity is responsible for more than 160,000 "excess" deaths a year, according to a study in the Journal of the American Medical Association. The average obese person costs society more than $7,000 a year in lost productivity and added medical treatment, say researchers at George Washington University. Lifetime added medical costs alone for a person 70 pounds or more overweight amount to as much as $30,000, depending on race and gender.

All this lends urgency to the question: Why are extra pounds so difficult to shed and keep off? It doesn't seem as though it should be so hard. The basic formula for weight loss is simple and widely known: consume fewer calories than you expend. And yet if it really were easy, obesity would not be the nation's number-one lifestyle-related health concern. For a species that evolved to consume energy-dense foods in an environment where famine was a constant threat, losing weight and staying trimmer in a modern world of plenty fueled by marketing messages and cheap empty calories is, in fact, terrifically difficult. Almost everybody who tries to diet seems to fail in the long run—a review in 2007 by the American Psychological Association of 31 diet studies found that as many as two thirds of dieters end up two years later weighing more than they did before their diet.

Science has trained its big guns on the problem. The National Institutes of Health has been spending nearly $800 million a year on studies to understand the metabolic, genetic and neurological foundations of obesity. In its proposed plan for obesity research funding in 2011, the NIH lists promising research avenues in this order: animal models highlighting protein functions in specific tissues; complex signaling pathways in the brain and between the brain and other organs; identification of obesity-related gene variants; and epigenetic mechanisms regulating metabolism.

This research has provided important insights into the ways proteins interact in our body to extract and distribute energy from food and produce and store fat; how our brains tell us we are hungry; why some of us seem to have been born more likely to be obese than others; and whether exposure to certain foods and toxic substances might modify and mitigate some of these factors. The work has also given pharmaceutical companies numerous potential targets for drug development. What the research has not done, unfortunately, is make a dent in solving the national epidemic.

Maybe someday biology will provide us with a pill that readjusts our metabolism so we burn more calories or resets our built-in cravings so we prefer broccoli to burgers. But until then, the best approach may simply be to build on reliable behavioral-psychology methods developed over 50 years and proved to work in hundreds of studies. These tried-and-true techniques, which are being refined with new research that should make them more effective with a wider range of individuals, are gaining new attention. As the NIH puts it in its proposed strategic plan for obesity research: "Research findings are yielding new and important insights about social and behavioral factors that influence diet, physical activity, and sedentary behavior."

How We Got Here

The desperation of the obese and overweight is reflected in the steady stream of advice pouring daily from sources as disparate as peer-reviewed scientific journals, best-selling books, newspapers and blogs. Our appetite for any diet twist or gimmick that will take the pounds off quickly and for good seems to be as insatiable as our appetite for the rich food that puts the pounds on. We, the public, love to believe in neat fixes, and the media oblige by playing up new scientific findings in headline after headline as if they are solutions.

It doesn't help that the scientific findings on which these headlines are based sometimes appear to conflict. For example, a study in September's *American Journal of Clinical Nutrition* found a link between increased dairy intake and weight loss, although a meta-analysis in the May 2008 *Nutrition Reviews* discovered no such link. A paper in the *Journal of Occupational and Environmental Medicine* in January 2010 postulated a connection between job stress and obesity, but in October a report in the journal *Obesity* concluded there was no such correlation. Part of the problem, too, is that obesity researchers are in some ways akin to the metaphorical blind men groping at different parts of the elephant, their individual study findings addressing only narrow pieces of a complex puzzle.

When the research is taken together, it is clear that the obesity fix cannot be boiled down to eating this or that food type or to taking any other simple action. Many factors contribute to the problem. It is partly environment—the eating habits of your friends, what food is most available in your home and your local stores, how much opportunity you have to move around at work. It is partly biology—there are genetic predispositions for storing fat, for having higher satiety thresholds, even for having more sensitive taste buds. It is partly economics—junk food has become much cheaper than fresh produce. And it is marketing, too—food companies have become masterful at playing on human social nature and our evolutionary "programming" to steer us toward unhealthy but profitable fare. That is why the narrow "eat this" kinds of solutions, like all simple solutions, fail.

When we go on diets and exercise regimens, we rely on willpower to overcome all these pushes to overeat relative to our activity level. And we count on the reward of getting trimmer and fitter to keep us on the wagon. It *is* rewarding to lose the weight, of course. Unfortunately, time works against us. As the weight comes off, we get hungrier and develop stronger cravings and become more annoyed by the exercise. Meanwhile the weight loss inevitably slows as our metabolism tries to compensate for this deprivation by becoming more parsimonious with calories. Thus, the punishment for sticking to our regimen becomes increasingly severe and constant, and the expected reward recedes into the future. "That gap between the reinforcement of eating and the reinforcement of maybe losing weight months later is a huge challenge," says Sung-Woo Kahng, a neurobehaviorist who studies obesity at the Johns Hopkins University School of Medicine and the Kennedy Krieger Institute.

We would be more likely to stick with the regimen if it remained less punishing and more reliably rewarding. Is there a way to make that happen?

From Biology to Brain

The most successful way to date to lose at least modest amounts of weight and keep it off with diet and exercise employs programs that focus on changing behavior. The behavioral approach, tested over decades, involves making many small, sustainable adjustments in eating and exercise habits that are prompted and encouraged by the people and the rest of the environment around us.

The research in support of behavioral weight-loss approaches extends back more than half a century to Harvard University psychologist B. F. Skinner's development of the science of behavioral analysis. The field is founded on the notion

---

Advances in the Lab

The Biology of Obesity

The National Institutes of Health has spent nearly $800 million a year on studies to understand the neurological, metabolic and genetic foundations of obesity. In the process, scientists have uncovered complex biochemical pathways and feedback loops that connect the brain and digestive system; a new appreciation for the regulatory functions of fat tissues; subtle hereditary changes that make some groups more prone to obesity than others; and the strong possibility that exposure to certain foods and toxic substances might modify and mitigate some of these factors. Given that it will likely take decades to understand the various causes of obesity, more surprises are no doubt in store.

- **Brain:** Scientists have long known that the hypothalamus and brain stem help to regulate feelings of hunger and fullness. Over the past several years researchers have found that the pleasure-reward centers of the limbic system and the evaluating functions of the prefrontal cortex are also heavily involved. Indeed, chronic overeating bears biochemical similarities to drug addiction.

- **Metabolism:** The ability to burn and store energy varies greatly from cell to cell. In 2009 three studies in the *New England Journal of Medicine* demonstrated that at least some women and men continue to benefit well into adulthood from small stores of brown fat, which, unlike white fat, is associated with being lean. Brown fat helps to generate heat and is apparently more closely related to muscle than to white fat, whose primary purpose is to store excess energy.

- **Genes:** Researchers have confirmed variations in 20-odd genes that predispose people to gaining weight easily. But further investigation shows that the effects are modest at best and cannot account for the current obesity epidemic. Genes may still play a role, however, through the environment's influence on which ones get turned on or off. So far most such genetic switches for obesity have been identified in mice, although a few likely human candidates are known.

---

that scientists cannot really know what is going on inside a person's brain—after all, even functional MRIs, the state of the art for peering into the mind, are crude, highly interpretable proxies for cognition and emotion that reduce the detailed firing of billions of neurons in complex circuits to a few blobs of color. But researchers can objectively and reproducibly observe and measure physical behavior and the immediate environment in which the behavior occurs, allowing them to identify links between environment and behavior. That typically includes trying to spot events or situations that may be prompting or triggering certain behaviors and noting what may be rewarding and thus reinforcing of some behaviors or punishing and thus inhibiting of others.

The effectiveness of behavioral interventions has been extensively documented for a wide variety of disorders and problem behaviors. A 2009 meta-analysis in the *Journal of Clinical Child & Adolescent Psychology* concluded that "early intensive behavioral intervention should be an intervention of choice for children with autism." A systematic review sponsored by the U.S. Preventive Services Task Force found that even brief behavioral counseling interventions reduced the number of drinks taken by problem drinkers by 13 to 34 percent for as long as four years. Review studies have found similar behavioral-intervention successes in challenges as diverse as reducing stuttering, increasing athletic performance and improving employee productivity.

To combat obesity, behavioral analysts examine related environmental influences: Which external factors prompt people to overeat or to eat junk food, and which tend to encourage healthful eating? In what situations are the behaviors and comments of others affecting unhealthful eating? What seems to effectively reward eating healthfully over the long term? What reinforces being active? Behavior-focused studies of obesity and diets as early as the 1960s recognized some basic conditions that seemed correlated with a greater chance of losing weight and keeping it off: rigorously measuring and recording calories, exercise and weight; making modest, gradual changes rather than severe ones; eating balanced diets that go easy on fats and sugar rather than dropping major food groups; setting clear, modest goals; focusing on lifelong habits rather than short-term diets; and especially attending groups where dieters could receive encouragement to stick with their efforts and praise for having done so.

If these strategies today sound like well-worn, commonsense advice, it is because they have been popularized for nearly half a century by Weight Watchers. Founded in 1963 to provide support groups for dieters, Weight Watchers added other approaches and advice in keeping with the findings of behavioral studies and used to bill itself as a "behavior-modification" program. "Whatever the details are of how you lose weight, the magic in the sauce is always going to be changing behavior," says nutrition researcher and Weight Watchers chief science officer Karen Miller-Kovach. "Doing that is a learnable skill."

Studies back the behavioral approach to weight loss. A 2003 review commissioned by the U.S. Department of Health and Human Services found that "counseling and behavioral interventions showed small to moderate degrees of weight loss sustained over at least one year"—a year being an eon in the world of weight loss. An analysis of eight popular weight-loss programs published in 2005 in the *Annals of Internal Medicine* found Weight Watchers (at that time in its pre-2010 points-overhaul incarnation) to be the only effective program, enabling a 3 percent maintained body-weight loss for the two years of the study. Meanwhile a 2005 *JAMA* study found that Weight Watchers, along with the Zone diet (which, like Weight Watchers, recommends a balanced diet of protein, carbohydrates and fat), achieved the highest percentage (65 percent) of one-year diet adherence of several popular diets, noting that

"adherence level rather than diet type was the key determinant of clinical benefits." A 2010 study in the *Journal of Pediatrics* found that after one year children receiving behavioral therapy maintained a body mass index that was 1.9 to 3.3 lower than children who did not. (BMI is a numerical height-weight relation in which 18.5 is held to be borderline underweight and 25 borderline overweight.) The *Pediatrics* report noted that "more limited evidence suggests that these improvements can be maintained over the 12 months after the end of treatments." A 2010 study in *Obesity* found that continuing members of Take Off Pounds Sensibly (TOPS), a national, nonprofit behaviorally focused weight-loss organization, maintained a weight loss of 5 to 7 percent of their body weight for the three years of the investigation. The UK's Medical Research Council last year declared that its own long-term study had shown that programs based on behavioral principles are more likely to help people take and keep the weight off than other approaches. (The study was funded by Weight Watchers, but without its participation.)

Mass-market programs tend to fall short when it comes to enlisting a full range of behavioral techniques and customizing them to meet the varied needs of individuals.

But Weight Watchers and other mass-market programs tend to fall short when it comes to enlisting a full range of behavioral techniques and customizing them to meet the varied needs of individuals. They cannot routinely provide individual counseling, adapt their advice to specific challenges, assess environmental factors in a member's home, workplace or community, provide much outreach to members who do not come to meetings, or prevent their members from shooting for fast, dramatic, short-term weight loss or from restricting food groups. As a for-profit company, Weight Watchers sometimes even mildly panders to these self-defeating notions in its marketing. "Some people join us to drop 10 pounds for a high school reunion," says Weight Watchers's Miller-Kovach. "They achieve that goal, then stop coming."

To close that gap, a number of researchers have turned their attention in recent years to improving, expanding and tailoring behavioral techniques, with encouraging results. For example, Michael Cameron, head of the graduate behavioral analysis department at Simmons College and a faculty member at Harvard Medical School, is now focusing his research on behavioral weight-loss techniques. He is one year into a four-person study—behavioral analysts generally do very small group or even single-subject studies to more closely tailor the intervention and observe individual effects—in which the subjects meet together with him via online videoconferencing for reinforcement, weigh themselves on scales that transmit results via wireless networks, and have their diets optimized to both reduce caloric density and address individual food preferences.

Favorite foods are used as a reward for exercise. So far the subjects have lost between 8 and 20 percent of their body weight.

Matt Normand, a behavioral analyst at the University of the Pacific, has focused on finding ways to more precisely track subjects' calorie intake and expenditure by, for example, collecting receipts for food purchases, providing food checklists to record what is eaten, and enlisting various types of pedometers and other devices for measuring physical activity. He then provides participants with daily detailed accounts of their calorie flow and in one published study showed three of four subjects reduced calorie intake to recommended levels. Richard Fleming, a researcher at the University of Massachusetts Medical School's Shriver Center, has in *Obesity* looked at ways to encourage parents to steer their children to healthier choices. He has found, among other techniques, that showing parents in person what appropriate serving sizes of foods look like on plates is helpful. Another successful Fleming trick: letting children pick out a small treat at a food store—as long as they walk there. "Kids can really respond to that reward for being active," he says.

Our environment is one in which ubiquitous, sophisticated marketing efforts prey on our need for sensory gratification as well as our vulnerability to misinformation.

Why are behavioral interventions effective? Laurette Dubé, a lifestyle psychology and marketing researcher at McGill University's Faculty of Management, notes that our environment is currently one in which ubiquitous, sophisticated marketing efforts prey on our need for sensory gratification as well as our vulnerability to misinformation. In addition, the poor eating and exercise habits we observe in our friends, family and colleagues encourage us to follow suit. In essence, behavioral interventions seek to reconfigure this environment into one in which our needs for information, gratification and social encouragement are tapped to pull us toward healthy food and exercise choices rather than away from them. "When we are getting the right messages in enough ways, we have a better chance of resisting the urge to eat more than we need," Dubé says.

Changing Policy

There is no one-size-fits-all solution, behavioral or otherwise, to the problem of obesity. But although behavioral interventions work best when they are customized to individuals, mass-market behavioral approaches such as Weight Watchers and TOPS are at least fairly effective. Why don't more people lose weight with them? The main reason is that people simply do not sign up for them, often because would-be weight losers are chasing fad diets or supplements or have read that obesity is locked into our genes. Weight Watchers, by far the most popular behavioral weight-loss program, counts only 600,000 meeting-attending members in its ranks in North America. That means that fewer than one out of 100 obese people in the U.S.

What Works?

Four Steps to Losing Weight

Behavior-focused studies of obesity and diets have identified some basic conditions that seem correlated with a greater chance of losing weight and keeping it off: setting clear, modest goals and focusing on lifelong habits, among others. Most of these behavior changes fall into four main categories.

Initial Assessment

Research underscores the need to determine baseline measurements. How much does an individual weigh? What rituals and routines contribute to overeating (eating under stress) or underexercising (unrealistic expectations)? A physician, a nurse practitioner or a nutrition counselor can help with the assessment.

Behavior Shifts

Many people find it is easier to make small changes at first—such as taking the stairs instead of an elevator. Studies show that surveying the entire buffet before serving themselves will help people put less food on their plate.

Self-Monitoring

Recording body weight, counting the calories eaten and logging steps taken provide objective feedback on how well individuals are changing their habits. Behavior studies have found both low-tech paper logs and wireless monitoring systems to be of benefit.

Support Groups

Studies document the benefits of encouragement by others. Being part of a group—whether an exercise group, a formal support group or even a virtual group—lets participants share triumphs, bemoan setbacks and strategize solutions.

and about one out of 200 overweight people are part of a formal behavioral-modification program.

Public policy may be changing, however. The U.S. Surgeon General's office and the CDC have both publicly lined up behind behavioral approaches as the main weapon in what is becoming a war on obesity. First Lady Michelle Obama's high-profile Let's Move campaign against childhood obesity consists almost entirely of behavioral weight-loss wisdom—that is, find ways to encourage children to eat less-calorie-dense foods, to become more active, and to enjoy doing it. The recent proposed ban of toys in Happy Meals in San Francisco suggests that more officials may be getting ready to pressure the food industry into easing up on contaminating the environment with what are essentially obesity-supportive marketing tactics. To make it easier and more tempting to buy healthier food in poorer, disproportionately overweight communities, the White House has proposed subsidizing the costs of fruits and vegetables. Approaching the problem from the other direction, New York City Mayor Michael Bloomberg is among those who have advocated modifying food-assistance programs to restrict the purchase of high-sugar beverages, and last year Washington, D.C., enacted a 6 percent tax on sugary drinks. New York City has also offered vouchers for buying produce at farmers' markets to low-income families and incentives to stores to offer healthier fare.

Some experts are trying to push the government to rewrite zoning and building codes to ensure that neighborhoods and buildings become friendlier to walkers, bikers and stair climbers. A 2009 study by researchers at Louisiana State University Medical School found that a mere 2.8 percent increase in a person's stair usage alone would keep off almost a pound a year. "The correlation between activity levels and healthy weight is one of the best-established ones in all of obesity research," says William M. Hartman, a psychologist and director of the behavioral program of the highly regarded Weight Management Program of the California Pacific Medical Center in San Francisco.

Increasing access to behavior therapy would help, too. Many overweight people might only need online behavioral monitoring, support and progress-sharing tools, which have proved moderately effective in studies. Others may need much more intensive, more personal interventions of the kind Cameron is developing. Given that obesity especially plagues the economically disadvantaged, fees for these programs may have to be heavily subsidized by the government and health care insurers. A weekly session with a behavioral therapist costing $50 would amount to $2,500 a year, or a bit more than a third of the $7,000 per year societal and medical costs of obesity—and the sessions might only be needed for a year or two to establish new, permanent eating and exercise habits, whereas the savings would continue on for a lifetime.

It is too soon to say whether the public will accept government efforts to push it toward healthier choices. In San Francisco, a community known to be especially friendly to public health initiatives, the plan to ban Happy Meals has provoked angry reactions, and Mayor Gavin Newsom vetoed it. Efforts by Let's Move to bring healthier food to school cafeterias have been intensely criticized by some as overly intrusive. Even if these efforts are eventually fully implemented nationwide, there is no way of being sure they will significantly reduce obesity. The current rate of obesity is far beyond any ever seen before on the planet, and thus a large-scale solution will necessarily be an experiment in mass behavior change. But the research suggests that such a grand experiment would be our best shot at fixing obesity and that there is reason to be hopeful it will succeed. Given that more and more scientists, public policy experts and government officials seem eager to get it off the ground, we may well have early findings within this decade.

More to Explore

About Behaviorism. B. F. Skinner. Vintage, 1974. A classic in behavior modification. You on a Diet: The Owner's Manual for Waist Management. Michael F. Roizen and Mehmet C. Oz. Free Press, 2006. Good layperson's guide to various aspects of weight management.

Determining the Effectiveness of Take Off Pounds Sensibly (TOPS), a Nationally Available Nonprofit Weight Loss Program. Nia S. Mitchell et al., in *Obesity*. Published online September 23, 2010. www.nature.com/oby/journal/vaop/ncurrent/full/oby2010202a .html

The entry portal to the range of NIH research on obesity: obesityresearch.nih.gov.

Critical Thinking

1. Describe the neurological, metabolic, and genetic causes of obesity.

2. Describe the behavioral approach to weight loss and why it is so effective.

3. How do the rewards/punishments for positive lifestyle modification change over time?

DAVID H. FREEDMAN has been covering science, business and technology for 30 years. His most recent book, *Wrong*, explores the forces that lead scientists and other top experts to mislead us.

The Fat Plateau

Americans are no longer getting fatter, it appears.

The Economist

A few years ago, Burger King, a fast-food chain, conducted a study of the eating habits of some of its most frequent customers. A few dozen "SuperFans", as the firm calls them, recorded and photographed everything they ate for two weeks. The results were collected in a book called "Food for Thought". Unsurprisingly, this book is not publicly available: amateur photos of heaps of junk food are hardly an enticing advertisement for a firm that supplies the stuff. Nonetheless, "Food for Thought" gives an insight into why some Americans have such poor diets.

The fast-food fans in the book typically lead chaotic lives. They often toil long, irregular hours for not much money. They grab food when they can, skipping many meals and gorging at unorthodox times. They favour whatever is quick, convenient and comforting. ("I selected the pie because it was easy to grab out of the fridge," says one.) They often have an imperfect grasp of nutritional science. ("I am eating chocolate muffins at work because they are not too heavy," says another.) Oddly for a piece of corporate research, the book contains passages that are quite moving. One single dad's diary shows him eating nothing but junk for days on end. Then, one evening, he visits his aunt's house and she cooks him a feast of real food: pork, okra stew, collard greens and corn bread.

At 33.8%, America's obesity rate is ten times higher than Japan's. In all, 68% of Americans are either obese or overweight. (Some studies yield lower numbers, but since they typically ask people how much they weigh, rather than weighing them, scepticism is in order.) Few problems, besides death, afflict more people. Americans are more likely to be overweight than to pay federal income tax.

But the good news is that the nation may have stopped getting fatter. A study published this month in the *Journal of the American Medical Association (JAMA)* found that American women were no more likely to be obese in 2008 than they were nearly a decade before. For men, there was a small rise in obesity over the same period, but no change in the past three years. Among children, too, there was no change in obesity rates except among the very heaviest boys, whose numbers increased slightly. Could it be that the American obesity epidemic has reached a plateau?

If the national girth really has stopped expanding, that would be a blessing, though of course it is a big fall in obesity that is really required. Although a little extra heft is no big deal, many Americans are so ample that it ruins their health. That places a burden on the health-care system: each obese American racks up medical bills 42% higher than an American of normal weight, according to Eric Finkelstein and Justin Trogdon, writing in *Health Affairs*. Add to that the indirect costs of obesity, such as lost productivity due to sickness or premature death.

The startling Republican victory in Massachusetts this week throws Barack Obama's health reforms up in the air. But the issue will not go away. And a plateau in the obesity rate would make some kind of reform a bit less expensive. It will not lead to a sudden dip in health-care costs, predicts Mr Trogdon. But it could substantially slow the rate at which they are rising. Previous projections typically assumed that Americans would keep on ballooning. As a thought experiment in 2008, Youfa Wang of the Johns Hopkins Centre for Global Health drew a line from recent trends and projected that 100% of Americans would be over-weight by 2048. By 2030, his model showed health-care costs attributable to excess weight approaching a trillion dollars a year.

The latest numbers remind us how little is known about public health. Of course, people put on weight when they consume more calories than they burn off. But no one knows for sure why America's obesity has trebled since 1960. Plausible theories abound. As people grow richer food becomes relatively cheaper. Time grows more precious: hence the lure of fast food. Desk work burns fewer calories than spadework. And labour-saving devices do just that if we still washed dishes and clothes by hand, we would burn off five pounds of flesh each year, reckons Barry Popkin, the author of a book called "The World is Fat". All this is no doubt true, but it does not explain why Americans are fatter than people in other rich countries, nor why they appear to have stopped getting fatter.

No to Nannies

Kathleen Sebelius, the health secretary, says that "fighting obesity is at the heart" of health reform. But telling people to eat more healthily is like telling them not to have risky sex. Americans are suspicious of the nanny state at the best of times, let alone when it nags them to curb their most basic instincts. Some regulations help: forcing restaurants to post calorie counts on dishes, for example, prompts diners to pick less calorific treats. But politicians are reluctant to attack voters' favourite vices too vigorously. A recent proposal to tax sugary drinks, for example, went nowhere. Opponents argued that it would disproportionately affect the poor. True enough, but the poor are disproportionately likely to be overweight.

The constant barrage of pro-vegetable propaganda in schools may have raised awareness of the need for a balanced diet, reckons Mr Trogdon. And popular pressure has prompted many fast-food outlets to offer salads and other wholesome fare. But even if good food were freely available, losing weight is hard. Every year, 25% of American men and 43% of American women attempt it. "[F]ailure rates are exceedingly high," notes a *JAMA* editorial. But there is hope. Eating is social. Studies suggest that people guzzle more if they have overweight friends and relatives, and less if they don't. So if Americans have stopped getting fatter, their children have a better shot at staying trim.

Critical Thinking

1. What are the primary factors that have contributed to the obesity epidemic in the United States?

2. What is the latest percentage of obese or overweight Americans? How does this percentage differ from the obesity rate percentage?

3. Describe the typical fast food fan depicted in the book, *Food for Thought*.

Obesity Rates in U.S. Appear to Be Finally Leveling Off

After three decades of climbing steadily, obesity rates appear to be stabilizing nationwide. Increases among certain demographic groups are still evident, however.

SHARI ROAN

After a 30-year, record-shattering rise, U.S. obesity rates appear to be stabilizing.

New statistics cited in two papers report only a slight uptick since 2005—leaving public health experts tentatively optimistic that they may be gaining some ground in their efforts to slim down the nation.

Many obesity specialists say the new data, from the Centers for Disease Control and Prevention, are a sign that efforts to address the obesity problem—such as placing nutritional information on food packaging and revising school lunch menus—are beginning to have an effect in a country where two-thirds of adults and one-third of children and teens are overweight or obese.

"A good first step is to stop the increase, so I think this is very positive news," said James O. Hill, director of the Center for Human Nutrition at the University of Colorado Health Sciences Center in Denver. "It may suggest our efforts are starting to make a difference. The bad news is we still have obesity rates that are just astronomical."

Historically, there was little change in Americans' sizes from 1960 through 1980. But obesity rates soared through the end of the century, for reasons that are still debated.

The new studies reflect 2009–10 data, the most recent available, from the government's National Health and Nutrition Examination Survey, which examined 6,000 adults and 4,111 children, measuring their body mass index, among other items. Though a number of organizations measure obesity rates, the survey's data are considered among the most accurate.

The statistics showed that more than 35 percent of U.S. adults (78 million people) are obese, defined as having a body mass index of 30 or greater. That is similar to the 2005–06 rate. Calculated as weight in kilograms divided by height in meters squared, the BMI is not a perfect measure of fatness but is still viewed as the gold standard in assessing population-wide trends.

An additional third of adults are overweight, the analysis found, also similar to the rates in 2005–06.

Likewise, data in children and teenagers from birth to age 19 reflect little change from the survey's 2007–08 data, according to the reports, which were published online Tuesday in the Journal of the American Medical Assn. Almost 17 percent are obese and 32 percent are overweight or obese.

But though obesity rates may be flattening overall, increases and disparities can still be found in specific racial and ethnic groups.

Rates have risen to 58.5 percent among non-Hispanic black women and to nearly 45 percent among Mexican American women since 2004, for example. And among children and teens, about 21 percent of Hispanics and 24 percent of blacks are obese compared with 14 percent of non-Hispanic whites.

The report also found that gender differences appear to be fading, with percentages of overweight males catching up with or even overtaking those of females.

Among males under 19, obesity rose from 14 percent in 1999–2000 to 18.6 percent in the latest survey; in adult men, the rate jumped from 27.5 percent to 35.5 percent.

In addition, more adult men are now overweight or obese as compared with women—73.9 percent to 63.7 percent. Severe obesity remains more common in women, however.

"We found no indication that the prevalence of obesity is declining in any group," the authors wrote in one of the papers, which looked at obesity rates among adults.

It's not clear why obesity rates are still rising in some groups while stabilizing in others, said Cynthia L. Ogden, a coauthor of the two papers and a researcher at the CDC. But the best bet of some leading obesity experts is that obesity prevention initiatives in some pockets of the country are paying off.

The Let's Move! program founded by First Lady Michelle Obama has raised national awareness through actions such as persuading Wal-Mart to stock more healthful foods and working with professional sports organizations to create public service announcements encouraging children to exercise.

Certain states, including California, have made obesity prevention a major health goal through measures to reduce access to sugary drinks and high-calorie, unhealthful snacks in schools.

A UCLA study released in November showed obesity rates ticking down in some parts of the state between 2005 and 2010, including a decline of 2.5 percent in Los Angeles County. And research published last month found obesity rates in New York City children fell 5 percent between the 2006–07 and 2010–11 school years.

"The places that are making serious changes in the schools and communities can take hope that these changes are starting to have an effect," said Dr. James S. Marks, senior vice president and director of the health group for the Robert Wood Johnson Foundation, a private organization aimed at improving health of Americans.

But, he added, a reduction in obesity rates will probably take many more years and more than the smattering of programs and initiatives so far underway.

The best hope for lowering rates, he said, is to stop people from getting fat to begin with: Experience and studies show that it is difficult for obese adults to permanently shed fat and that children who are already overweight or obese are highly likely to be overweight as adults.

Only one prescription anti-obesity medication is currently approved for long-term use, and researchers have stalled in their efforts to find more. Moreover, most obesity is untreated or under-treated.

Since obesity contributes to joint damage as well as diseases such as diabetes, heart disease and certain cancers, the epidemic truly is a national crisis, said Patrick M. O'Neil, president of the Obesity Society and director of the weight management center at the Medical University of South Carolina in Charleston.

"Even if the statistics stay at current prevalence rates, I see little good news in that," O'Neil said.

People should look to their own lives and individual experiences, and strive for progress by eating more healthfully and exercising more, he said.

"On a population basis you are trying to turn an aircraft carrier, and it's going to take a long time for it to change," he said.

Critical Thinking

1. Interpret the most recent obesity rate data from the National Health and Nutrition Examination Survey (NHANES).

2. Identify the two subgroups that have experienced an increase in obesity since 2005.

3. Define the classifications of obesity and overweight based on body mass index.

The Hungry Brain

The urge to eat too much is wired into our heads. **Tackling obesity may require bypassing the stomach** and short-circuiting our brains.

DAN HURLEY

At 10:19 P.M. on a Monday evening in October, I sat in a booth at Chevys Fresh Mex in Clifton, New Jersey, reviewing the latest research into the neurobiology of hunger and obesity. While I read I ate a shrimp and crab enchilada, consuming two-thirds of it, maybe less. With all this information in front of me, I thought, I had an edge over my brain's wily efforts to thwart my months-long campaign to get under 190 pounds. But even as I was taking in a study about the powerful lure of guacamole and other salty, fatty foods, I experienced something extraordinary. That bowl of chips and salsa at the edge of the table? It was whispering to me: *Just one more. You know you want us. Aren't we delicious?* In 10 minutes, all that was left of the chips, and my willpower, were crumbs.

I am not alone. An overabundance of chips, Baconator Double burgers, and Venti White Chocolate Mochas have aided a widespread epidemic of obesity in this country. Our waists are laying waste to our health and to our health-care economy: According to a study published by the Centers for Disease Control and Prevention in 2010, nine states had an obesity rate of at least 30 percent—compared with zero states some 10 years earlier—and the cost of treatment for obesity-related conditions had reached nearly 10 percent of total U.S. medical expenditure. So-called normal weight is no longer normal, with two-thirds of adults and one third of children and adolescents now classified as overweight or obese. Dubbed the "Age of Obesity and Inactivity" by the *Journal of the American Medical Association,* this runaway weight gain threatens to decrease average U.S. life span, reversing gains made over the past century by lowering risk factors from smoking, hypertension, and cholesterol. We all know what we should do—eat less, exercise more—but to no avail. An estimated 25 percent of American men and 43 percent of women attempt to lose weight each year; of those who succeed in their diets, between 5 and 20 percent (and it is closer to 5 percent) manage to keep it off for the long haul.

The urgent question is, why do our bodies seem to be fighting against our own good health? According to a growing number of neurobiologists, the fault lies not in our stomachs but in our heads. No matter how convincing our conscious plans and resolutions, they pale beside the brain's power to goad us into noshing and hanging on to as much fat as we can. With that in mind, some scientists were hopeful that careful studies of the brain might uncover an all-powerful hormone that regulates food consumption or a single spot where the cortical equivalent of a neon sign blinks "Eat Heavy," all the better to shut it off.

After extensive research, the idea of a single, simple cure has been replaced by a much more nuanced view. The latest studies show that a multitude of systems in the brain act in concert to encourage eating. Targeting a single neuronal system is probably doomed to the same ill fate as the failed diets themselves. Because the brain has so many backup systems all geared toward the same thing—maximizing the body's intake of calories—no single silver bullet will ever work.

The brain's prime directive to eat and defend against the loss of fat emerged early in evolution.

"I call it the 'hungry brain syndrome'," says Hans-Rudolf Berthoud, an expert in the neurobiology of nutrition at the Pennington Biomedical Research Center in Baton Rouge, Louisiana. The brain's prime directive to eat and defend against the loss of fat emerged early in evolution, because just about every creature that ever trotted, crawled, swam, or floated was beset by the uncertainty of that next meal. "The system has evolved to defend against the slightest threat of weight loss, so you have to attack it from different directions at once."

With the obesity epidemic raging, the race for countermeasures has kicked into high gear. Neuroscientists are still seeking hormones that inhibit hunger, but they have other tactics as well. One fruitful new avenue comes from the revelation that hunger, blood sugar, and weight gained per calorie consumed all ratchet up when our sleep is disrupted and our circadian rhythms—the 24-hour cycle responding to light and dark—[are] thrown into disarray. All this is compounded by stress, which decreases metabolism while increasing the yen for high-calorie food. We might feel in sync with our high-tech world, but the obesity epidemic is a somber sign that our biology and lifestyles have diverged.

Seeking Silver Bullets, Shooting Blanks

The path forward seemed so simple back in 1995, when three papers in *Science* suggested a panacea for the overweight: A hormone that made animals shed pounds, rapidly losing body fat until they were slim. Based on the research, it seemed that doctors might soon be able to treat obesity the way they treat diabetes, with a simple metabolic drug.

Fat cells release that "diet" hormone—today named leptin, from the Greek *leptos,* meaning thin—to begin a journey across the blood-brain barrier to the hypothalamus, the pea-size structure above the pituitary gland. The hypothalamus serves as a kind of thermostat, setting not only body temperature but playing a key role in hunger, thirst, fatigue, and sleep cycles. Leptin signals the hypothalamus to reduce the sense of hunger so that we stop eating.

In early lab experiments, obese mice given extra leptin by injection seemed sated. They ate less, their body temperature increased, and their weight plummeted. Even normal-weight mice became skinnier when given injections of the hormone.

Once the pharmaceutical industry created a synthetic version of human leptin, clinical trials were begun. But when injected into hundreds of obese human volunteers, leptin's effect was clinically insignificant. It soon became clear why. In humans, as in mice, fat cells of the obese already produced plenty of leptin—more in fact than those of their thin counterparts, since the level of leptin was directly proportional to the amount of fat. The early studies had worked largely because the test mice were, by experimental design, leptin-deficient. Subsequent experiments showed that in normal mice—as in humans—increases in leptin made little difference to the brain, which looked to *low* leptin levels as a signal to eat more, essentially disregarding the kind of high levels that had caused deficient mice to eat less. This made leptin a good drug for maintaining weight loss but not a great candidate for getting the pounds off up front.

Despite that disappointment, the discovery of leptin unleashed a scientific gold rush to find other molecules that could talk the brain into turning hunger off. By 1999 researchers from Japan's National Cardiovascular Center Research Institute in Osaka had announced the discovery of ghrelin, a kind of antileptin that is released primarily by the gut rather than by fat cells. Ghrelin signals hunger rather than satiety to the hypothalamus. Then, in 2002, a team from the University of Washington found that ghrelin levels rise before a meal and fall immediately after. Ghrelin (from the Indo-European root for the word "grow") increased hunger while jamming on the metabolic brakes to promote the body's storage of fat.

So began another line of attack on obesity. Rather than turning leptin on, researchers began exploring ways to turn ghrelin off. Some of them began looking at animal models, but progress has been slow; the concept of a ghrelin "vaccine" has been floated, but clinical trials are still years off.

Seeking a better understanding of the hormone, University of Washington endocrinologist David Cummings compared ghrelin levels in people who had lost considerable amounts of weight through diet with those who shed pounds by means of gastric bypass surgery—a technique that reduces the capacity of the stomach and seems to damage its ghrelin-producing capacity as well. The results were remarkable. For dieters, the more weight lost, the greater the rise in ghrelin, as if the body were telling the brain to get hungry and regain that weight. By contrast, the big losers in the surgical group saw ghrelin levels fall to the floor. Surgical patients never felt increases in appetite and had an easier time maintaining their weight loss as a result. (A newer weight-loss surgery removes most of the ghrelin-producing cells outright.)

Based on such findings, a ghrelin-blocking drug called rimonabant was approved and sold in 32 countries, though not in the United States. It remained available as recently as 2008, even though it also increased the risk of depression and suicidal thinking; it has since been withdrawn everywhere. The verdict is still out on a newer generation of combination pharmaceuticals, including one that contains synthetic versions of leptin and the neurohormone amylin, known to help regulate appetite. In a six-month clinical trial, the combination therapy resulted in an average weight loss of 25 pounds, or 12.7 percent of body weight, with greater weight loss when continued for a full 52 weeks; those who stopped taking the drug midway regained most of their weight.

The Circadian Connection

The limited results from tackling the hypothalamus sent many scientists looking at the other gyres and gears driving obesity in the brain, especially in regions associated with sleep. The first big breakthrough came in 2005, when *Science* published a landmark paper on mice with a mutated version of the Clock gene, which plays a key role in the regulation of the body's circadian rhythms. The mutant mice not only failed to follow the strict eat-by-night, sleep-by-day schedule of normally nocturnal mice, they also became overweight and developed diabetes. "There was a difference in weight gain based on when the food was eaten, whether during day or night," says the study's senior author, endocrinologist Joe Bass of Northwestern University. "That means the metabolic rate must differ under those two conditions."

Could *my* late-night hours be the undoing of my weight-loss plans? Four days after my humiliating defeat by a bowl of tortilla chips, I met with Alex Keene, a postdoctoral researcher at New York University with a Matisse nude tattooed on his right forearm and a penchant for studying flies. His latest study asked whether a starved fly would take normal naps or sacrifice sleep to keep searching for food. He found that like humans (and most other creatures), flies have a neurological toggle between two fundamental yet incompatible drives: to eat or to sleep. "Flies only live a day or two when they're starved,"

Keene told me as we walked past graduate students peering at flies under microscopes. "If they decide to sleep through the night when they're starved, it's a bad decision on their part. So their brains are finely tuned to suppress their sleep when they don't have food and to sleep well after a meal."

For a major study published last year, Keene bred flies with dysfunctional mutations of the Clock gene and also of Cycle, another gene involved in circadian rhythms. He found that the genes together regulate the interaction between the two mutually exclusive behaviors, sleep and feeding, kicking in to suppress sleep when a fly is hungry.

Even when fed, flies without working versions of the Clock and Cycle genes tended to sleep poorly—about 30 percent as much as normal flies. "It was as if they were starving right away," Keene explains. Keene went even further, pinpointing where, amid the 100,000 or so neurons in the fly brain, the Clock gene acts to regulate the sleeping-feeding interaction: a region of just four to eight cells at the top of the fly brain.

"My father is an anthropologist," Keene told me as we stood in the fly room, its air pungent with the corn meal and molasses the flies feed on. "It's ironic, right? He looks at how culture determines behavior, while I look at how genes determine behavior. I used to get him so mad he'd storm out of the house."

Perhaps it takes an anthropologist's son to see that the excess availability of cheap, high-calorie chow cannot fully explain the magnitude and persistence of the problem in our culture. The rebellion against our inborn circadian rhythms wrought by a 24-hour lifestyle, lit by neon and fueled by caffeine, also bears part of the blame. The powerful effect of disordered sleep on metabolism has been seen not just in flies but also in humans. A 2009 study by Harvard University researchers showed that in just 10 days, three of eight healthy volunteers developed prediabetic blood-sugar levels when their sleep-wake schedule was gradually shifted out of alignment.

"It's clear from these types of studies that the way we're keeping the lights on until late at night, the way in which society demands that we stay active for so much longer, could well be contributing to aspects of the metabolic disease we're seeing now," says Steve Kay, a molecular geneticist at the University of California, San Diego.

These insights have fostered collaboration between once-diverse groups. "Physicians who specialized in obesity and diabetes for years are now discovering the importance of circadian effects," Kay says. At the same time, "basic research scientists like me, who have been studying the circadian system for so many years, are now looking at its metabolic effects. When so many people's research from so many areas starts to converge, you know we're in the midst of a paradigm shift. This is the slow rumbling before the volcano blows."

This past April, the National Institute of Diabetes and Digestive and Kidney Diseases (NIDDK) of the National Institutes of Health organized a first-ever national conference focused solely on how circadian rhythms affect metabolism. "What has become obvious over the past few years is that metabolism, all those pathways regulating how fats and carbohydrates are used, is affected by the circadian clock," says biochemist Corinne Silva, a program director at the NIDDK. Her goal is to find drugs

that treat diabetes and obesity by targeting circadian pathways. "The mechanisms by which circadian rhythms are maintained and the cross talk with metabolic signaling are just beginning to be elucidated," she says, but they should lead to novel therapeutic approaches in the years ahead.

In Keene's view, the newfound link between sleep and obesity could be put to use right now. "People who are susceptible to diabetes or have weight issues might just get more sleep. I get only about six hours of sleep myself. I usually run in the middle of the night. I'm not a morning person," the enviably thin, 29-year-old Keene states.

My visit to his fly room convinced me to try a new angle in my quest to get under 190 pounds: Rather than focus on *how much* food I put in my mouth, I would focus on *when* I eat. I decided I would no longer eat after 10 P.M.

The Pleasure Factor

Timing may be everything for some folks, but it wasn't for me. No wonder: The brain has no shortage of techniques to goad us into eating. Another line of evidence suggests that the brains of overweight people are wired to feel more pleasure in response to food. Sleep deprived or not, they just enjoy eating more. To study such differences, clinical psychologist Eric Stice of the Oregon Research Institute mastered the delicate task of conducting fMRI brain scans while people were eating. The food he chose to give the volunteers inside the tunnel-like scanners was a milk shake. And let the record show, it was a *chocolate* milk shake.

Brains of the overweight are wired to feel more pleasure in response to food.

Obese adolescent girls, Stice found, showed greater activation compared with their lean peers in regions of the brain that encode the sensory experience of eating food—the so-called gustatory cortex and the somatosensory regions, archipelagoes of neurons that reach across different structures in the brain. At the same time, the obese girls sipping milk shakes showed decreased activation in the striatum, a region near the center of the brain that is studded with dopamine receptors and known to respond to stimuli associated with rewards. Stice wondered whether, even among normal-weight girls, such a pattern might predict an increased risk of overeating and weight gain.

To test his hypothesis, he followed a group of subjects over time, finding that those with reduced activation in the dorsal (rear) region of the striatum while sipping a milk shake were ultimately more likely to gain weight than those with normal activation. The most vulnerable of these girls were also more likely to have a DNA polymorphism—not a mutation, per se, but a rather routine genetic variation—in a dopamine receptor gene, causing reduced dopamine signaling in the striatum and placing them at higher risk. "Individuals may overeat," Stice and his colleagues concluded, "to compensate for a hypofunctioning dorsal striatum, particularly those with genetic polymorphisms thought to attenuate dopamine signaling in this region."

Stice was initially surprised by the results. "It's totally weird," he admits. "Those who experienced less pleasure were at increased risk for weight gain." But his more recent studies have convinced him that the reduced pleasure is a result of years of overeating among the obese girls—the same phenomenon seen in drug addicts who require ever-greater amounts of their drug to feel the same reward. "Imagine a classroom of third graders, and everyone is skinny," he says. "The people who initially find that milk shake most orgasmic will want more of it, but in so doing they cause neuroplastic changes that downregulate the reward circuitry, driving them to eat more and more to regain that same feeling they crave."

Even among people of normal weight, individual differences in brain functioning can directly affect eating behaviors, according to a 2009 study by Michael Lowe, a research psychologist at Drexel University. He took fMRI brain scans of 19 people, all of them of normal weight. Nine of the volunteers reported following strict diets; the other 10 typically ate whenever and whatever they wanted. Lowe had all of them sip a milk shake immediately before getting scanned. The brains of the nondieters, he found, lit up just as one would expect, showing activations in areas associated with satiation and memory, as if saying, "Mmmm, that was good." The chronic dieters showed activations in areas of the brain associated with desire and expectation of reward, however. If anything, the milk shake had made them hungrier.

"What we have shown is that these chronic dieters may actually have a reason to restrain themselves, because they are more susceptible than average to overeating," Lowe says.

Yet inborn differences in hunger and desire, too, turn out to be only part of the weighting game. Eating behaviors are also linked to areas of the brain associated with self-control (such as the left superior frontal region) and visual attention (such as the right middle temporal region). A recent fMRI study led by Jeanne McCaffery, a psychologist at Brown Medical School, showed that successful weight losers had greater activation in those regions, compared with normal-weight people and obese people, when viewing images of food.

The effects of stress on eating behaviors also has a neurobiological basis, according to University of Pennsylvania neurobiologist Tracy Bale. She showed that neural pathways associated with stress link directly to areas of the brain associated with seeking rewards. "Few things are more rewarding evolutionarily than calorie-dense food," Bale told me a few days after presenting a seminar on the subject at last fall's Society for Neuroscience meeting in San Diego. "Under stress people don't crave a salad; they crave something high-calorie. It's because those stress pathways in the limbic system feed into the reward centers, and they drive reward-seeking behaviors. What that tells us is that in addition to drug companies' trying to target appetite, they need to look at the reward centers. We're not necessarily fat because we're hungry but because we're looking for something to deal with stress."

Aha! Perhaps it was stress that was messing with my latest, clock-based diet. Back in March 2010, a tree had fallen on my family's home during a major storm, crushing the roof, destroying half the house, and forcing us to flee to a nearby apartment. By November, as I researched this story, we had finally moved back into our rebuilt house. With nerves fully frayed, I found myself drawn as never before to the Tick Tock Diner, where the motto literally is "Eat Heavy," and where the french fries never tasted better. Instead of losing a few pounds to get under 190, by Thanksgiving I had hit 196.

How to Fix a Hungry Brain

Neuroscience has yet to deliver a weight-loss elixir for paunchy 53-year-old journalists like me, much less for those suffering from serious obesity. But that day will come, Steve Kay asserts, once researchers figure out the correct combination of drugs that work simultaneously on multiple triggers of eating and metabolism, just as hypertension is now routinely treated with two- or three-drug combinations.

Some scientists think a more radical approach is called for. Since the triggers of obesity lie in the brain, neurosurgeons at West Virginia University Health Sciences Center are attempting to rewire those triggers directly using deep brain stimulation (DBS). Since 2009 they have performed surgery on three obese patients to implant electrodes that emit rhythmic electric shocks into the hypothalamus. Having failed other medical therapies for obesity, the three agreed to volunteer for DBS, a treatment already approved for treating the tremors and dystonia of Parkinson's disease. "These patients weren't eating all that much; it was mainly a problem of having very slow metabolisms," says Donald M. Whiting, one of the neurosurgeons leading the study. "Our goal was to speed it up." On the basis of successful animal studies, he adds, "we thought we'd switch on the energy and collect our Nobel Prize."

All three patients experienced significantly less hunger when the electrodes were switched on, and all regained their normal hunger when the electrodes were switched off. Unfortunately, none lost a significant amount of weight in the study's first year. The problem, Whiting concludes, is that there are many ways to adjust DBS. With four contact points on the electrodes, each placed half a millimeter apart and each adjustable for voltage, frequency, and pulse width, the research team has been seeking the combination of settings that most effectively rev up metabolism. So far they have found settings that work only temporarily.

"The brain is really pretty smart," Whiting says. "It tends to want to reboot to factory settings whenever it can. We find that we can reset things for a week or two, but then the brain gets back to where it wants." Despite the challenges, Whiting remains convinced that finding a safe and effective medical treatment for weight control will be essential to turn the obesity epidemic around—and that no amount of preaching from Oprah, no behavior program from Weight Watchers nor food from Jenny Craig, will ever suffice.

"This mystification that obesity is caused by a lack of willpower or just eating the wrong foods is simply a misconception," Joe Bass of Northwestern told me. "There is so much social stigma attached to weight that we make a lot of value judgments. The effort in science is to peel back those layers of belief and try to understand things in an experimental, rational mode. Just as we have made progress against heart disease with statins and blood pressure drugs, we will find medications that can safely and substantially lower weight."

Months after my investigation of the brain-gut connection began, I faced the acid test. In early March I stepped back onto my bathroom scale for a final weigh-in. Rather than slip below 190, for the first time in my life I had tipped, by a single pound, over 200. You might blame it on insufficient exercise or on the cheese and crackers I failed to remove from my late-night work ritual. I'm blaming it on my brain.

Critical Thinking

1. Describe the hormones that impact food intake and explain their actions in the body.

2. Explain how sleep and circadian rhythms influence feeding behavior and metabolism.

3. How does the limbic system dictate the types of foods that we crave during stress?

In Your Face
How the Food Industry Drives Us to Eat

BONNIE LIEBMAN AND KELLY BROWNELL

Excess pounds raise the risk of diabetes, heart disease, stroke, cancer (of the breast, colon, esophagus, kidney, and uterus), gallbladder disease, arthritis, and more. And once people gain weight, the odds of losing it and keeping it off are slim.

"Estimates are that this generation of children may be the first to live fewer years than their parents," says Kelly Brownell. "Health care costs for obesity are now $147 billion annually."

What are we doing about it? Not enough.

"The conditions that are driving the obesity epidemic need to change," says Brownell. Here's why and how.

Q: *Why do you call our food environment toxic?*
A: Because people who are exposed to it get sick. They develop chronic diseases like diabetes and obesity in record numbers.

Q: *How does the environment influence what we eat?*
A: When I was a boy, there weren't aisles of food in the drugstore, and gas stations weren't places where you could eat lunch. Vending machines in workplaces were few and far between, and schools didn't have junk food. Fast food restaurants didn't serve breakfast or stay open 24 hours. Today, access to unhealthy choices is nearly ubiquitous.

Burgers, fries, pizza, soda, candy, and chips are everywhere. Apples and bananas aren't. And we have large portion sizes—bigger bagels, burgers, steaks, muffins, cookies, popcorn, and sodas. We have the relentless marketing of unhealthy food, and too little access to healthy foods.

Q: *Does the price structure of food push us to buy more?*
A: Yes. People buy a Value Meal partly because that large burger, fries, and soft drink cost less than a salad and bottle of water. A large popcorn doesn't cost much more than a small. A Cinnabon doesn't cost much more than a Minibon.

Q: *And most stores are pushing junk food, not fresh fruit?*
A: Yes. There's a Dunkin' Donuts at our Stop 'n Shop supermarket and at the Wal-Mart near us. And if you look at retail stores, they're set up in ways that maximize the likelihood of impulse purchases.

For example, the candy is on display at the checkout line at the supermarket. And when you go to a modern drugstore, the things you usually go to a drugstore to buy—like bandages, cough medicine, pain reliever, your prescriptions—are all at the back. People typically have to walk by the soda, chips, and other junk food to navigate their way there and back.

Old Genes, New World

Q: *You've said that our biology is mismatched with the modern world, How?*
A: Thousands of years ago, our ancestors faced unpredictable food supplies and looming starvation. Those who adapted ate voraciously when food was available and stored body fat so they could survive times of scarcity.

Our bodies were programmed to seek calorie-dense foods. They were exquisitely efficient calorie-conservation machines, which matched nicely with a scarce food supply.

But now we have abundance. And there's no need for the extreme physical exertion that our ancestors needed to hunt and gather food. It's a mismatch.

Q: *How do ads encourage overeating?*
A: Overeating is written into the language that companies use—names like Big Gulp, Super Gulp, Extreme Gulp. At one point, Frito-Lay sold dollar bags of snack foods called the Big Grab. The burger companies describe their biggest burgers with words like the Monster Burger, the Whopper, the Big Mac. The industry capitalizes on our belief that bigger is better and promotes large amounts of their least healthy foods.

Q: *Why do we want a good deal on a bad food?*
A: Everybody likes value. Getting more of something for your money isn't a bad idea. You like to do that when you buy an automobile or clothing or laundry detergent or anything.

But when the incentives are set up in a way that offers value for unhealthy food, it's a problem. If you buy the big bag of Cheetos, you get a better deal than if you buy the little bag. A big Coke is a better deal than a little Coke. But if you buy six apples, you don't always get a better deal than if you buy three.

Q: *Is indulgence a code word for overeating?*
A: Right. You deserve a reward and we're here to offer it to you. And ads describe foods as sinful. Or we make light of eating too much, like the ad that said "I can't believe I ate the whole thing."

Are We Irresponsible?

Q: *How does the food industry blame people for the obesity epidemic?*

A: The two words it uses most frequently are personal responsibility. It plays well in America because of this idea that people should take charge of their own lives and because some people have the biological fortune to be able to resist our risky environment.

But it also serves to shift blame from the industry and government to the individuals with a weight problem. It's right out of the tobacco-industry playbook.

Q: *What else is in the food industry's playbook?*

A: Industry spokespeople raise fears that government action usurps personal freedom. Or they vilify critics with totalitarian language, characterizing them as the food police, leaders of a nanny state, and even food fascists, and accuse them of trying to strip people of their civil liberties.

They also criticize studies that hurt the food industry as "junk science." And they argue that there are no good or bad foods—only good or bad diets. That way, soft drinks, fast foods, and other foods can't be targeted for change.

Q: *So people think it's their fault?*

A: Many people who struggle with weight problems believe it's their own fault anyway. So exacerbating that is not helpful. But removing the mandate for business and government to take action has been very harmful.

For example, if you look at funding to reduce obesity, it has lagged far behind the extent of the problem. It's because of this idea that people are responsible for the way they are, so why should government do anything about it?

Q: *Are people irresponsible?*

A: There's been increasing obesity for years in the United States. It's hard to believe that people in 2010 are less responsible than they were 10 or 20 years ago. You have increasing obesity in literally every country in the world. Are people in every country becoming less responsible?

We looked into the literature to find data on other health behaviors like mammograms, seat belt use, heavy drinking, and smoking. All those other behaviors have remained constant or have improved in the U.S. population.

If irresponsibility is the cause of obesity, one might expect evidence that people are becoming less responsible overall. But studies suggest the opposite.

So if people are having trouble acting responsibly in the food arena, the question is why? There must be enormous pressure bearing down on them to override their otherwise responsible behavior.

Q: *It's not as though society rewards obesity.*

A: No. Obesity is stigmatized. Overweight people, especially children, are teased and victimized by discrimination. Obese children have lower self-esteem and a higher risk of depression. They're less likely to be admitted to college. And obese adults are less likely to be hired, have lower salaries, and are often viewed as lazy and less competent. So the pressure to overeat must be overwhelming.

Q: *Are the pressures worse for children?*

A: Yes. Kids don't have the natural cognitive defenses against marketing. And they're developing brand loyalty and food preferences that can last a lifetime.

To allow the food industry to have free range with our children has come at a tremendous cost. A third of kids are now overweight or obese. And when you project ahead to the adult diseases that will cause, it's incredible. Someday, our children may wonder why we didn't protect them from the food companies.

Q: *Do we do anything to protect kids?*

A: We do some nutrition education in schools, but it's a drop against the tidal wave of what the food industry is doing to educate those children.

The Robert Wood Johnson Foundation is by far the biggest funder of work on childhood obesity, and it's now spending $100 million a year on the problem. The food industry spends that much every year by January 4th to market unhealthy food to children. There's no way the government can compete with that just through education.

If parents ate every meal with their children, that would amount to 1,000 teaching opportunities per year. Yet the average child sees 10,000 food ads each year. And parents don't have Beyoncé, LeBron, and Kobe on their side.

Q: *So if irresponsibility isn't to blame, what is?*

A: When you give lab animals access to the diets that are marketed so aggressively in the United States, they become obese. We have abundant science that the environment is the causative agent here. So the environment needs to be changed.

That's what public policy is all about. We require that children get vaccinated and ride in child safety seats. We have high taxes on cigarettes. Your car has an air bag. The government could educate us to be safe drivers and hope for the best. Or it could just put an air bag in every car. Those are examples of government taking action to create better defaults.

Keeping It off

Q: *Why is it so important to prevent obesity?*

A: Because it's so difficult to fix. The results of studies on treating obesity are very discouraging, especially if one looks at long-term results. The exception is surgery, but that's expensive and can't be used on a broad scale. So this is a problem that screams out to be prevented.

Q: *Why is it so hard to keep weight off?*

A: There's good research, much of it done by Rudolph Leibel and colleagues at Columbia University, that shows that when people are overweight and lose weight, their biology changes in a way that makes it hard to keep the weight off.

Take two women who weigh 150 pounds. One has always weighed 150 and the other was at 170 and reduced down to 150. Metabolically, they look very different. To maintain her 150-pound weight, the woman who has dropped from 170 is going to have to exist on about 15 percent fewer calories than the woman who was always at 150.

Q: *Why?*

A: It's as if the body senses that it's in starvation mode so it becomes more metabolically efficient. People who have lost weight burn fewer calories than those who haven't, so they have to keep taking in fewer calories to keep the weight off. That's tough to do day after day, especially when the environment is pushing us to eat more, not less.

And Leibel and others have shown that there are changes in hormones, including leptin, that explain why people who lose weight are hungry much of the time.

Q: *Are you saying that our bodies think we're starving when we lose just 10 percent of our body weight?*

A: Right. It's not hopeless, but the data can be discouraging. The results of weight-loss studies are clear. Not many people lose a significant amount of weight and keep it off. All these environmental cues force people to eat, and then this biology makes it hard to lose weight and keep it off.

Q: *Does genetics play a role in obesity?*

A: Yes. Genetics can help explain why some people are prone to gain weight and some are not. But genetics can't explain why there are so many overweight people. The reason we have more obesity than Somalia, let's say, is not because we're genetically different. The fact that so many people are overweight is all environment.

Addictive Foods

Q: *Are some foods addictive?*

A: My prediction is that the issue of food and addiction will explode onto the scene relatively soon, because the science is building almost by the day and it's very compelling. I think it's important to put the focus on the food, rather than the person. There are people who consider themselves food addicts, and they might be, but the more important question is whether there's enough addictive properties in some foods to keep people coming back for more and more. That's where the public health problem resides.

Q: *What are those properties?*

A: What's been studied most so far is sugar. There are brain-imaging studies in humans and a variety of animal studies showing that sugar acts on the brain very much like morphine, alcohol, and nicotine. It doesn't have as strong an effect, but it has a similar effect on reward pathways in the brain. So when kids get out of school and they feel like having a sugared beverage, how much of that is their brain calling out for this addictive substance? Are we consuming so many foods of poor nutrient quality partly because of the addictive properties of the food itself?

Q: *What do you mean by reward pathways?*

A: There are pathways in the brain that get activated when we experience pleasure, and drugs of abuse like heroin hijack that system. The drugs take over the system to make those substances extremely reinforcing and to make us want those things when we don't have them.

The drugs do that by setting up withdrawal symptoms when we don't have them. The drugs set up the addiction by creating tolerance, so you need more over time to produce the same effect. The drugs set us up to have cravings. The same reward system is activated by foods, especially foods high in sugar.

Q: *Do we need more research in people?*

A: Yes, but we already have animal and human studies, some done by highly distinguished researchers. I think this is a top priority because if we get to the point where we say that food can be addictive, the whole landscape can change.

Think of the morality or legality of marketing these foods to children. Could the industry ever be held accountable for the intentional manipulation of ingredients that activate the brain in that way? The stakes are very high.

Q: *How much does exercise matter to losing weight?*

A: Exercise has so many health benefits that it's hard to count them. It lowers the risk for cancer, heart disease, and cognitive impairment as people age. There's a very long list of reasons to be physically active, but weight control may not be one of them. Recent studies have suggested that the food part of the equation is much more important than the activity part.

Q: *Because you can undo an hour of exercise with one muffin?*

A: Yes. The food industry has been front and center in promoting exercise as the way to address the nation's obesity problem. The industry talks about the importance of physical activity continuously, and they've been quite involved in funding programs that emphasize physical activity. The skeptics claim that that's the way to divert attention away from food.

Answers

Q: *So what's the answer to the obesity epidemic?*

A: The broad answer is to change the environmental conditions that are driving obesity. Some of the most powerful drivers are food marketing and the economics of food, so I would start there. I don't think we have much chance of succeeding with the obesity problem unless the marketing of unhealthy foods is curtailed.

Q: *Not just to kids?*

A: No, but children would be a great place to start. Second would be to change the economics so that healthy food costs less and unhealthy food costs more. So a small tax on sugar-sweetened beverages—say, one penny per ounce—would be part of that effort.

Ideally, the tax revenues would be used to subsidize the cost of fruits and vegetables. That creates a better set of economic defaults. Now, especially if you're poor, all the incentives are pushing you toward unhealthy foods.

Q: *Like zip codes where there are no grocery stores?*

A: That's a great example of a bad default. Another, which applies not just to the poor, would be what children have available in schools. You can sell a lot of junk in schools and then try to educate your way out of it. Or you can just get rid of the junk food and kids will have healthier defaults. They'll eat healthier food if that's what's available. You can inspire that just by changing the default.

Imagine the optimal environment to combat obesity. We would have affordable and healthful food, especially fresh fruits and vegetables, easily accessible to people in low-income neighborhoods. TV commercials for children would encourage them to eat fresh fruits and vegetables rather than pushing processed snacks that are associated with TV and movie characters. And every community would have safe sidewalks and walking trails to encourage physical activity.

Q: *So people wouldn't have to struggle to avoid eating junk?*

A: Right. We have a terrible set of defaults with food: big portions, bad marketing, bad food in schools. These conditions produce incentives for the wrong behaviors. So the question is: can we create an environment that supports healthy eating, rather than undermines it?

If you count the number of places where you can buy sugared beverages and salty snack foods and candy, it's enormous. If you count the number of places where you can buy baby carrots and oranges, it's a fraction of that.

So if you were creating an environment from scratch, you would do the opposite of what we have. The population deserves a better set of defaults.

Critical Thinking

1. What is meant by the quote, "our biology is mismatched with the modern world"?
2. What types of foods are considered addictive?
3. The author talks about the U.S. food defaults. What are the U.S. food defaults that are causative factors in our toxic food environment?

KELLY BROWNELL is a professor in the Department of Psychology at Yale University. He is also a professor of epidemiology and public health. Brownell co-founded and directs Yale's Rudd Center for Food Policy and Obesity, which works to improve the world's diet, prevent obesity, and reduce weight stigma. Brownell, who is a member of *Nutrition Action*'s scientific advisory board, has published more than 300 scientific articles and chapters and 14 books including *Food Fight: The Inside Story of the Food Industry, America's Obesity Crisis, and What We Can Do About It* (McGraw-Hill). He spoke to *Nutrition Action*'s Bonnie Liebman from New Haven.

The Subtle Knife

After weight-loss surgery, strange things start happening to people's minds. Samantha Murphy found out for herself.

Samantha Murphy

It had been so long since I had had anything to drink but water. Finally, the day I had been waiting for arrived and I mixed a glass of my favourite peach iced tea. Anticipating its tart sweetness, I took a big swig of the drink, holding it in my mouth to savour the flavour. My euphoria turned to horror. It tasted like fish.

I spat the foul brew into the sink and tried the raspberry flavour. Fish, again. I slumped dejectedly onto the sofa. Why had no one warned me about this?

Two weeks earlier, I had had surgery to help me lose weight. Eating and drinking had been a struggle ever since: my new hypersensitivity to sweetness was surpassed only by the nausea that hit me when I smelled cooking meat. What was going on?

I hunted for answers in online forums. While my turncoat taste buds seemed to be a common phenomenon after weight-loss or bariatric surgery, no one offered a convincing explanation. But I soon realised that I had got off lucky: the forums were filled with horror stories detailing side effects, from memory loss and anxiety to auditory hallucinations. Even more puzzling were the unexplained mental boosts. About three months after surgery, a significant number of people experienced a sudden burst of "mental clarity".

No obvious thread linked these effects—but it seemed that when surgeons operated on our stomachs, something had happened in our brains, too. Even more intriguing, the surgery seems to work precisely because it creates fundamental changes in the brain. How can this be happening?

For me, surgery was a last resort. I had struggled with my weight since early childhood, and last year I finally opted to have a surgical procedure called a duodenal switch.

Surgery offers many ways to reduce the size of the stomach. Least invasive is a band that constricts it, but if you want to surgically restrict the stomach, the most popular option is Roux-en-Y or "gastric bypass". All such bariatric surgeries work on the same principle: they reduce the amount of food the body can absorb. In the US, where 36 per cent of the population is classified as obese, at least 200,000 people sign up to have the surgery every year, and that number keeps climbing.

Keeping the Weight Off

That's because surgery works. Whatever procedure people have, most find that their excess weight melts away within 18 months (*Obesity Surgery*, vol 6, p 651). For at least 50 per cent of those who choose the more invasive methods like Roux-en-Y, the weight stays off, demolishing the abysmal long-term success rates of diets and pills (*Annals of Surgery*, vol 254, p 272).

Initially, this success was thought to be down to the mechanics—constricting the stomach simply meant a person ate less. There was just one problem with that logic. If it were so simple, 50 per cent of people wouldn't regain their weight, for example by eating high-calorie, liquid foods like heavy cream-based soups and ice cream milkshakes. Those who kept the weight off did so in spite of the availability of such workarounds. There had to be another reason for their success.

The first clue lay in my taste buds' bizarre behaviour and how that affected my food preferences. Most doctors will tell you that long-term weight loss is only possible with sweeping lifestyle changes: eating foods with less fat and fewer calories. Unfortunately, by definition, most weight-loss methods foster a temporary "dieting" mentality, which is quickly discarded when the goal is reached or when disappointment overtakes motivation.

One reason it is so hard to keep weight off is that we are fighting our very nature. We are all hard-wired to crave unhealthy foods, and these cravings only intensify after we have lost weight by dieting.

But a strange thing was happening after bariatric surgery—food cravings were immediately, massively dampened. "People who have lost weight after surgery don't report a compensatory increase in food cravings or hunger the way dieting people do," says Stephen Benoit, a behavioural neuroscientist at the University of Cincinnati, Ohio, who studies obesity. Quite the opposite: they tend to report reduced levels of hunger, fewer food cravings and an overall altered relationship with food.

Food cravings aren't simply reduced, they are transformed. Within hours of any weight-loss surgery, many people can't stand the taste of sugar or fat and sometimes find the very smell offensive, says Carel le Roux, a bariatric endocrinologist at the Imperial Weight Centre in London. For Roux-en-Y, the effects linger. "In the long-term, we find people shifting their food preferences and going for the salad bar instead of a burger and fries," he says.

Might the switch be psychological? Perhaps, after expensive and physically demanding surgery, people convince themselves they crave only healthy foods. So le Roux and his team devised a test to tease out what lay behind these behavioural changes. They performed Roux-en-Y surgery on rats and then tested their subsequent food preferences. Like so many of their human counterparts, the rats almost instantly shifted their tastes to favour lower-fat, lower-sugar items. "These rats had never met a dietician," says le Roux, "so it wasn't as though they were suddenly more motivated to make healthier choices because they had surgery."

Le Roux had confirmed that these changes were physiological. But what could be causing them? An obvious starting point would be the hormones generated by the digestive system. The upper stomach, for example, produces a powerful hunger-promoter

called ghrelin. The small intestine releases a number of appetite-suppressing hormones that promote satiety, including glucagon-like peptide-1 (GLP-1) and peptide YY, or PYY. Even fat cells play a part in regulating appetite, releasing leptin, a hormone that inhibits the desire to eat and regulates metabolism.

Weight-loss surgery cuts into these major hormone manufacturing areas, radically altering their production. "Gastrointestinal hormones and leptin levels change after Roux-en-Y, and do so in a favourable direction," says Lauren Beckman, a researcher at the University of Minnesota in Minneapolis who is studying hormonal changes in people who have had bariatric surgery.

Rearranging the stomach also lowers the production of appetite-stimulating ghrelin, which might explain why many surgery recipients have to force themselves to eat (*Journal of Parenteral & Enteral Nutrition,* vol 35, p 169). Leptin, too, is affected, spiking immediately to damp down hunger (*Journal of Clinical Investigation,* vol 118, p 2380).

Could it be that these hormone changes were triggering the weight loss? Beckman thinks so. If it were the other way around, she explains, "elevated hormone levels would not be expected to occur until at least one month later". Instead, she and other researchers are finding that concentrations of appetite-suppressing GLP-1 and PYY increase within about two days. Not only do these changes happen immediately, but they stay that way, Beckman found, for at least one to two years after surgery.

Intriguingly, the effects of GLP-1 and ghrelin seem to reach beyond the metabolism. Recent animal studies have shown that both hormones can disrupt the nervous system and synaptic plasticity—the very mechanisms that create structural and functional changes in the brain. For example, ghrelin alters the wiring of mouse neurons (*The Journal of Clinical Investigation,* vol 116, p 3229).

Researchers are not completely sure what these fluctuating hormones do to the human brain, but they have a ready-made experimental pool: people who have had weight-loss surgery.

"Super Normal"

The post-surgical flood of GLP-1, for example, immediately creates changes in the brain's reward centres in the orbitofrontal cortex, says le Roux. Could this explain the permanent shift in food preferences? To test the connection, last year, he and his colleagues at Imperial College London used MRI scanners to look at the brains of people before and after they had Roux-en-Y surgery. The results were staggering. Before surgery, pictures of cakes or burgers caused large areas of their reward centres to light up. But when the experiment was repeated just four days after surgery, their reward centres were impervious to the sight of the tempting foods. "Their exaggerated satiation makes the patient in effect 'super normal'," le Roux says, which accounts for the permanent weight loss. Their brains' circuits were being rewired to make them think like thin people.

That's not all. There is also evidence that changing the gut hormones' balance explains the improved brain function people reported on the weight-loss surgery forums.

GLP-1 is a particularly strong candidate for this effect. Because it suppresses the appetite by lowering blood sugar, it appears to have a strong effect on insulin, whose production

---

Change Your Stomach, Change Your Brain

After weight-loss surgery, the production of hormones by the digestive system is immediately altered, which seems to affect the way the brain responds to food

Appetite Regulators

Several hormones produced in the gut affect the brain's satiety centres, particularly the hypothalamus and potentially the thalami.

Ghrelin
Appetite-stimulating hormone
Released by stomach

Glucagon-like peptide-1 (GLP-1):
Appetite-suppressing hormone
Released by small intestine

Peptide YY (PYY)
Appetite-suppressing hormone
Released by small intestine

Leptin
Inhibits the desire to eat
Released by fat cells

Surgery Variants

The three irreversible types of stomach surgery all work on the same principle: reduce the amount of food that can be eaten and absorbed, often by making the stomach smaller

Roux-en-Y

The stomach is stapled to leave only a small pouch at the top, which is then connected directly to the small intestine.

Vertical Sleeve Gastrectomy

The stomach is cut so that only a long, narrow tube remains.

Duodenal Switch

As in VSG, the stomach is cut into a tube. The intestine is also shortened so it can absorb fewer nutrients.

drops dramatically within hours of surgery. Lower insulin levels, in turn, reduce the insulin resistance caused by excess weight, which has itself been tied to neurological problems (*Neuroepidemiology,* vol 34, p 222).

Although we don't understand exactly why, most researchers agree that obese volunteers tend to perform less well than leaner people on some learning and memory tasks, specifically ones that measure what is called inhibitory control. This is a subtle measure: your ability to remember where you parked your car this morning depends on your short-term memory. But distinguishing where you parked your car this morning from where you parked it yesterday morning requires inhibitory control, which involves suppressing yesterday's information. So while it is certainly not true that obese people are less smart, it seems they aren't able to distinguish this information as well.

Some researchers think the simple act of balancing insulin levels lifts this cognitive burden. In 2010, Gladys Strain, an obesity researcher at Cornell University's medical college in Ithaca, New York, found that just three months after weight-loss surgery, people scored better on cognitive tests than they did prior to surgery. One year later their test scores were even better (*Surgery for Obesity and Related Diseases,* vol 4, p 465). Benoit says his group is also finding evidence of cognitive improvements after weight-loss surgery.

But there is a stinging caveat to evidence that the brain is permanently altered by surgery: not all of the changes are positive.

Keith Josephs made the connection by accident. Several years ago, Josephs, a neurologist at the Mayo Clinic in Rochester, Minnesota, began seeing a steady increase in patients with a variety of cognitive problems. Frustrated when batteries of tests revealed nothing amiss, they had turned to him. "They were coming to me with issues like having trouble finding the right word, difficulty concentrating at work, being slow to respond to people talking to them and short-term memory issues," he says. Initially, he was nonplussed. Then he began to see a pattern. All of them had had Roux-en-Y surgery.

"Four days after surgery to lose weight, people were impervious to the sight of tempting food"

Josephs set to work pulling participant records from the hospital database and comparing them against two control groups: obese people who had not had surgery, and people of a normal weight. His results, published late last year, were alarming.

MRI scans revealed that those reporting cognitive problems had 24 per cent less volume in the thalamus, a small area of the brain associated with memory, attention, concentration and sensory information about taste (*Journal of Clinical Neuroscience,* vol 18, p 1671). In particular, the thalamus contains binding sites for ghrelin and GLP-1 (*Brain Research Reviews,* vol 58, p 160).

Large changes in these hormones could affect this brain area in the same way they alter the reward centres. And just as the positive changes in food preference appear not to be temporary, so do these negative changes. "Once the thalami have shrunk, there is nothing we can do to regrow these nerve cells," Josephs says.

Josephs is cautious about the results of his small study, and acknowledges that it needs to be replicated. Nonetheless, he can't ignore or dismiss the results. The group was thorough about checking for confounding factors. For example, because the average age of the participants was 54, they screened for signs of Alzheimer's disease. They also tested rigorously for surgery-related vitamin deficiencies, and found none. Only hormonal changes could explain the shrinkage, he says: "The probability that this occurred just by chance is at best 1 in 1000."

These cognitive problems indicate that the effects of bariatric surgery are far more complicated than most surgeons currently imagine. Even my comparatively harmless fish tea defies explanation. "Taste changes after bariatric surgery in strange ways," le Roux says. "Something is scrambling the signal from the taste buds to the brain."

Are certain populations more susceptible to the positive effects of bariatric surgery? Is one kind of surgery more likely to lead to cognitive decline than the others? Questions like these are only now being asked. The US National Institutes of Health, for example, has just funded a series of longitudinal studies to track the long-term health of people who have had different kinds of bariatric surgery. Some researchers are beginning to wonder whether these changes point to a "knifeless solution" that makes use of these hormonal fluctuations to combat obesity at the neurological level (*International Journal of Obesity,* vol 35, p 40).

Seven months and 45 kilograms later, I find myself benefiting from some of these effects. I still encounter the occasional unexpected cup of fish tea, so I find myself drinking a lot more water. Chocolate remains a joy, but only less sweet dark chocolate, and only in small doses.

There's no question that the possibility of neurological problems is scary. But for me, at least, they are easy to put into perspective. Weight-loss surgery is a life-saving procedure: with a few well-placed cuts, it knocks out diabetes, high blood pressure and sleep apnea, among others. In the context of my new mental clarity, healthier future, and all the small ways my everyday life has been improved, the threat of permanent cognitive effects seems to me a fair trade. Even with the occasional cup of fish tea.

Critical Thinking

1. Differentiate between the three main forms of bariatric weight loss surgery: Roux-en-Y, Vertical Sleeve Gastrectomy, and Duodenal Switch.

2. Identify the hormone appetite regulators that are produced by the gastrointestinal system and fat cells.

3. Evaluate the possible reasons for changes in taste preferences, food cravings, and mental functions that have been reported by individuals who have bariatric surgery.

SAMANTHA MURPHY is a freelance writer based in Pennsylvania.

From *New Scientist Magazine,* May 19, 2012, pp. 43–45. Copyright © 2012 by Reed Business Information, Ltd, UK. Reprinted by permission via Tribune Media Services.

Eating Disorders in an Obesogenic Environment

Joyce A. Corsica, PhD and Megan M. Hood, PhD

An obesogenic environment is an environment that produces and supports overweight and obesity through several intersecting mechanisms. Obesogenic environments and behavior, particularly in the context of genetic susceptibility to obesity, are believed to account for the increased prevalence of overweight and obesity in the world today. Such an environment includes decreased physical activity, increased energy intake, heavy promotion of energy-dense foods, greater number of overweight people, biological predisposition to weight difficulties, food addiction and changes in neurochemistry, and impact of both social discrimination and media manipulation of the ideal body image. Together these factors pose substantial problems for individuals with disordered eating behaviors, as will be discussed in this article. Although the development of eating disorders is complex and multifactorial, the combination of these factors in the obesogenic environment has the potential to contribute to the disordered eating behavior and cognitions to which some young people are vulnerable.

The Obesogenic Environment

Contributors to the obesogenic environment include the current physical environment, behavior (including energy intake and decreased physical activity), and the social environment, as well as a biological predisposition to positive energy balance (1). In the past 3 decades, environmental changes have reduced physical activity via labor-saving devices such as cars, elevators, escalators, motorized walkways, and remote controls, which have had a cumulative impact in decreasing daily energy expenditure (2,3). At the same time, energy expended in leisure-time physical activities has decreased as people spend more time sitting passively in front of computers, televisions, DVD players, and video games rather than participating in physical activities that require movement and greater amounts of energy expenditure. National statistics confirm that fewer than one third of Americans engage in the recommended amounts of physical activity of at least 30 minutes most days (4). There is no federal standard or education mandate for physical education in schools (5), and physical activity programs are among the first areas to succumb to budget cuts (6).

Obesogenic behavior includes the consumption of larger portions of food, particularly high-fat, high-sugar foods, often combined with greater time spent in passive or sedentary activity. The current environment promotes the overconsumption of energy-dense, nutrient-poor food (7,8), which is typically considered obesogenic. Processed foods in particular pose difficulties for weight management. Comprised of primarily refined grains, sugars, and preservatives, processed foods (most packaged foods) are generally inexpensive, highly palatable, energy-dense, and convenient. When the diet includes higher amounts of processed foods, higher levels of hunger are reported (9). Excess consumption of processed food can also displace the consumption of healthier, whole foods and promote repeated cycles of eating (and craving) more processed, highly palatable foods. Moreover, these high-calorie and low-cost items are readily available at convenience stores, drug stores, and 24-hour service stations, in addition to fast-food restaurants, grocery stores, and food courts (7). In addition, more sugar-sweetened beverages are being consumed than ever before (10), which has been shown to be an independent risk factor for obesity in children (11). Lastly, many of these problematic foods are being served and consumed in increasingly large portion sizes, particularly in restaurants. Eating away from home, especially at fast-food restaurants, is associated with higher energy and higher fat intake (12) and is a significant contributor to weight gain and the increasing prevalence of overweight (13–15).

The obesogenic social environment includes constant advertising as well as opportunities and pressure to eat. Unhealthy foods, including many breakfast cereals and pastries, are often marketed selectively to children and vulnerable populations. The average child watches 10,000 advertisements for food each year, an astonishing 95 percent of which are for sugared cereals, candy, fast foods, and soft drinks (16). Television-watching is often accompanied by snacking on energy-dense foods (which are often being advertised) and is associated with higher body weight (17).

Finally, it is recognized that all of these environmental factors occur on a foundation of biology. Biological factors include a genetic predisposition to positive calorie balance, which was formerly an adaptive and protective response to environmental changes in energy availability. Several convergent lines of evidence support that there are individual differences in the predisposition to weight gain and suggests that genetic variation has much to do with the risk of becoming obese (18). In summary, the obesogenic environment is characterized as a confluence of highly palatable, readily available, heavily advertised foods; larger portion sizes; increased pressure to eat; and significantly decreased work and leisure activity, all in the context of biology that predisposes many to weight gain.

The Impact of the Media

The media's portrayal (and some would say, idealization) of a very thin female body type has long been viewed as an important socio-cultural risk factor for eating disorders (19,20). The media's impact on potential body dissatisfaction, disordered eating, and obesity is actually twofold. Media sources, including television shows, commercials, movies, and fashion magazines, encourage a generally unattainable, very thin ideal body image. For example, the average fashion model weighs 24 percent less than the average female today (21). Viewing of such images in fashion magazines seems to be associated with increased eating disorder symptomatology in adolescent girls (22,23). Yet, at the same time that a thin body is idealized, media-based advertising reinforces the availability and even the sex appeal of high-energy-dense foods. Taken together, the average woman faces conflicting messages: very thin equals beautiful, but eating energy-dense foods is attractive and desirable. The combination of what many perceive as an unhealthy, unattainable, but highly valued body image perpetuated in the media, with the realities of the obesogenic environment, sets up a virtually no-win situation that can lead to feelings of learned helplessness, psychological distress, and potential self-dislike/hatred and increased rates of both disordered eating and obesity. Although the media's influence has been longstanding, it has a far greater presence now than ever before (24).

Psychosocial Consequences of Obesity: Impact on Disordered Eating and Dieting

The obesogenic environment, by definition, promotes obesity, and obesity can and does result in considerable social discrimination and psychological distress. Social consequences associated with obesity (which result from the widespread but mistaken belief that overweight people lack self-control) include bias, stigmatization, and discrimination, consequences that can be highly detrimental to psychological well-being (25). Negative attitudes toward obese people have been reported by children as well as adults, by health care professionals as well as the general public, and by overweight individuals themselves (26,27). Discrimination due to obesity may well be the last socially acceptable form of widespread prejudice. The impact of this prejudice on young people, in terms of their body image, food choices, and behaviors, cannot be understated. Discrimination or bias may compel more restriction in the current environment, and the high rates of obesity make this more likely. Exposure to critical comments by family about shape, weight, or eating behaviors, as well as weight-related teasing, have been identified as risk factors for a range of eating disordered behaviors (28,29).

Up to one in four 11-year-olds has already tried to diet once (30). This is concerning because children who diet may actually end up gaining more weight in the long term compared with children who do not diet due to the fact that dieting may cause a cycle of restrictive eating followed by overeating or binge-eating (31). The risk for obesity may be more than 300 percent higher for adolescent girls who describe themselves as dieters compared with those who do not diet (32). Adolescent girls who are obese or at risk for becoming obese are also more likely to use unhealthy weight practices, such as vomiting and using diet pills or laxatives (33).

Notably, an obesogenic environment confers more potential for parents to be overweight. Rates of overweight in this county have now reached 68 percent (34), which means it is likely that a child will have at least one parent who is overweight. In some children and adolescents, a combination of genetics and environmental factors related to having an overweight parent may increase perception/risk for eating disorders (22). This is especially true if overweight parents allow energy-dense foods in the diet (and in the house), promote the use of food to modulate mood states, promulgate weight and shape biases, make critical comments about shape or weight, and do not tend to encourage leisure-time physical activity.

Newer Research: Food Addiction and External Food Sensitivity as Contributors to Intake Regulation Difficulties and Disordered Eating

Many people report addiction-like symptoms, including cravings and loss of control over eating, related to eating the very foods previously discussed as contributing to the obesogenic environment (high-sugar, high-fat, processed foods) (35,36). Recent research suggests that addiction-like processes may underlie some intake regulation difficulties in some people and may contribute to disordered eating and weight-control difficulties (37). For example, sugar is thought to have addiction potential as a highly palatable food that releases opioids and dopamine (38), but researchers have demonstrated in animals that it is a pattern of restriction alternated with brief availability that seems to produce an addictive pattern of eating. Recent evidence suggests that behavioral and neural pathway changes may be induced by the restriction/exposure pattern, including tendency to self-medicate, restricting/bingeing pattern, or tendency to eat certain foods while hungry. It has been suggested that some disordered eating behaviors, including the frequently seen pattern of daytime restriction and nighttime overeating/loss of control, binge eating, or even diet cycling, may replicate the restriction/exposure pattern found in animal studies, resulting in food addiction symptoms (36).

Another recently identified factor that may encourage increased energy intake is susceptibility to environmental cues (known as external food sensitivity), which has been demonstrated via functional resonance imagery to serve as a predisposing factor to food cravings and food intake (39). This means that the sight, smell, or suggestion of food can serve as a potent eating trigger in susceptible people. Given the obesogenic environment, replete with easily available, heavily advertised, and palatable foods, this increased exposure may induce cravings, loss of control, and binge cycling as early as childhood and adolescence in those who are susceptible to these environmental cues, which, as previously discussed, are pervasive in our current environment.

Eating Disorders in the Obesogenic Environment

Rates of eating disorders in women are increasing (40), and eating disorders are being diagnosed at younger ages and with greater frequency (41). Although most teens do not suffer from a diagnosable eating disorder or from obesity, many engage in disordered eating behaviors such as binge-eating, purging, and dieting that are sustained across the next decade of life (42). These behaviors can be associated with serious physical and emotional difficulties, as well as ongoing and unremitting symptomatology across many years.

In an obesogenic environment, it is a far greater challenge to maintain healthy eating habits in light of the environmental and biological factors discussed thus far. Exposure to this environment, with its energy-dense food choices that are constantly available, low levels of physical activity, greater likelihood of overweight parents, bias/discrimination either received or observed, and very early dieting, combined with conflicting messages in the media can together, or even in isolation, lead to feelings of loss of control, food restriction, bingeing, and weight gain. Considering that those with binge-eating behaviors are more susceptible than non–binge-eaters to the variety of processed, sweetened, high-fat foods that are available (as they report receiving greater enjoyment out of the taste, smell, and texture of food [43] and tend to have lower dietary restraint than those with restricting eating disorders), this environmental onslaught of food availability poses considerable and constant challenges to those who engage in binge-eating behavior (44).

Even in very young children, there is a substantial impact of the environment on the development of obesity and disordered eating. Binge-eating episodes have been reported in 2 percent of children age 5 to 6 years and presence of these episodes is associated with obesity (45). Moreover, the presence of binge-eating in these children is strongly associated with eating disturbances in their mothers. Warning signs of possible disordered eating behavior in children include eating in the absence of hunger, eating to modulate strong or negative affect, eating in secret, or hiding food (46).

Prevention: Changing the Obesogenic Environment

Efforts toward prevention of weight- and eating-related problems must occur on multiple levels, including, perhaps most importantly, changes in the obesogenic environment (47). Current efforts at prevention, such as taxes on soda and processed foods, and reduced availability of sugar-sweetened soft drinks and vending machines in schools, have the potential to reduce exposure to some especially obesogenic foods. Interventions targeting the school environment are particularly important given the potential to dramatically impact awareness and eating habits for children and adolescents during key developmental periods (see references [48–51] for reviews of obesity-prevention programs). To improve the obesogenic environment, we offer the following suggestions (adapted from reference [52]), which lend themselves to reducing the potential for disordered eating in this environment.

Continue to Intervene in Schools

Schools are in a unique position to support the promotion of healthy lifestyles. Interventions in the school environment can result in beneficial changes in both diet and physical activity. School-based physical activity programs that provide for enjoyable and regular exercise participation for all students are a necessity. In addition, schools should promote healthy eating patterns by ensuring that cafeterias and vending machines offer a variety of low-cost, nutritious foods and snacks. Continuing to address processed food availability, including fast-food operations on school premises, is necessary. It is imperative that we decrease access to high-calorie, nutritionally poor foods and provide greater opportunities for students to select healthy foods. In addition, an effective school-based intervention may require multiple components, including a behavioral curriculum, parent involvement, changes in the school food program, and support from the food industry.

Regulate Advertising of Junk Foods

Restaurant, soft drink, and candy companies spend more than $400 billion per year to advertise their products, often targeting their messages to young people, whereas very little is spent on advertising to promote healthy dietary practices (7). This dramatic inequity requires attention, and more stringent regulation is needed to decrease the advertising of unhealthy foods, particularly during children's shows. It may be helpful to require TV commercials to disclose prominently the nutrient values (eg, calories, calories from fats, serving size) of advertised products, particularly snack foods. The concept of food addiction makes a strong case for reducing, limiting, or controlling foods with addiction potential in the environment (36).

Impose a "Sugared Beverage Tax"

For many years, Brownell and his colleagues (53,54) have recommended adopting a tax on unhealthy foods, with the revenues from such a tax used to fund public health initiatives to promote healthy eating and exercise habits. A modest tax per 12-oz soft drink or per pound of snack foods would go toward subsidizing healthier food choices, underwriting the cost of a national campaign to improve the nation's eating habits, or reducing health care costs. A recent national survey showed that 60 percent to 70 percent of adults would support such a tax if the revenues were used to reduce health care costs (55).

Prevention in the Home: Helping Adolescents Develop Healthy Eating Attitudes and Behaviors in an Obesogenic Environment

Adults can serve as positive role models for their children. Because children of overweight parents are more likely to be overweight, and daughters of mothers who diet are more likely to diet than other girls, it is critical that adults, particularly women, model healthy eating attitudes and behaviors. The following guidelines are adapted from BodyWise and Bodyworks, which are initiatives of the US Department of Health and Human Services Office on Women's Health (56).

- Assist children in attaining a positive relationship with food. Serve and eat a variety of foods and balanced meals, plan meals in advance, and keep healthy snacks available. Skipping meals should be discouraged, and food should not be used as a reward.
- Help children learn control of their own eating behaviors. Avoid forcing food on children and adolescents (including cleaning the plate) and avoid forbidding or restricting certain foods. Studies show that when mothers restrict their children's food, the children tend to eat more when unsupervised (57). Encourage eating until satisfied, and discourage eating outside of hunger.
- Encourage family meals and eating breakfast. Eating meals as a family has emerged as a possible buffer against the development of eating disorders in adolescent girls (33). Likewise, breakfast-eating may also play a role in preventing the development of eating problems (58) and improving dietary quality and physical activity among adolescents (59).
- Be aware of children's emotional health. Depression, anxiety, and the use of food to cope with emotional states may signal both the need for intervention and increased risk for disordered eating patterns.

- Provide opportunities for children to participate in a variety of physical activities, including sporting activities, dancing, hiking, swimming, and anything that is enjoyable and gets them moving. Encourage both a wide range of activities and mindful physical activity choices (eg, stairs vs elevator). Parents and other adults and older siblings should model increased activity so that it is a natural part of the environment. At the same time, exposure and opportunity for sedentary activities, such as computer use and television-viewing, should be limited.

- Discuss unrealistic media messages about females' bodies as well as the mixed messages conveyed in the media. It is important to discuss how media images are manipulated by computers and airbrushing and how they are not real images of real females. Create a positive focus on health and health-promoting behaviors and activities to build and foster self-esteem. It may be particularly important to address the internalized aesthetic standards that produce faulty weight-related expectations, to resist the social pressure to achieve an "ideal" body, to adopt non-derogatory self-statements about large body size, and to uncouple the association between body weight and self-esteem (60).

References

1. Bouchard C, Rankinen T. Exciting advances and new opportunities. In: Clement K, Sorensen T (eds). *Obesity: Genomics and Postgenomics.* New York, NY: Informa Healthcare; 2008. 549–562.

2. Hill JO, Wyatt HR, Melanson EL. Genetic and environmental contributions to obesity. *Med Clin North Am.* 2000;84:333–346.

3. James WP. A public health approach to the problem of obesity. Int J Obes. 1995;19(suppl 3):S37–S45.

4. US Department of Health and Human Services, Centers for Disease Control and Prevention. Vital and Health Statistics Summary. Health Statistics for US Adults: National Health Interview Survey, 2009. US Department of Health and Human Services, Centers for Disease Control and Prevention. 2010. www.cdc.gov/nchs/data/series/sr_10/sr1_249.pdf. Accessed March 31, 2011.

5. Plaza C. School nutrition & physical education legislation: An overview of 2005 state activity. Robert Wood Johnson Foundation Web site. www.rwjf.org/files/research/NCSL%20-%20April%202005%20Quarterly%20Report.pdf. Accessed March 31, 2011.

6. Lee SM, Burgeson CR, Fulton JE, Spain CG. Physical education and physical activity: Results from the School Health Policies and Programs Study 2006. *J Sch Health.* 2007;77:435–463.

7. Battle EK, Brownell KD. Confronting a rising tide of eating disorders and obesity: Treatment vs prevention and policy. *Addict Behav.* 1996;21:755–765.

8. Kant AK. Consumption of energy-dense, nutrient-poor foods by adult Americans: Nutritional and health implications. The Third National Health and Nutrition Examination Survey, 1988–1994. *Am J Clin Nutr.* 2000;72:929–936.

9. Fuhrman J, Sarter B, Glaser D, Acocella S. Changing perceptions of hunger on a high nutrient density diet. *Nutr J.* 2010;9:51.

10. Nielsen SJ, Popkin BM. Changes in beverage intake between 1977 and 2001. *Am J Prev Med.* 2004;27:205–210.

11. Ludwig DS, Peterson KE, Gortmaker SL. Relations between consumption of sugar-sweetened drinks and childhood obesity. *Lancet.* 2001;357:505–508.

12. French SA, Harnack L, Jeffery RW. Fast food restaurant use among women in the Pound of Prevention study: Dietary, behavioral and demographic correlates. *Int J Obes.* 2000;24:1353–1359.

13. Binkley JK, Eales J, Jekanowski M. The relation between dietary change and rising U.S. obesity. *Int J Obes.* 2000;24:1032–1039.

14. McCrory MA, Fuss PJ, Hays NP, Vinken AG, Greenberg AS, Roberts SB. Overeating in America: Association between restaurant food consumption and body fatness in healthy adult men and women ages 19 to 80. *Obes Res.* 1999;7:564–571.

15. Pereira M, Kartashov AI, Ebbeling CB, Van Horn L, Slattery ML, Jacobs Jr. M, Ludwig DS. Fast-food habits, weight gain, and insulin resistance (The CARDIA Study): 15-year prospective analysis. *Lancet.* 2005;365:36–42.

16. Brownell K. The environment and obesity. In: Fairburn CG, Brownell KD, eds. *Eating Disorders and Obesity,* 2nd ed. New York, NY: Guilford Press; 2002:433–438.

17. Harris JL, Bargh JA, Brownell KD. Priming effects of television food advertising on eating behavior. *Health Psychol.* 2009;28:404–413.

18. Bouchard C. The biological predisposition to obesity: Beyond the thrifty gene scenario [commentary]. *Int J Obes.* 2007;31:1337–1339.

19. Levine M, Harrison K. Media's role in the perpetuation and prevention of negative body image and disordered eating. In: Thompson JK, ed. *Handbook of Eating Disorders and Obesity.* Hoboken, NJ: John Wiley & Sons, Inc; 2004:695–717.

20. Stice E, Schupak-Neuberg E, Shaw H, Stein RI. Relation of media exposure to eating disorder symptomatology: An examination of mediating mechanisms. *J Abnorm Psychol.* 1994;103:836–840.

21. Kilbourne J. *Deadly Persuasion: Why Women Must Fight the Addictive Power of Advertising.* New York, NY: Free Press, 1999.

22. Bulik CM. Genetic and biological risk factors. In: Thompson JK, ed. *Handbook of Eating Disorders and Obesity.* Hoboken, NJ: John Wiley & Sons, Inc; 2004:3–16.

23. Vaughan K, Fouts G. Changes in television and magazine exposure and eating disorder symptomatology. *Sex Roles.* 2003;49:313–320.

24. Derenne, JL, Eugene V. Beresin, EV. Body Image, Media, and Eating Disorders. *Acad Psychiatry.* 2006;30:257–261.

25. Stunkard AJ, Sobal J. Psychosocial consequences of obesity. In: Brownell KD, Fairburn CG, eds. *Eating Disorders and Obesity: A Comprehensive Handbook.* New York, NY: Guilford Press; 1995;417–421.

26. Crandall CS, Biernat M. The ideology of antifat attitudes. *J Appl Soc Psychol.* 1990;20:227–243.

27. Rand CS, Macgregor AM. Morbidly obese patients' perceptions of social discrimination before and after surgery for obesity. *South Med J.* 1990;83:1390–1395.

28. Wade T, Gillespie N, Martin NG. A comparison of early family life events amongst monozygotic twin women with lifetime anorexia nervosa, bulimia nervosa, or major depression. *Int J Eat Disord.* 2007;40:679–686.

29. Fairburn C, Doll HA, Welch SL, Hay PJ, Davies BA, O'Connor ME. Risk factors for binge-eatingdisorder: A community-based, case-control study. *Arch Gen Psychiatry.* 1998;55:425–432.

30. Hill AJ. Prevalence and demographics of dieting. In: Fairburn CG, Brownell KD eds. *Eating Disorders and Obesity,* 2nd ed. New York, NY: Guilford Press; 2002:80–83.

31. Field AE, Austin SB, Taylor CB, Malspeis S, Rosner B, Rockett HR, Gillman MW, Colditz GA. Relation between dieting and weight change among preadolescents and adolescents. *Pediatrics.* 2003;112:900–906.

32. Stice E, Cameron RP, Killen JD, Hayward C, Taylor CB. Naturalistic weight-reduction efforts prospectively predict growth in relative weight and onset of obesity among female adolescents. *Consult Clin Psychol.* 1999;67:967–974.

33. Neumark-Sztainer D, Eisenberg ME, Fulkerson JA, Story M, Larson NI. Family meals and disordered eating in adolescents: Longitudinal findings from project EAT. *Arch Pediatr Adolesc Med.* 2008;162:17–22.

34. Flegal KM, Carroll MD, Ogden CL, Curtin LR. Prevalence and trends in obesity among US adults, 1999–2008. *JAMA.* 2010;303:235–241.

35. Bjorvell H, Ronnberg S, Rosner S. Eating patterns described by a group of treatment seeking overweight women and normal weight women. *Scand J Behav Trier.* 1985;14:147–156.

36. Gearhardt AN, Corbin WR, Brownell KB. Preliminary validation of the Yale Food Addiction Questionnaire. *Appetite.* 2008;52:430–436.

37. Corsica JA, Pelchat ML. Food addiction: True or false? *Curr Opin Gastroenterol.* 2010;26:165–169.

38. Avena NM, Rada P, Hoebel BG. Evidence for sugar addiction: Behavioral and neurochemical effects of intermittent, excessive sugar intake. *Neurosci Biobehav Rev.* 2008;32:20–29.

39. Passamonti L, Rowe JB, Schwarzbauer C, Ewbank MP, von dem Hagen E, Calder AJ. Personality predicts the brains response to viewing appetizing foods: The neural basis of a risk factor for overeating. *J Neurosci.* 2009;29:43–51.

40. Borzekowski DL, Bayer AM. Body image and media use among adolescents. *Adolesc Med.* 2005;16:289–313.

41. Field AE, Carmargo, CA, Taylor, CB. Peer, parent, and media influences on the development and frequent dieting among preadolescent and adolescent girls and boys. *Pediatrics.* 2001;107:54–60.

42. Neumark-Sztainer D, Wall, M, Larson, NI, Eisenberg, ME, Loth, K. Dieting and disordered eating behaviors from adolescence to young adulthood: Findings from a 10-year longitudinal study. *J Am Diet Assoc.* 2011;111:1004–1011.

43. Mitchell JE, Mussell MP, Peterson CB, Crow S, Wonderlich SA, Crosby RD, Davis T, Weller C. Hedonics of binge eating in women with bulimia nervosa and binge eating disorder. *Int J Eat Disord.* 1999;26:165–170.

44. Wilfley DE, Schwartz MB, Spurrell EB, Fairburn CG. Using the eating disorder examination to identify the specific psychopathology of binge eating disorder. *Int J Eat Disord.* 2000;27:259–269.

45. Lamerz A, Kuepper-Nybelen J, Bruning N, Wehle C, Trost-Brinkhues G, Brenner H, Hebebrand J, Herpertz-Dahlmann B. Prevalence of obesity, binge eating, and night eating in a cross-sectional field survey of 6-year-old children and their parents in a German urban population. *J Child Psychol Psychiatry.* 2005;46:385–393.

46. Marcus MD, Kalarchian MA. Binge eating in children and adolescents. *Int J Eat Disord.* 2003;34(suppl 1):S47–S57.

47. Brownell K. The humbling experience of treating obesity: Should we persist or desist? *Behav Res Ther.* 2010;48:717–719.

48. Baranowski T, Cullen KW, Nicklas T, Thompson D, Baranowski J. School-based obesity prevention: A blueprint for taming the epidemic. *Am J Health Behav.* 2002;26:486–493.

49. Doak CM, Visscher TM, Renders CL, Seidell J. The prevention of overweight and obesity in children and adolescents: A review of interventions and programmes. *Obes Rev.* 2006;7:111–136.

50. Kropski JA, Keckley PH, Jensen GL. School-based obesity prevention programs: An evidence-based review. *Obesity.* 2008;16:1009–1018.

51. Stice E, Shaw H, Marti CN. A meta-analytic review of obesity prevention programs for children and adolescents: The skinny on interventions that work. *Psychol Bull.* 2006;132:667–691.

52. Corsica JA, Perri MG. Obesity. In: Nezu A. ed. *Handbook of Psychology.* Vol 9. 2nd ed. Hoboken, NJ: John Wiley & Sons, Inc. In press.

53. Brownell KD. Get slim with higher taxes. *The New York Times.* Dec 15, 1994;A29.

54. Jacobson MF, Brownell KD. Small taxes on soft drinks and snack foods to promote health. *Am J Public Health.* 2000;90:854–857.

55. Center for Science in the Public Interest. Taxing sugared beverages would help trim state budget deficits, consumers' bulging waistlines, and health care costs. Center for Science in the Public Interest Web site. www.cspinet.org/new/pdf/state_budget_report_-_sugar_tax.pdf. 2010. Accessed March 31, 2011.

56. US Department of Health and Human Services Office on Women's Health. US Department of Health and Human Services Web site. www.4woman.gov. Accessed March 15, 2011.

57. Birch L. Acquisition of food preferences and eating patterns in children. In: Fairburn CG, Brownell, KD eds. *Eating Disorders and Obesity,* 2nd ed. New York, NY: Guilford Press; 2002:75–79.

58. Fernández-Aranda F, Krug I, Granero R, Ramon JM, Badia A, Giménez L, Solano R, Collier D, Karwautz A, Treasure J. Individual and family eating patterns during childhood and early adolescence: An analysis of associated eating disorder factors. *Appetite.* 2007;49:476–485.

59. Timlin M, Pereira MA, Story M, Neumark-Sztainer D. Breakfast eating and weight change in a 5-year prospective analysis of adolescents: Project EAT (Eating Among Teens). *Pediatrics.* 2008;121:e638–e645.

60. Foster GD, Kendall PC. The realistic treatment of obesity: Changing the scales of success. *Clin Psychol Rev.* 1994;14:701–736.

Critical Thinking

1. Describe the obesogenic environment in the United States.

2. Explain how negative stigmas and prevalence of negative messages regarding obesity can potentiate the development of eating disorders.

2. List five ways adults can address the impact of the obesogenic environment on the development of eating disorders.

J. A. CORSICA AND M. M. HOOD are assistant professors, Rush University Medical Center, Chicago, IL.

How to Count a Calorie

An apple and a cookie can have the same number of calories. But which should you eat? Until recently, Weight Watchers couldn't say. The company's solution was to totally revamp its formula and ask a million members to change their diet.

JEFFREY M. O'BRIEN

Like many weight watchers members, David Kirchhoff has a before picture and an after picture.

In the Before, he looks jolly but hefty, all cheeks and jowls, the result of years of eating obliviously. A 32-year-old with a biomedical engineering degree from Duke, an MBA from the University of Chicago, and a job as a management consultant, he's clearly been paying more attention to his studies and advancement than his appearance or health. Things aren't so bad that he would get the Kevin Smith treatment from Southwest Airlines, but it's easy to imagine him breaking into a sweat carrying a pint of Ben & Jerry's up a flight of stairs. He'll soon be diagnosed with high blood pressure and high cholesterol. His doctor suggests a statin.

Now the After, more than a decade later: close-cropped blond hair, 34-inch waist, and 15 percent body fat on his 6' 3" frame. In a form-fitting suit, the 45-year-old father of two cuts the figure of a Marine sergeant 20 years his junior. This is a picture of a man in control.

Kirchhoff's tale of weight gain is a common one. Between the end of high school and his midthirties, a slowing metabolism, changing lifestyle, and some disposable income all conspired to reshape his body. Looking back, it's not hard to see where things went wrong. "In college, it was all-you-can-eat—10,000 gallons of beer, pizza, the whole thing," he recalls. "Then I got a job with a lot of traveling. There was life on the road, room service. It became really easy to have any kind of awesome food any time I wanted. Take-out Chinese, delivery Chinese, deep-dish Chicago pizza, barbecue, huge breakfasts. There was literally no restraint. If you look at my swing from high school to my peak, it's about 75 pounds."

Unlike most, however, Kirchhoff found his way back to fighting trim. He entirely credits Weight Watchers. Walking the aisles of a mom-and-pop grocery store in Manhattan's Flatiron District, he parses the contents of the shelves to demonstrate what the company taught him about the effect of various foods

on his body. Chips, pretzels, prepared meals loaded with oils and butter, blue cheese dressing: all obviously evil. Orange juice, sun-dried tomatoes, and hummus: surprisingly bad. Then there's the good stuff: any (nonprocessed) fruit and (non-starchy) vegetables, shellfish, and whole-grain bread, as well as chicken sausage, flank steak, skinless turkey breast, and pork tenderloin. "You know what's funny? People tend to run away from bacon, but it's not bad," he says, picking up a vacuum-sealed package in the meat case and tapping the nutritional information into a calculator app on his iPhone. "And turkey bacon is a great deal."

If Kirchhoff sounds like the perfect spokesperson for Weight Watchers, it's no accident. He's not just one of the dieting giant's million-odd members around the globe, he's the guy in charge: In 2006, he became the company's president and CEO. And lately he's been guiding the sprawling enterprise through a sort of renaissance.

In the past year, Kirchhoff has crafted a corporate After picture as impressive as his own. In the midst of protracted economic malaise, he's boosted online membership by 64 percent and increased attendance at North American meetings by 14 percent. He's breathed new life into the brand, posted impressive revenue and profit growth, and doubled the company's market cap to, as of mid November, roughly $5 billion.

The story of how he's managed to do all this starts with Kirchhoff ripping out the foundation of Weight Watchers in the name of science. Actually, it starts with a hunch that the science underlying the company's venerable weight-loss formula—the very formula that helped Kirchhoff lose all that weight and made his own After picture possible—was flawed.

In 1980, 15 percent of adult Americans were obese, defined as having a minimum body mass index of 30, or roughly 200 pounds on a 5' 8" frame. Today, more than a third of us qualify. Throw in the pudgy and portly—a BMI of 25 or more, or 165 pounds on that 5' 8" frame—and the Centers for Disease Control and Prevention estimates that two-thirds of us are overweight. The downsides aren't just aesthetic. Our corpulence is making us sick, and we're all paying the bill. Treatments for obesity-related conditions such as diabetes, chronic joint pain, asthma, heart disease, and several types of cancer account for an estimated $147 billion annually, or roughly 10 percent of the nation's total health care outlay. That's 50 percent more than the cost of smoking-related treatments.

A fat and sickly society has many fathers, including agricultural subsidy policies, traffic, screen time, sedentary lifestyles, and the increased energy density of our foods. But on an individual level, obesity, at least among adults, is a disease of choice. For most of us, obesity comes from repeatedly making the wrong decisions about what to eat. And whatever your preconceptions about Weight Watchers, its rah-rah tactics, or its bubbly celebrity spokespeople, it's a provably effective tool for making better choices.

The program works, and peer-reviewed science has repeatedly shown this. Most recently, the medical journal *The Lancet* detailed the findings of a one-year randomized clinical trial initiated in 2007 by researchers from the Medical Research Council in Cambridge, the Technical University of Munich, and the University of Sydney. Eight hundred overweight or obese subjects were split into two camps. One group went to general practice MDs for weight-loss advice, and the other went to Weight Watchers. In all three countries, the medical counsel group showed an average weight loss of about 5 pounds at the one-year mark. Going for medical counseling worked. But members of the Weight Watchers group did better: On average, they lost 11 pounds.

This makes it all the more strange that Kirchhoff decided it was time for the program to change. Until the end of 2010, members participated in a dieting regimen called Points, in which all foods and drinks were assigned a numeric value, based primarily on their caloric content. Members received a daily allocation of points based on their height, weight, age, and gender. They also got a weekly stipend of extra points to use at their discretion and could earn more points through exercise. This system, which boiled down to a formula for caloric restriction, had been in place for close to a decade when Kirchhoff took the helm. Despite his personal success with Points, the program's agnostic approach to calories nagged at him. A member could theoretically go on an all-donut diet and still be in the program's good graces. "Think about it. It's 3 o'clock in the afternoon, and under the old program, we'd have a member who is thinking, 'I can have an apple, which is two points, or a cookie snack pack, which is also two points,'" Kirchhoff says. "It didn't feel right,"

So when Kirchhoff became CEO, one of his first official actions was to call a meeting of his top lieutenants, including his chief scientific officer, Karen Miller-Kovach. At the meeting he asked a simple question. "If we knew everything we know now when we developed Points, would it look exactly the way it does?" he remembers saying. "And Karen being Karen, because she has no filter, looked back at me and said, 'No.'"

As part of her job, Miller-Kovach and her team constantly follow the latest trends in nutritional science. A few years before the meeting, for example, they had explored a concept called the glycemic index, or GI, which establishes a hierarchy of carbohydrates based on their effect on blood glucose. The body converts some carbs—like those found in fruits, vegetables, whole grains, and nuts—into glucose slowly. They tend not to cause blood sugar spikes and are thus said to have a low GI quotient. In 2004, Miller-Kovach commissioned a clinical trial in France in which subjects followed a Points program that also pushed them toward low GI foods. The study showed that the dual system resulted in higher levels of satiety. "One of the key factors that can derail people who are trying to lose weight is that they're hungry," says the 56-year-old dietitian who also has an MBA from Baldwin-Wallace College. "They feel deprived. It's difficult to sustain a behavior change for a long time if it's uncomfortable." Unfortunately, the modified system didn't increase weight loss.

But combining the broad notion of satiety with other new ideas in nutrition might. One promising avenue of research was a concept known as the thermic effect of food. This describes how the body works to metabolize various types of calories. It takes more effort to metabolize protein calories, for example, so you store fewer of these. Meanwhile, Miller-Kovach knew that a calorie of protein also provides the greatest degree of satiety, followed by a calorie of fiber-containing carbohydrate, nonfiber carbs, and finally, a calorie of fat. So eating protein means you absorb fewer calories, but also feel full longer. All this meshes well with another concept called energy density, which had played a role in the original Points system. The notion of energy density holds that people tend to eat the same volume of food no matter the caloric content, so an effective weight-loss strategy is to fill up on foods that are less dense with energy. Miller-Kovach felt that together these concepts collectively represented an important advancement in our understanding of how the human body processes food. Simply put, not all calories are equal, and so, for the first time in Weight Watchers' history, she felt the organization needed to develop a system that moved radically beyond just counting calories.

Weight Watchers CEO David Kirchhoff lost 35 pounds on the original Points program. Despite this success, he felt the system could be improved.

After the meeting with Kirchhoff, Miller-Kovach and her team started looking for ways to combine all this research and make it scale for a million members. "We take science, pools of evidence, and we distill it, we simplify it," she says. "I spend my life translating science to businesspeople and business to scientists. I consider myself bilingual."

To show how surprising food values can be, newbies are shown a poster with a croissant on one side and a ham-and-egg breakfast on the other. Points-wise, the pastry and the full breakfast are roughly the same.

The result is found in U.S. Patent Application 2010/0055271:

$$P = \frac{\begin{bmatrix} (PROm \times Cp \times Wpro) \\ + (CHOm \times Cc \times Wcho) \\ + (FATm \times Cf \times Wfat) \\ + (DFm \times Cdf \times Wdf) \end{bmatrix}}{D}$$

This new formula distinguishes among calories and ascribes values to a given food based on its makeup of protein, carbohydrates, fiber, and fat. From an eater's perspective, the formula brings both good and bad news. Members receive more points under the new system. But many foods cost more points now, including alcohol. The name change—from Points to PointsPlus—may have made the program sound like a minor upgrade, but the kernel underneath is entirely new. The program has effectively declared war on processed foods, which include obvious targets like breakfast pastries and fast food. But it also makes enemies of seemingly benign (or even healthy) foods, like orange juice.

Oranges, on the contrary, are encouraged. In fact, they're absolutely "free," zero points, as are all other fruits and most vegetables. That's because they offer a lot of food per calorie and are loaded with fiber, which makes us feel full even though it passes through the body essentially unprocessed. This somewhat radical move to free fruit drew criticism in the nutritional community, but Kirchhoff dismisses the hand-wringing. He explains the rationale while holding a quart of OJ, which contains the juice of eight oranges. "You could drink this. You may not feel great, but if you ate all the oranges that are in this, you'd feel horrible," he says. "When we made fruit zero points, a few dietitians said, 'Fruit has real sugar in it. People can really abuse fruit.' But there's so little evidence that people abuse fruit. It takes a while to eat. It's filling. Could you eat 12 bananas and count it as zero points? Yes. But how would you feel afterward?"

Weight watchers was founded in the early 1960s by a Queens, New York, homemaker named Jean Nidetch, who had a key insight: Sustainable weight loss is more achievable with emotional support. She prescribed a simple calorie-deficient diet developed by the New York Board of Health to some overweight neighbors and gathered them at her house for weekly commiseration, progress reports, and empathy. In effect, she took a system based in nutritional science and, instinctively, added a helping of behavioral science. Half a century later, this remains the Weight Watchers fundamental approach: a sound diet backed up by support meetings.

Which is not to say there haven't been bumps along the way. The company's darkest days came after its acquisition in 1978 by packaged foods giant H. J. Heinz, which turned the meetings into shill sessions for prepackaged meals. But unlike competitors Jenny Craig and Nutrisystem, Weight Watchers didn't require attendees to purchase the food. Low uptake and high overhead including the cost of freezers and distribution made for a weak business model. Membership dwindled, and in the mid-'90s, meeting attendance hit bottom.

A few years later, Weight Watchers introduced Points, and the company's fortunes began to turn. Although it was 95 percent based on calories, with a slight penalty for fat and a slight reward for fiber, the program had simplicity going for it. Rather than counting, say, 1,900 calories in a day, members could track 35 points. It made keeping tabs on food intake easy and even fun—almost gamelike. Membership and meeting attendance jumped as a result. With the company healthy, Heinz was able to sell Weight Watchers to private equity firm Invus for $750 million while retaining a royalty-free license to produce prepared meals, which are available in frozen-food cases. The sale, Miller-Kovach says, was "the best thing that ever happened to the company, in my opinion. We weren't pickles, baked beans, or soup. It was always like they didn't know what to do with us."

At a time when Americans were rushing to embrace fad diets, from Atkins to South Beach, the private equity firm instilled a more analytical mindset that was focused on market testing and peer review analysis, says Miller-Kovach, who joined the company in the early '90s. Weight Watchers went public in 2001, but the quantitative culture instilled by Invus lives on.

Kirchhoff and Miller-Kovach knew that moving to PointsPlus would tamper with all the success and goodwill the company had engendered since introducing Points. But Kirchhoff decided the time was right. Since its founding, Weight Watchers has been based on a combination of nutrition science and behavior modification. The nutritional science had evolved, so the company needed to as well. "On some level, you operate with belief. We believed it was the principled thing to do," he says. "We didn't imagine ourselves being on a calorie-dependent system 10 years from now."

The transformation required a radical, stealth operation. The company's more than 12,000 leaders, the emcees who guide the local meetings, were put on PointsPlus so they'd have it mastered before the switch. This meant they were practicing one program while preaching another. Meanwhile, marketing and brochures needed to be updated, new smartphone apps, calculators, and cookbooks had to be developed, and the website needed to be overhauled. Miller-Kovach's team compiled a new database of some 47,000 foods. All while, even in the executive

---

THEN *and* NOW

For years, Weight Watchers has been helping people track how much they eat by assigning point values to various foods. In 2010, the company radically altered how it determines these values with a new system called PointsPlus. The result: Some foods suddenly got a lot more expensive. Here's a look at how things changed.

	Points	PointsPlus
Banana	2	0
Wine (6-ounce glass)	3	5
Filet mignom (3 ounces)	10	7
Glazed doughnut	6	7
Orange juice (1 cup)	2	3
Domino's sausage pizza (1 slice)	4	8

ranks, people were questioning such a wholesale change. "Do I think at least 90 percent of the people who worked for Weight Watchers regretted Dave asking me that question? Yes," says Miller-Kovach, referring to the initial meeting with Kirchhoff. "The business had at least quadrupled since the introduction of Points, and very few people in areas of responsibility had been through a program transition. When reality hit, it was big."

Just after Thanksgiving 2010, Weight Watchers flipped the switch. Says Kirchhoff: "It was as though we went from dollars to euros overnight."

Considering the plight of the euro lately, there are those who consider the metaphor especially apt. Kirchhoff maintains a fist-pounding but eminently entertaining blog called Man Meets Scale, in which he damns the siren call of M&Ms and breakfast burritos while providing members a way to get his attention. In the weeks after the transition, Man Meets Scale received hundreds of comments. Some accused Kirchhoff of ripping away a security blanket. "Why change a plan that was working?" wrote one commenter. "It seems to me that this is a marketing plan to win over those people who are using other eating plans like South Beach, Zone, Atkins and also a way to sell more products." And another: "I hate it. I hate learning the new points and losing all my foods that I've put in over the last three years. I'm completely annoyed that microwave popcorn is three points now!!!!"

Then there are the experts who are dubious about the scientific validity of PointsPlus. Among them is Gary Taubes, the best-selling author of *Good Calories, Bad Calories* and *Why We Get Fat*. He evangelizes and consumes a high-fat, low-carb diet that he contends causes a reduction in insulin levels, which signal the body to burn fat. From his perspective, any system designed to restrict dieters from overeating is flawed. Taubes argues that as long as you're eating the right foods, you can eat as much as you'd like and stay thin. "What you want to do is to pay attention to fat metabolism and lower insulin levels, not lower calories," he says. "By building something on calories, you end up being in a constant state of hunger."

Taubes is especially incredulous about the move to make fruit free, which he says can definitely contribute to weight gain, especially among the obese. "I'm skeptical of the science in any program that allows you to eat as much fruit as you want," he says.

I tell Taubes that in 12 weeks of researching this story, I've lost more than 20 pounds, mostly thanks to PointsPlus. He asks about my diet, and I tell him I eat a lot more vegetables than I did previously and often four or more servings of fruit a day. He shares a story about how he once added five to six pears a day to his diet and gained 15 pounds in six months. "I got rid of the pears and the weight went away," he says. "Your body would prefer a certain amount of energy to run it. If you feed it less food, you're going to burn less calories. Your weight loss is very good, but the key is always long-term weight loss. If you do exactly what you're doing now, will the weight loss maintain—particularly if it requires deprivation?"

It's the right question. Taubes could be wrong about everything else and still be right to suggest that my pendulum will swing back. The odds are stacked against me and everyone else who has succeeded in shedding a few pounds. According to a study published in late October in *The New England Journal of Medicine,* weight loss causes a troubling hormonal shift. When deprived of enough calories to shed weight, the body fights back by increasing hunger pangs. Put the same plate of food in front of a 182-pound man who lost 22 pounds (me) and another who has been 182 pounds all along, and in all likelihood, I'll be the one calling for seconds.

So does Weight Watchers really help people succeed for the long term? Even one of the company's successful partners isn't sure. Cleveland Clinic, one of the country's premier heart hospitals, began a program in 2008 to pay for employee memberships to Weight Watchers and fitness centers in the hope of promoting health and reducing health care costs. The results have been impressive. "We had thousands of people join in the first year; the total number who have signed up is now over 16,000," says Paul Terpeluk, Cleveland Clinic's medical director of employee health services. The ones who joined Weight Watchers have lost a total of 128,411 pounds over three years, and "we've started to slow the rate of increase of our costs," he says.

But Terpeluk worries that the program is basically a crutch. "Successful weight management is going to be more than Weight Watchers. What if you fall off the wagon and don't count your points, do you gain the weight back and spiral downward?" he asks. "That's good business for Weight Watchers. But weight maintenance has more to do with behaviors and less to do with nutrition. It's a life-transformation approach. People have to take responsibility for their behaviors."

An hour north of San Francisco, surrounded by Sonoma's wine country, Santa Rosa, California, offers great weather and enviable access to both culture and nature. But other than that, this medium-size city is not unlike other places in the US. It has traffic jams, big-box stores, budget issues, and a serious weight problem. In the southern part of the city, 65 percent of the adult population is overweight or obese.

It's 9:30 am on a Tuesday at the Mendocino Avenue strip mall and nearly 60 locals have run, OK, walked, a gauntlet of caloric temptations (Panda Express, Five Guys, Cold Stone Creamery, Starbucks) to squeeze into a Weight Watchers meeting room. This is the company's nod to Terpeluk's assertion about lifestyle change and, more directly, its founder's original insight about the effectiveness of group therapy.

Members pay $42.95 a month to attend regular meetings. That fee also gives them access to Weight Watchers' digital tools and smartphone apps. More than 43,892 pounds were shed at this location during the first 10 months of 2011. The company knows this because every member steps on a scale upon crossing the threshold.

Today's session leader is Adrienne Bacigalupi, a cheerful woman who stands at the front of the room in a loud-patterned dress. Handing out medallions, hawking branded water bottles and fitness kits, consoling members about inevitable setbacks: She does it all with a smile. And like all leaders, she's on the program. After 14 years, she has lost and kept off 50 pounds and proudly displays her before and after photos.

The 30-minute meeting features plenty of cheerleading support for PointsPlus to bring along the newbies and any remaining skeptics. The gathering is short on whining and self-pity and long on accolades, tips, tricks, and laughter. Bacigalupi generously praises everyone who speaks up. "I just gotta say," she tells one, "you look hot!"

A few attendees offer advice. "For me, walking is so meditative. It just soothes my soul," says one woman. Adds another, knitting in the front row, "This week I bought almond milk and made a banana shake. That's one point! Even if you add the banana, that's still one point!" (The four men in attendance, outnumbered about 15 to 1, are all comparatively silent. Online memberships, which for about $20 a month provide access to online tools but no meetings, also skew female, but at about 85/15, rather than a meeting's average 90/10.)

After the meeting adjourns, Bacigalupi instructs three tire-kickers on the basics of PointsPlus. She's holding a poster displaying a croissant on one side and a ham, egg, and toast breakfast on the other. It demonstrates that the pastry costs seven points while the full breakfast costs six. The newbies are flummoxed. She nods empathetically and wades into an explanation of how the body processes different types of calories differently. She tells them this will become more intuitive over time. "The Weight Watchers approach is to change our behaviors and habits," Bacigalupi says. "This isn't a diet that you're going to go through. It's a new way of life." The pep talk is remarkably in sync with Kirchhoff's message, which is pretty impressive given the 3,000-mile separation between the boss and his frontline soldier.

Back in Manhattan, Kirchhoff says the company never could have pulled off the transition without leaders like Bacigalupi. They're carrying out the vision in a way that makes him feel as good about the company as he does about the new dieting regimen. "Weight Watchers is not a Harvard MBA organization," he says. "It's different, funky, and people are really passionate about what they do."

Kirchhoff's praise of his leaders is a nod to what makes the original notion behind Weight Watchers hold up even today. The real secret to the company's success isn't as much about dissecting the relationship between fat and carbs and protein as it is understanding the links between nutrition, weight gain, and psychology. Not everyone needs a weekly meeting to lose weight, but for many the commiseration and general back-slapping helps. That's been the Weight Watchers formula from day one. And for now, it seems to be working better than ever. Profits are up. Pounds are down.

Critical Thinking

1. Distinguish between the original Points system and "Points Plus" developed by Weight Watchers
2. Define glycemic index and explain why it was incorporated into the Points Plus system.
3. Define the basic principles of the thermic effect of food.
4. Critique the philosophy, "a calorie is a calorie; all calories are equal."

JEFFREY M. O'BRIEN (jeffrey.obrien@gmail.com) *is a former* Wired *senior editor.*

UNIT 6

Health Claims

Unit Selections

Learning Outcomes

After reading this unit, you will be able to:

- Defend the claim that chocolate is good for the heart and cardiovascular system.

- Identify the three flavanols (phytochemicals) found in chocolate.

- Compare the effects of the dietary components that are touted to increase brain function.

- Discuss the challenges of evaluating the "brain-boosting power" of dietary substances.

- List the nutrients that are required to be included on the Nutrition Facts panel.

- Contrast the types of health claims that can be published on product labels: nutrient content claims and structure/function claims.

- Identify the form of omega-3 fatty acid found in flax.

- Explain why fish oil is considered the more potent source omega-3 fatty acids compared to flax oil.

- List the beneficial characteristics of flax, other than containing omega-3 fatty acids.

Student Website
www.mhhe.com/cls

Internet References

Federal Trade Commission (FTC): Diet, Health & Fitness
   www.ftc.gov/bcp/menus/consumer/health.shtm
Food and Drug Administration (FDA)
   www.fda.gov/default.htm
National Council against Health Fraud (NCAHF)
   www.ncahf.org
Office of Dietary Supplements: Health Information
   http://ods.od.nih.gov/Health_Information/Health_Information.aspx
QuackWatch
   www.quackwatch.com

Technological advances in the 21st century have resulted in high-speed communication of results from scientific research and the possibility for miscommunication. Even if the scientific protocol, study, design, data collection, and analysis are impeccable, it is still possible to report the findings in a confusing and biased manner. According to a survey conducted by the Academy of Nutrition and Dietetics (formally the American Dietetic Association), 90 percent of consumers polled get their nutrition information from television, magazines, and newspapers. Health claims of food is a topic that grasps the attention of readers even if the health claims seem to good to be true. Health claims of food are all over the Internet and communication of a new health claim spreads quickly without much regard to the validity or reliability of the message.

Some Americans are so confused and overwhelmed by the controversies surrounding food and health that they have stopped paying attention to the contradictory claims reported by news media. Which one is better, butter or margarine? Are eggs good or bad for health? The media very frequently misinterpret results, simplify the message, and do not provide the proper context to accurately interpret the information. In addition, the media are eager to publish sensational information and not wait for evidence to be evaluated for validity and reliability. However, some popular heath claims are supported by reputable scientific research. Several of these topics are presented in this chapter: the overall health benefits of dark chocolate and omega-3 fatty acids and certain foods and herbs for brain health.

One of the most popular health messages held in high regard and followed by many is that chocolate is good for the cardiovascular system. Research that supports this theory refers to dark chocolate, which is lower in saturated fat and higher in phytochemicals from the high cocoa content. Milk chocolate, the form most commonly consumed in the United States does not provide the health benefits of dark chocolate. The article by Hara Estroff Marano summarizes the research that supports chocolate as a heart healthy brain food and also provides a brief, interesting history of chocolate as a health food.

The health claims of omega-3 fatty acids are based on its beneficial effect on the inflammatory system. Omega-3 fatty acids have been shown to reduce the risk of chronic diseases such as heart disease, certain cancers, and arthritis. Since so many people in the United States suffer from these chronic diseases, the health claims of omega-fatty acids have captured the attention of the United States population. Demand for supplements and fortified foods containing omega-3s has culminated in a vast number of products on the market. The information marketed on omega-3 may be confusing to most Americans. Since the metabolic pathways of these PUFAs are complex, there is a great deal of confusion about the best and safest source of omega-3 fatty acids.

Flax meal, flax seeds, and flax oil are all products derived from flax, which contains omega-3 fatty acids. Flax has been

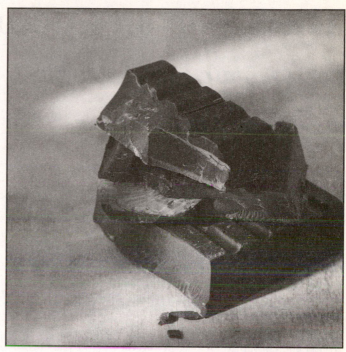

© ULTRA.F/Getty Images

reported to lower heart disease risk, reduce inflammation, diabetes, depression, and anxiety among other health benefits. Consumers are increasingly interested in purchasing and using flax for its health-promoting properties. "The Benefits of Flax" from *Consumer Reports on Health* discusses the difference between omega-3s from flaxseed oil versus fish oil.

Interest in nutrition's impact on brain function and energy level has become a hot topic for the aging "baby boomer" population. Producers of dietary supplements have responded to this increase in demand by introducing a vast number of dietary supplements to the market that supposedly improve cognitive function and provide energy. "Brain Boosters," by Janet Raloff, provides advice on how to intelligently interpret the claims about nutritional supplements touted to enhance brain function. This article provides information on foods, food components, and other products that are thought to improve mental performance and energy level. Caffeine, caffeine derivatives, glucose, ginkgo biloba, Chinese ginseng, and cocoa flavanols are on the "mental menu" as improving brain function in the article by Janet Raloff.

Articles in this unit were selected based on the common interests in the topics. Our society is inundated with health claims of foods and dietary supplements. People want an easy fix and the next greatest product that will make them healthy without all the troublesome work of diet and physical activity. The articles in Unit 6 provide a few items of good news as well as practical information to follow.

The Scoop on Chocolate

Is chocolate really healthy?

Hara Estroff Marano

The cocoa bean formally belongs to the genus *Theobroma,* or food of the gods. Not many mortals would disagree. And science now rewards their taste. Researchers are finding that consumption of cocoa-rich chocolate, loaded with classy antioxidants, offers a growing array of benefits to brain and body. Most surprising is that, when processed to preserve its fullest complement of natural antioxidants, cocoa may have therapeutic benefits against cardiovascular ills that take a special toll on the aging brain.

Native to South America, the bean of *Theobroma cacao* was ground and consumed as a warm beverage 2,000 years ago by Mayans and, later, by the Aztecs, who called it "bitter water." Columbus was the first European to sample the beverage, often spiced with pepper, but it was only after Cortes conquered the Aztecs that it became a prized drink in Spain, despite the fact that the hot and spicy drink was considered morally dangerous. Mixing it with milk and sugar made it more palatable to Europeans.

Long before chocolate was transformed into a dessert, it was valued for promoting health. Cortes wrote to King Carlos I of Spain that he had found a "drink that builds up resistance and fights fatigue" and brought tons of beans back with him. When Thomas Jefferson got his first sip in France, he wrote John Adams: "The superiority of chocolate, both for health and nourishment, will soon give it the same preference over tea and coffee in America which it has in Spain." European doctors recommended cacao for angina, respiratory problems, dysentery, indigestion, weakness, gout, liver and kidney disease, and general revitalization.

Long before chocolate was transformed into a dessert, it was valued for promoting health.

Cacao begins its transcendence into chocolate with fermentation after harvesting. The large, rugby-ball-shaped fruit of *Theobroma* contain about 40 cocoa beans embedded in a sticky, white pulp. The beans are scooped out and placed in trays for open-air fermentation, during which the pulp sugars alter the chemical composition of the bitter beans. Then the beans are dried, typically outdoors. An average tree produces 30 viable pods a year—yielding two pounds of chocolate.

Shipped off to factories, the dried beans undergo roasting for flavor development—at high temperatures for a short time, which boosts chocolate flavor, or lower temperatures for a longer time, believed to preserve more subtle flavors and more of the antioxidants. Then they are ground.

The resulting chocolate liquor may—with the variable addition of sugar, vanilla, and powdered milk—head straight for molding into chocolate bars or undergo pressing to separate the fatty cocoa butter from the cocoa solids, which are pulverized into cocoa powder. The cocoa butter—about a third of which is oleic acid, the same fat found in olive oil—is typically mixed back into chocolate as it later undergoes kneading and hot-and-cold tempering to further develop flavor and impart gloss. Cocoa butter also contains saturated fats, primarily stearic acid, which does not raise cholesterol levels.

During processing, cocoa beans may be washed to neutralize acids and decrease bitterness. Such so-called Dutch processing darkens the cocoa but halves its naturally high antioxidant level.

Cocoa and cocoa-laden dark chocolate have been identified as rich sources of antioxidants known as flavanols. Cocoa has more cardioprotective proanthocyanidins than blueberries, more brain-saving catechins than green tea, more heart-healthy phenols than red wine. Two tablespoons of cocoa have more antioxidants than four cups of green tea.

For over two decades, chocolate has been linked to protecting the cardiovascular system, and especially to lowering blood pressure, shielding the brain from stroke and the heart from overwork.

Researchers at Johns Hopkins have shown that a few squares of chocolate—the equivalent of two tablespoons of dark cocoa—can halve the risk of heart attack by decreasing the tendency of blood platelets to clot. The effect is similar to that of aspirin. Italian investigators have found that a small square of chocolate two or three times a week reduces levels of C-reactive protein, an inflammatory substance that is a risk factor for heart attack and stroke.

How to Choose [and Eat] Your Treat

What makes chocolate so appealing to you and me is what excites scientists about the health value of chocolate: People don't have to retrain habits to partake of the merits. They just have to make sure to buy a cocoa-rich version, but not too much. A square of dark chocolate a day will do it. More promotes weight gain, which offsets cardiovascular benefits. And the milk in milk chocolate interferes with antioxidant absorption.

The finest cocoa beans come from the tropics of Madagascar and the Americas, but Africa is the bulk producer; the single largest supplier of cocoa is the Ivory Coast.

Look for a product with the highest cocoa content (above 70 percent) and the fewest other ingredients. The best chocolate, says Jacques Torres, renowned New York chocolatier, contains only cocoa, sugar, cocoa butter, and lecithin, an emulsifier.

In a German study, a mere 30 calories worth of dark chocolate significantly lowered both systolic and diastolic blood pressure in middle-age and older men and women—without adding weight. Prevalence of hypertension dropped from 86 to 68 percent over 18 weeks of chocolate-eating, which, by boosting flavanols in blood, stimulated production of arterial nitric oxide, a compound known to relax blood vessels and increase blood flow through them (it's the source of Viagra's power). Swedish researchers have found that dark chocolate also biochemically mimics the first-choice drugs for hypertension by inhibiting the ACE enzyme known to raise blood pressure.

A German study that followed nearly 20,000 men and women age 35 to 65 for 10 years observed a 39 percent decrease in risk of stroke and heart attack among those who ate a small square of chocolate daily. Canadian researchers determined that eating 50 grams of dark chocolate a week markedly reduces the risk of death in those who have already suffered a stroke. What's more, chocolate seems to protect against heart failure and to lower the risk of death among those already diagnosed with the condition.

By increasing blood flow to the brain, chocolate also significantly protects against cognitive decline among those over 60, a separate study found. And Oxford University researchers who tested older chocolate eaters confirmed that they perform significantly better on a range of cognitive tests than those who do not partake.

But chocolate's benefits are not limited to any age group. "If you're going to have a treat," says Murray Mittelman, who directs a cardiovascular research unit at Harvard, "dark chocolate is probably a good choice, as long as it's in moderation."

Critical Thinking

1. Describe the processing of cocoa beans.

2. Why does "Dutch chocolate" have half of the antioxidant content?

3. Name the three flavanols (phytochemicals) found in chocolate.

4. Discuss how chocolate is good for the heart and cardiovascular system.

The Benefits of Flax

Flax products have been popping up all over grocery-store shelves lately, with claims such as "special protection for women's health" and "fights the blues." Here's our take on the seed's potential benefits, as well as some advice on how to incorporate it into your diet.

As Good as Fish Oil?

Flax products come in three forms: supplements, oil, and the seed itself. All of those, like fish oil, contain omega-3 fatty acids. In fish oil, those substances protect the heart in several ways, notably thinning the blood and lowering levels of LDL (bad) cholesterol and triglycerides. Moreover, those fatty acids might offer other health benefits, including protection against mild depression, Alzheimer's disease, and macular degeneration.

But it's unclear if the fatty acids in flax, which come in the form of alpha-linolenic acid (ALA), provide the same benefits. That's because the body has to convert ALA into the two fatty acids, eicosapentaenoic acid (EPA) and docosahexaenoic acid (DHA), found in fish oil. And to get meaningful amounts of those compounds you may have to consume lots of flax, according to a September 2008 study in the American Journal of Clinical Nutrition. It found that even large doses of flax oil—four to six 600-milligram capsules—boosted blood levels of EPA by only about 35 percent and had no effect on DHA.

Benefits Beyond the Heart

Still, flax oil might provide at least some coronary protection. And flaxseeds, especially crushed or ground, may offer certain benefits that fish oil does not. For example, they are rich sources of lignans, compounds that alter the way the body handles estrogen. That may explain why preliminary research hints that flaxseed can lower the risk of breast cancer. And one small study of women with mild menopausal symptoms found that about 3 tablespoons of flaxseed a day eased their hot flashes and night sweats as effectively as supplemental estrogen. Finally, the seeds contain lots of fiber, protein, magnesium, and thiamin.

How to Get More into Your Diet

- Add a tablespoon of crushed or ground flaxseed to your hot or cold breakfast cereal or yogurt.
- Add a teaspoon of crushed or ground flaxseed to mayonnaise or mustard when making a sandwich.
- Use crushed or ground flaxseed in place of eggs in baking. Mix 1 tablespoon with 3 tablespoons of water as a substitute for 1 large egg, and let it sit for a few minutes. Note that this will change the texture of the food.
- Look for products that contain flax, including cereals, granola bars, and breads.

Recommendation

Flax-oil supplements might be worth a try for people who want some of the benefits of fish oil but don't like the taste of fish or fish-oil pills, or avoid fish because they're vegetarians. But the supplements aren't good for people who can't take fish oil for safety reasons, because they may interact with the same blood-thinning drugs. And women with a history of breast, ovarian, or uterine cancers, as well as endometriosis or fibroids, should talk with their doctor before consuming flaxseeds because of their possible effect on estrogen. But most other people can safely add flaxseed to their diet.

Critical Thinking

1. Define alpha-linolenic acid (ALA), eicospentaenoic acid (EPA), and docosahexaenoic acid (DHA).

2. Explain why fish oil is considered the more potent source of omega-3 fatty acids compared to flax oil.

3. Describe the beneficial characteristics of flax, other than containing omega-3 fatty acids.

Brain Boosters

Some Nutritional Supplements Provide Real Food for Thought

Janet Raloff

On his third consecutive evening of air combat, a military pilot closes in on the night's quarry, a suspected Taliban fuel depot in Afghanistan. Fatigued, his alertness flagging, the pilot throws some chewing gum into his mouth. Laced with caffeine, it's the cockpit alternative to a cup of coffee.

This pilot would probably suspect that the gum is just a perk-me-up. But several caffeinated military rations—including this relatively new one—do more than stave off sleepiness. Emerging data indicate that these rations boost not only attention but also cognitive performance, features that do not necessarily climb in lockstep.

The U.S. Department of Defense has been investigating such supplements to improve the ability of U.S. armed forces to maintain sustained periods of intense vigilance and focus, explains Harris Lieberman, a psychologist at the Army Research Institute of Environmental Medicine in Natick, Mass. Another hope, he notes: These dietary aids might minimize the risk of "friendly fire."

Army researchers at the institute, including Lieberman, are at the forefront of a small but growing cadre of investigators exploring how to boost what they call mental energy. This rather fuzzy phrase embraces wakefulness, but also includes mood, motivation and the capacity to perform key mental tasks.

Increasing mental energy is important for those enervated because of a lack of sleep or for those whose jobs, like those of fighter pilots, require vigilance even in the face of sleep deprivation. Compounds that keep you awake, it turns out, can also boost other aspects of mental performance. Improved cognition is emerging as a quantifiable side benefit of many of these substances—in some cases, even for those folks who aren't sleepy to begin with.

But the data can be hard to interpret, primarily because no test exists to directly measure mental energy, explains Patrick O'Connor of the University of Georgia in Athens. It must be inferred from other indicators. Still, it is fair to view fatigue and mental energy as anchoring opposite poles of a common spectrum, he says.

Similarly, caffeine anchors the stimulatory end of a spectrum of natural products exhibiting promise in hiking or sustaining cognitive aspects of mental energy. Others include L-theanine in tea, guarana, cocoa constituents and ginseng.

Learning how these compounds work, at what doses and under what circumstances, is important, argues O'Connor, because "mental energy underlies everything in our lives." It's key, he says, to achieving goals at home and work—and even to the success of the economy.

Perky Brews

More data has emerged on caffeine's role in promoting mental energy than on any other dietary constituent. The stimulant blocks the activity of adenosine, a molecule that slows heart rate and induces drowsiness. Caffeine perks people up, Lieberman says, "by blocking something that normally slows you down."

At the Experimental Biology 2010 meeting in April in Anaheim, Calif., he described how, some 25 years ago, his team found that as little as 32 milligrams of caffeine—equivalent to what's in a 12-ounce can of cola or less than a cup of regular coffee—improved attentiveness for auditory and visual cues.

People had thought that any improved performance from caffeine might be limited to people who were tired. Here, though, the young men in the study were well rested, suggesting broader benefits.

Lieberman's more recent work has tested caffeine's effects on tasks especially relevant to the military. For instance, a study conducted during the training of 68 Navy SEALs assayed the effects of caffeine after 72 hours of sleep deprivation and round-the-clock exposure to cold and other stressors. The men were taking part in a weeklong test of endurance known as Hell Week.

Not surprisingly, the exhausted trainees didn't do nearly as well on tests of vigilance and other measures of cognitive performance three days into Hell Week as they had before the training marathon began. But those who got between 100 and 300 milligrams of caffeine an hour before a battery of mental tests made fewer mistakes and responded more quickly.

One task asked SEALs to scan for faint images that appeared for a couple of seconds on a computer monitor. Trainees who got no caffeine scored an average of 7.9 correct hits out of 20, while those given caffeine averaged between 10.6 and 12.2 correct responses. Caffeine recipients also had nearly 30 percent shorter response times. Scores on several other tasks, including a test of marksmanship, were unaffected.

Other scientists have been exploring caffeine's impacts on the brain. Andrew Smith of Cardiff University in Wales, for instance, asked 118 students to watch a computer screen where three-digit numbers appeared at a rate of 100 per minute. When two consecutive numbers matched, participants were to note it with a keystroke. Before the tests, 84 students were given chewing gum; roughly half (41) got gum laced with 40 milligrams of caffeine.

Students reported feeling substantially more alert after chewing the caffeinated gum. They also performed better on some tests, including the one in which they had to identify repeated numbers. Those given caffeine were 4.4 percent faster than those who worked gum-free and 4 percent faster than noncaffeinated-gum chewers. The stimulant also appeared to speed up people's ability to learn new information, Smith reported in the April 2009 *Human Psychopharmacology.*

Tea's Bonus

Tea, which people worldwide drink more of than any other beverage except water, is a major dietary source of caffeine. Unlike coffee, it contains another potentially powerful ingredient for brain activity: L-theanine, an amino acid that can alter alpha brain wave rhythms, inducing wakeful relaxation.

In 2008 in *Nutrition Reviews,* Janet Bryan of the University of South Australia in Adelaide observed that alpha wave activity has been linked to "increased performance under stress and improved learning and concentration" and reduced anxiety. L-theanine seems to enhance caffeine's mental benefits, she noted.

Unilever, which owns Lipton, is actively investigating L-theanine's effects. Neither caffeine nor tea's caffeine-theanine combo augment performance on all types of mental tests, says Eveline De Bruin, a cognitive neuroscientist with Unilever's R&D facility in Vlaardingen, the Netherlands. The biggest impacts, she says, are in enhancing what's known as executive function—the ability to perform complex tasks that rely on planning or decision making.

For instance, in an upcoming issue of *Appetite,* De Bruin's team reports that tea brings boosts in executive function that increase with dose. On each day of a two-day study, 26 volunteers drank either strong tea or a tealike placebo before testing. One test asked participants to listen to rules on how to respond to sounds or images on a computer screen—and the rules changed every few seconds during each five-minute session. The men and women responded correctly in the auditory test almost twice as often (around 15 to 20 percent of the time versus 8 or 9 percent) after drinking tea rather than the placebo. Participants were also marginally—but reliably—more accurate after tea on a test that looked at the ability to plan and execute decisions.

While Unilever has demonstrated that tea enriched with triple the normal amount of L-theanine improves attention, De Bruin says Lipton has no plans to market such a product. "It is an interesting idea," she concedes, "but at present Lipton is proud of producing an all-natural leaf-tea product that is unmodified yet capable of noticeably improving attention and alertness."

Sweet Paradox

Thinking, calculating, planning, learning, remembering—such mental tasks consume plenty of energy. Because glucose, better known as blood sugar, fuels body and brain, it might seem that a good dose of something sweet would be just what Mother Nature ordered to kick-start your neural hardware. Yet people with diabetes and high blood sugar levels can suffer from cognitive impairments.

Studies have begun probing this seeming contradiction. Two papers in August in *Psychopharmacology,* for instance, report a boost in mental performance when healthy people down a drink fortified with at least 50 grams of glucose (about 10 teaspoons worth) following a 12-hour overnight fast.

Christine Gagnon of the University of Quebec at Montreal and colleagues showed that in 44 people age 60 and up, drinking the glucose 15 minutes before the start of testing led to better scores on some tests than did the sugar-free alternative. Those on a sugar rush performed faster and accrued fewer errors when asked to quickly read a color name or name the color of words (even if a color word, such as *green,* appeared in a different color, say red). Glucose appeared especially beneficial in tasks that required switching and dividing attention, the researchers observed.

Among 90 undergrads, a sugary drink improved immediate recall of words, not faces, compared with a sugar-free one, reported a team led by Lauren Owen of the Brain Sciences Institute at the Swinburne University of Technology in Melbourne, Australia. Recall of large numbers that had appeared in earlier math calculations also improved.

Doses given in each study were high and would be ill-advised for people with trouble controlling their blood sugar, such as those with diabetes or metabolic syndrome.

But David Benton of Swansea University in Wales has shown there may be a way to get the benefits of a glucose burst without overdoing sugary drinks. At the experimental biology meeting, he presented data indicating that for mental performance, it's actually better to deliver glucose parsimoniously. He does it by giving subjects foods containing carbohydrates that digest slowly.

In an early study, Benton's team gave cereals, breakfast bars or biscuits with roughly equal calories to 106 undergraduate women. The main difference between the meals was their glycemic index—how quickly the carbs break down into glucose.

Thirty minutes later and at regular intervals thereafter, the women took memory tests. Those who got the low-glycemic breakfast performed progressively better than those eating the rapidly digested meals. The difference was most dramatic for a later testing, 3.5 hours after breakfast, Benton says.

His group ran a similar test in rats, feeding them either quickly or slowly digested carbs. The rodents exhibited a similar improvement in learning when they got the slowly digested chow.

In a follow-up test, Benton's group administered breakfast to kids in an elementary school class for four weeks. Kids got a meal with high-glycemic carbs on one-third of the days, low-glycemic foods on another third, and carbs that broke down at an intermediate rate on the remaining days.

On various days throughout the trial, hidden cameras recorded the 19 children while they were supposed to be working independently on a reading or math assignment. The behavior of each child was recorded over a 30-minute period and scientists later logged what the youngster had been doing: working, looking around the room, talking to others, fidgeting, acting out or moving around the room. On days when the kids had eaten the low-glycemic breakfast, they were much more likely to remain on task—26 percent of the time versus 18 percent or less on the other days.

The kids also took simple memory tests and played with a video game that was rigged to be frustratingly difficult to master. On days they had eaten the slow-to-digest breakfast, kids exhibited more initial patience with the game. Their recall was also better—"about 10 percent better," Benton says. It's a small difference, he acknowledges. "But if your child came home with 10 percent better scores on a test, would it matter to you? Most parents would say yes."

Herbal Therapies

Tea and coffee aren't the only natural stimulant-laced plant extracts to show energizing as well as brain-boosting attributes. There's also guarana. Seeds of this Amazonian plant are an especially potent source of caffeine, which can constitute 5 percent of dried extracts. But guarana may have more than caffeine going for it.

At the experimental biology meeting, David Kennedy of Northumbria University in Newcastle upon Tyne, England,

described cognitive benefits in young adults given small amounts of guarana—more benefits than when those volunteers received high doses. Indeed, Kennedy noted, guarana amounts needed to boost test scores and mood contained just 4 to 9 milligrams of caffeine. "That's only about a tenth as much as you'd find in a cup of coffee," Kennedy points out.

On the Mental Menu

Recent work suggests dietary substances such as caffeine and glucose may boost mental skills. Evidence for others ("Emerging substances") is preliminary.

Caffeine

Increases visual and auditory vigilance; speeds reaction times, improves accuracy and limits false positives on vigilance tasks; and increases learning and short-term memory on computer tests that require keystroke responses.

L-theanine

Increases speed and accuracy of pattern recognition that switches arbitrarily over time, increases relaxation, boosts accuracy of processing of rapidly delivered visual information and reduces susceptibility to distracting information during memory tests. May improve aspects of cognitive performance when delivered with caffeine, as in tea.

Glucose

Enhances memory of recent words or images, increases verbal fluency, improves pace of some types of serial subtraction, speeds decision times, enhances facial recognition and, among children, limits vulnerability to distraction when working alone.

Guarana

Increases alertness and the ability to recall words and images at a later point in time.

Emerging Substances

Ginkgo biloba

Improves pattern recognition and sustained attention, enhances delayed recall and memory of faces, and improves pace of serial subtraction and executive decision making.

Chinese ginseng

Enhances speed of recall, improves performance on simple arithmetic tasks and decreases false alarms on tests that require rapid processing of visual information.

Cocoa flavanols

Increase processing of rapid visual information and improve the ability to count backward (though have led to more errors in some serial subtractions).

— Janet Raloff

"So guarana was doing something that wasn't attributable to its caffeine"—although his team doesn't yet know what.

He and colleagues have also been investigating other natural products that might elevate energy, attention and mental performance. Among these: Chinese ginseng (*Panax ginseng*). Young adults scored better on a battery of mental tests—including serial subtraction of numbers in their heads—and exhibited less mental fatigue after getting this herbal supplement rather than a placebo.

How Chinese ginseng may improve performance is unknown, but Kennedy suspects the effect might have to do with ginseng's ability to moderate blood sugar levels. At least at the 200-milligram dose used by his group, this supplement caused a drop in blood-glucose levels one hour after consumption.

Researchers report that American ginseng (*P. quinquefolius*) also shows promise. Compared with a placebo, all doses improved some aspect of cognition, Swinburne's Andrew Scholey and colleagues report in October in *Psychopharmacology*. One difference: This herbal supplement had no effect on blood glucose.

The Northumbria researchers are also exploring the idea that some natural products bolster brain function by affecting blood flow. For instance, if they dilate vessels, the products might allow more fuel—glucose—in to power brain activities. Kennedy and colleagues tested the idea by giving 30 students a cup of cocoa on three mornings. Each day's formulation contained a different amount—46, 520 or 994 milligrams per serving—of cocoa flavanols, natural agents that have antioxidant and sometimes heart-healthy properties.

The cocoa packages used in the study were prepared by Mars, a candy company that has been exploring health attributes of some chocolate products.

Both higher-dose formulations, especially the middle one, improved performance during mentally challenging tests involving math and the visual processing of information, the scientists report. At the same time, the college students receiving the middle dose reported a reduction in mental fatigue. Maximum benefits showed up two hours into testing, which roughly corresponds to the expected peaks in concentrations of flavanols in the blood and in blood flow to the brain, Kennedy's team reported in the October *Journal of Psychopharmacology*.

Buyer Beware

The concept of mental energy is hardly new; recognition of it, on some level, dates back to Aristotle. But only during the last two decades has a steady trickle of studies begun quantifying how various dietary constituents battle fatigue and the fuzzy thinking that may accompany it.

The food industry has paid rapt attention to study findings (and, as is the case with Unilever and Mars, has even helped pay for some of the research). Indeed, O'Connor observes, hundreds of new products claim to boost mental energy. And

their appeal is understandable since mental energy helps motivate people not only to work but also to stick with it when the going gets hard.

"Unfortunately," he adds, product claims "rarely are supported by compelling, unbiased scientific evidence."

Michael Falk and colleagues at the Life Sciences Research Organization in Bethesda, Md., recently conducted a major review of supplements and ingredients (other than caffeine) that purport to boost attentiveness and mental performance in people. The researchers identified 265 research reports in the scientific literature that met certain criteria.

Falk's team focused on 35 dietary constituents or factors, such as meal timing and the number of calories consumed. Promising data exist for ginkgo, ginseng, glucose and a few others, Falk says. But overall, his team concluded, for most "insufficient evidence is available to evaluate mental energy claims."

Hundreds of products claim to boost mental energy, but few claims are supported by evidence.

Much of the problem may reflect how the testing was conducted, he points out. For about three-fourths of the substances, there were no more than 10 qualifying studies; for more than half, there were five or fewer, the team reported in the December 2010 *Nutrition Reviews*. And for any given nutrient, Falk notes, different trials often applied different tests to assess mood, motivation and mental prowess—which made comparisons difficult.

Many of the reports also tested very different populations (young adults in some, the elderly in others), had different criteria for whether subjects were healthy, and failed to establish baseline measures of mood and mental proficiency before administering a potential brain booster. Further complicating the picture: "You're looking at what are relatively small effects and hard to measure," he says. "And these are against a background of high methodological and statistical noise." Such variations "undermine our ability to make strong conclusions."

But Falk suspects that may change fairly soon. Researchers have been investigating what to measure and how to do it. And they've determined that agents with promise don't always point to common benefits. Some may aid memory. Others may sharpen mental focus or speed up reaction times. Still others might make decision making easier.

When scientists begin standardizing tests, "I'm betting they'll come out with stronger, more narrowly focused and more [scientifically] supportable conclusions," Falk says. Findings that he says should point to whom these dietary supplements will benefit—and under which real-world conditions.

Explore More

H.E. Gorby, A.M. Brownawell and M.C. Falk. "Do specific dietary constituents and supplements affect mental energy? Review of the evidence." *Nutrition Reviews,* December 2010.

Critical Thinking

1. Identify the challenges of evaluating the "brain boosting power" of dietary substances.

2. Compare the effects of the dietary substances that are touted to increase brain function.

3. List the three factors that are commonly evaluated when considering brain function.

From *Science News,* February 26, 2011, pp. 26–29. Copyright © 2011 by Society for Science & the Public. Reprinted by permission.

UNIT 7

Food Safety and Technology

Unit Selections

Learning Outcomes

After reading this unit, you will be able to :

- Describe how viruses can be used to curtail food-borne illness.

- Summarize the concept and the benefits of vertical farms.

- Define the potential "input traits" and "output traits" of genetically modified foods.

- Discuss the advantages and disadvantages of genetically modified crops.

- Define high-pressure processing in food preservation.

- Describe the responsibilities of the USDA in ensuring our food supply is safe.

- Identify foods that have been the culprits in the spread of *E. coli* 0157.

- Discuss the advantages and disadvantages to growing animal tissue in a lab.

- List the four most common biological contaminants (bacteria and viruses) found in our water supply.

- Identify the natural and man-made sources of lead and arsenic exposure.

- Describe how the FDA regulates arsenic and lead in U.S. food and beverages.

Student Website

www.mhhe.com/cls

Internet References

American Council on Science and Health (ACSH)
www.acsh.org
Centers for Disease Control and Prevention (CDC)
www.cdc.gov
FDA Center for Food Safety and Applied Nutrition
www.fda.gov/food/foodsafety/default.htm
Food Safety Project (FSP)
www.extension.iastate.edu/foodsafety
USDA Food Safety and Inspection Service (FSIS)
www.fsis.usda.gov

Food-borne illness constitutes an important public health problem in the United States. The United States Centers for Disease Control has reported 76 million cases of food-borne illness each year, out of which 5,000 end in death. The annual cost of losses in productivity ranges from $20 to 40 billion. Food-borne disease results primarily from microbial contamination (bacteria, viruses, and protozoa) and naturally occurring toxins, environmental contaminants, pesticide residues, and food additives.

The Food and Drug Administration (FDA) controls and regulates procedures dealing with food safety, including food service and production. The FDA has established rules (Hazard Analysis and Critical Control Points) to improve the control of food safety practices and to monitor the production of seafood, meat, and poultry.

Surveys show that over 95 percent of the time people do not follow proper sanitation methods when working with food at home. Thus our best defense is to incorporate safe food-handling practices at home. The United States government launched the Food Safety Initiative program to minimize food-borne disease and to educate the public about safe handling practices. An emphasis on improving food safety practices at home is also seen in the 2010 Dietary Guidelines. The subcommittees of the USDA and HHS recommend creating and offering food safety education programs for children in schools and preschools, along with improving education efforts with adults.

Agricultural trade between nations has led to a truly globalized food supply. This globalization meets the demand of wealthy nations for year-round access to foods grown in tropical environments and strengthens the economies of poorer, underdeveloped countries. One detriment of the global food supply is the translocation of biological contaminants via food. Estimations speculate that less than one percent of foods imported into the United States are inspected each year. Although United States demand for a variety of foods has driven the worldwide food trade, our nation has not established an effective method to regulate the safety of foods shipped in from other countries. The current regulatory agency for United States food, the Food and Drug Administration, is faced with many challenges of trying to regulate the United States food and pharmaceutical industries, much less the newly introduced challenges of the safety of food imports.

Imported foods are not the only concern for biological contaminants. Changes in food production and farming in the United States have led to an increase in the spread of bacterial contamination of our foods. Many conventional poultry and livestock farms raise their animals in crowded, unsanitary conditions. The crowded conditions make the spread of bacteria very likely; therefore, conventional farmers must inoculate their animals with antibiotics to prevent bacteria from spreading throughout the entire stock. An example of poor regulation of foods grown in the United States is the dramatic increase in *Salmonella* and *Campylobacter* bacteria in chickens over the past few years. Possible explanations for the increase in these two microorganisms could be due to the United States Department of Agriculture having no standards for *Campylobacter* and testing for *Salmonella* in a very small proportion of animals.

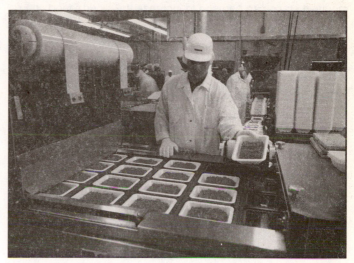

Concern for food safety also applies to the beverages that we drink. An estimated 19.5 million illnesses occur each year in the United States due to microorganisms in our water. The harmful effects may originate from viruses, bacteria, and protozoa or potential health consequences of chemical compounds and contaminants in our drinking water. Recent reports of high levels of arsenic and lead in juice have consumers concerned about the safety of drinking juice, especially by children. Although there is a federally enforced limit on the amount of arsenic and lead in drinking water, no limits exist for juices. Chronic low-level consumption of arsenic has been linked to slower cognitive development, various cancers, high blood pressure, diabetes, and infertility.

Advances in food technology are leading to radically different methods of producing and preserving food. Principles of genetic engineering, vertical farms, lab-grown meats, bacteriophages, and nanotechnology provide ways to increase production with less burden, enhance food safety, and keep foods fresh longer. Advancing technology in food preservation, most notably high pressure processing, is stretching the concept longer shelf life. The use of water-absorbing ingredients and edible polymers are also being used to create convenience foods that will not be soggy in the years that the food is on the shelf. These principles of food technology are shaping the future of food.

A controversial topic covered in this unit is the concept of growing meat for human consumption in a lab. Harvesting meat tissue grown in petri dishes to be grilled, sauteed, or broiled along with your favorite sauce is an ingenious idea to some and bizarre to others. Several labs are working to perfect techniques to grow beef, chicken, and lamb tissue in a chemistry lab. The concept would significantly impact agriculture and food supply. The article by Jeffrey Bartholet addresses this concept and provides a historical perspective of this practice.

Genetically modifying our food crops is another controversial topic. The topic has gained much attention from people who perceive the possible threats of genetically altered crops. The positions of people who oppose the practice are fueled by the actions of large agricultural companies that have genetically altered seeds to be resistant to herbicides, which allows for easier and heavy use of the herbicide on the crops. However, there are benefits to using genetically modified crops. Genetically modified crops can be used to increase the world's food supply to meet the demand of its growing population and increase the nutrient density of crops to provide the key nutrients missing in underdeveloped countries' food supply.

The articles in Unit 7 will be useful as a supplement to food safety sections of general nutrition courses. These article topics add a slightly different view of the future of food, food safety, an food technology that are not publicized as often.

The Future of Food: Five Frontiers

How nanotechnology, vertical farms, and lab-grown meat may change the way you eat.

ELIZABETH WEINGARTEN

Generations of kids have grown up forbidden to taste chocolate cake batter. The rationale for this quasi-torture: fear of salmonella poisoning.

And at the current rate of food technology, the kids of 2040 may be eating healthier cookie dough, too—gooey hunks infused with nano-sized nutrients, with chocolate chips engineered to be less fattening.

But future children may never know what salmonella is: A Dutch company is currently developing a consumer spray to kill the bacteria on contact. Salmonelex may sit next to Windex on future kitchen counters.

But most of the latest advancements in food technology go beyond dessert. Rather, scientists are motivated by an impending agricultural crisis: The world population will likely hit 9 billion by 2050, while climate change may render current agricultural systems and seeds inadequate. To stave off an agricultural doomsday, researchers are developing new techniques to transform our unsustainable practices.

For the month of June, Future Tense—a partnership of *Slate*, the New America Foundation, and Arizona State University—will look at the future of food in both the developed and developing world. We'll explore how we grow food, package it, genetically engineer it, and cook it at home.

To kick things off, here are five of the exciting food frontiers, some of which we'll be addressing more thoroughly in the weeks to come. *Bon appetit.*

1. Coding Corn

Some of the first genetically modified commercial crops in the '90s were tweaked to be tolerant to herbicides and resistant to plant diseases caused by viruses. Scientists built these superfoods by introducing certain genes into the plant's DNA.

Today, most genetically modified foods on the market are commodity crops used for animal feed or processed ingredients, like corn, soybeans, and sugar beets. Typically, they aren't manipulated to be more nutritious for human consumers. But that may soon change. A DuPont-owned company is currently marketing a "high oleic" heart-healthier soybean—meaning its oil has 20 percent less saturated fat than normal commodity soybean oil. Monsanto is also developing omega-3 enriched soybeans.

Researchers are working to enhance the nutrients in staple crops like sweet potatoes and cassava, which provide some populations in developing countires with the majority of their daily calories. That's a problem because though sweet potatoes, for example, are nutritious, they alone don't contain all the nutrients necessary for a balanced diet.

And for a couple of years, another corporation has been seeking FDA approval for genetically engineered salmon, dubbed AquAdvantage, that matures to its full size in half the time. But the process has been mired in controversy, particularly over concerns about the environment.

Gregory Jaffe, the director of the Biotechnology Project at the Center for Science in the Public Interest, says that there are other concerns about GM foods in general. For example, genetic modification could introduce a new gene that produces an allergen in a food, posing consumer health risks. Scientists also have to worry about introducing a new gene and, in the process, inadvertently activating an existing gene in the plant that could produce a harmful substance in the edible part.

2. Tiny Titans

Nanoparticles aren't new: The minuscule units appear naturally in some foods. But in the past decade, researchers have begun trying to use the particles to alter the taste and texture of food. Nanotechnology could be particularly useful for concocting diet-friendly foods: The particles can enhance the flavor and consistency of products without adding calories, sugar, or fat.

The Project on Emerging Nanotechnologies' comprehensive database of nano-products in the United States lists only four in the food and beverage category. Canola Active Oil uses nanoparticles to inhibit "the transportation of cholesterol from the digestive system into the bloodstream." Another product, Nanoceuticals' chocolate-flavored SlimShake, promises "enhanced flavor without the need for excess sugar." (If you've tried it, let us know how it tastes by weighing in in the comments.)

But some scientists worry that nanoparticles in food could pose a danger to human health, and that companies are releasing products without adequate safety testing. Todd Kuiken at the Project on Emerging Nanotechnologies, which is affiliated with the nonpartisan Woodrow Wilson Center and advocates for the advancement of nanotechnology, says he hasn't heard of much current research "on actual food products—what happens when [nanoparticles] get into the body, blood stream, and brain." The FDA says it's funding some research into the safety of nano-tech. But the paucity of testing means that right now, no one can be certain that ingesting these tiny particles won't come with big health consequences.

3. Lettuce Skyscrapers

Columbia University professor Dickson Despommier says Babylonians, with their hanging gardens, were first to pioneer the idea of vertical farms. But it was Despommier's 2010 book *The Vertical Farm*—and website, launched in 2004—that inspired the modern movement. Despommier defines a vertical farm as a building that's at least two stories with crops growing inside—stacked greenhouses, if you will. Back in 2010, there were none. Today, seven have sprouted around the world in places like South Korea, Japan, the Netherlands and Chicago.

Horizontal farmland can't grow enough food to sustain the swelling population, Despommier says. Not only do vertical farms do more with less land; they also allow food producers to grow crops in cities next to consumers, eliminating transportation costs. Cultivating food indoors with hydroponics (a system of growing plants without soil) uses 60 percent to 70 percent less water than traditional farming, and indoor crops aren't susceptible to drought, pests, diseases or floods.

PlantLab, based in the Netherlands, is a vertical farm that goes beyond Despommier. Rather than sunlight, it uses red, blue, and far-red LED lights to grow plants. But PlantLab isn't a food producer (though the researchers there do sometimes eat the tomatoes they grow). Rather, they glean information from the plants they grow to create growing recipes for food production companies. These formulas specify the temperature, humidity, carbon dioxide, airflow, nutrients, water, and LED light necessary to grow a crop most efficiently. Gertjan Meeuws, the managing partner of PlantLab, told me he's currently developing recipes of more than 40 crops for about 20 companies—most of which have traditional greenhouses. He guesses that in five to 10 years, retail houses like Wal-Mart will be producing their own vegetables and herbs.

But unlike outdoor farmers, vertical cultivators don't get government subsidies or tax breaks. "Indoor farmers aren't looked at as serious yet by the United States government—there are no major incentive programs to make vertical farming part of the landscape," Despommier says, stressing the vast size and influence of the American farm lobby. That means "the U.S. government will not be a big player in establishing vertical farming in the U.S.—but city governments might. If you talk to the mayor of Chicago or Philadelphia, you'll learn that they're passionate about this idea."

4. Lab Burgers

Dutch scientist Willem van Eelen imagined creating animal meat—or muscle tissue—in a laboratory back in the 1940s. Decades later, Mark Post, a stem cell scientist at the Netherlands' Maastricht University, is currently growing meat by capturing stem cells from cow muscles. His goal: to create a hamburger by November. But it's slow work, as he's forming the patty piece by piece. He's produced about 500 slivers of muscle tissue and estimates he needs 3,000. Once he's finished, Post estimates the hamburger will cost about 250,000 euros.

When will products from Post be on supermarket shelves? With sufficient funding, Post says, "we can probably make it happen in the order of 10 to 15 years." But, he says, "If the research continues to be funded the way it's funded now, it's never going to happen."

Another obstacle: Right now, cell division outside the body is induced with fetal bovine serum—liquid produced from the fetal blood of a dead cow. Not exactly PETA-friendly. Post tells me he would like to create a solution to replace the fluid. Alternative liquids that induce division in certain cells do exist—but so far, Post hasn't found them to work as well with skeletal muscle cells. Creating a replacement will be tough, he says, since fetal bovine serum contains about 10,000 individual proteins. But it's doable. The bottom line: You won't be chowing down on an in-vitro steak any time soon.

5. Salmonella-Fighting Soldiers

Bacteriophages (also referred to as "phages") are viruses that infect and kill bacteria. At Micreos, a company based in the Netherlands, researchers have created a phage spray to target particular bacteria that cause food-borne illnesses, like listeria and salmonella. (If you're keeping track at home—that's the third food technology incubated in the Netherlands.) The technology arose from research into antibiotic alternatives that began at the National Institute of Health in 1993. Micreos, a spinoff from the NIH project, was the first company to introduce phage spray technology—but others are entering the field, too. Recently, the FDA approved an American company's E. coli spray. Right now, its main customers are large scale food producers. But Micreos plans to release a consumer spray in the next year, CEO Mark Offerhaus told me. The industrial spray costs a penny per pound of meat, and Offerhaus guesses that the consumer spray will run about $10 per bottle.

Martin Loesser, a professor of food microbiology at the Institute of Food Science and Nutrition at the Federal Institute of Technology Zurich, has been researching the consumer safety effects of phage technology for 25 years. Though early critics of phage treatments worried that since phages contain proteins they could cause allergic reactions, Loesser dismisses this risk. He's confident because he can identify the proteins that comprise each phage through genetic sequencing and then test those proteins against a database of all known allergenic proteins—like those from wheat, soy, peanuts, and milk. He hasn't found a similarity between a phage protein and a known allergen yet. "The amount of protein that's in [these treatments] is still so low that even if that was allergenic, I doubt that this would cause any kind of reaction," he says.

A Nano-Grain of Salt

Pondering the future of food has long captivated the imaginations of science fiction writers and policymakers. But these visionaries are often way off the mark. Take the food pill. Matt Novak, writer of the Paleofuture blog for *Smithsonian* magazine, recently traced the pill's origins, finding that the premise—encapsulating a meal's worth of calories synthetically—harkens back to the 1893 World's Fair in Chicago. As part of an essay project to promote the fair, suffragette Mary Elizabeth Lease predicted that Americans would be eating synthetic food essences by 1993, freeing women from their kitchen shackles.

The food-pill prediction appeared again in various newspapers, magazines, TV shows (like *The Jetsons*) and in the 1933 Chicago World's Fair. We now know that cramming a meal into a pill isn't scientifically possible. Turns out that consuming 2,000 calories—what the average person needs daily—would mean swallowing about half a pound of pills per day.

Lease's prediction now sounds both quaint and sweeping: Cooks of the future, she wrote, "will take, in condensed form from the rich loam of the earth, the life force or germs now found in the heart of the corn, in the kernel of wheat, and in the luscious juices of the fruits. A small phial of this life from the fertile bosom of Mother Earth will furnish men with substance for days. And thus the problems of cooks and cooking will be solved."

Her prose offers an important reminder: Be wary of any scientist who suggests her technology is a food future panacea. Predicting which technology will radically change the food landscape is tough. For now, we'll have to be content with the promise of licking a safer cake batter spoon.

Critical Thinking

1. Describe how viruses that kill bacteria can be used to curtail outbreaks that cause food borne illness.

2. Critique the theory of providing a nutritious meal in pill form.

3. Define commodity crops.

4. Describe current research being conducted by corporations to develop genetically modified soybeans and salmon.

5. Summarize the concept and the benefits of vertical farms.

Genetic Engineering for Good

A researcher modifies crops to feed the hungry and cut pesticide use.

ERIK VANCE, FROM *CONSERVATION*

In the mid-1940s, Norman Borlaug started the Green Revolution on a small farm in Mexico. His idea was simple. As the human population skyrocketed, he would grow a new kind of wheat with a thicker stem and bigger seed heads, thus increasing yield and allowing farmers to grow more wheat—and feed more people—per acre.

The results were staggering. Within two decades, Mexico's wheat harvest had swollen sixfold, thanks to crops descended from Borlaug's modified wheat. Borlaug then turned his talents toward rice in the Philippines, and high-yield crops spread into almost every major food staple. All told, Borlaug's revolution helped feed millions of people in poor and developing countries—an achievement that earned him the 1970 Nobel Peace Prize.

But the Green Revolution wasn't "green" in the modern sense of the word. In fact, it exacted a huge environmental toll. Its crops require liberal use of fertilizer and pesticides that bleed into the land and sea, poisoning wildlife and creating nitrogen-rich dead zones in the oceans. Now, with climate change threatening to upend many of the world's crops, a new generation of researchers is poised to correct some of the original revolution's flaws.

Pam Ronald, a University of California, Davis, researcher, sees a future dominated not by Monsanto-like corporations but by small partnerships between farmers and scientists. By combining genetically modified crops with organic farming and other eco-friendly practices, Ronald believes, we can create a system that slashes pesticide use, insulates crops against floods and drought, and protects the livelihoods of poor farmers in the developing world. Using genetic engineering as a conservation tool sounds like an oxymoron to many people, but the scales may finally be tipping in Ronald's favor.

Her ideas have become a favorite of opinion makers such as Michael Pollan and Bill Gates. What's more, they serve as a stark reminder that genetically modified foods are here, whether we like it or not. Which means that, at a time when we need to reinvent the world's food supply, the critical question may be: Can we get it right?

Ronald is an unlikely genetic-engineering advocate. Pulling into her driveway, I see that her yard looks like that of any eco-foodie. Her pesticide-free garden—a tangled mix of herbs and native plants—has a happy, new age feel. Her barn sports a mural that she describes as "Diego Rivera meets Cesar Chavez." And her husband, Raoul Adamchak, is an organic farmer.

But Ronald, a plant geneticist, is also an unabashed supporter of genetically modified (GM) crops. Her book on the benefits of bioengineered organic crops, *Tomorrow's Table* (Oxford University Press, 2008), which she wrote with Adamchak, has started reshaping the way we look at GM foods.

While debate traditionally has been focused on genetically modified corn and other lucrative foodstuffs, Ronald has been doing pioneering work on a crop that is largely ignored: rice. In fact, while companies such as Monsanto pour billions into GM crops, rice research is almost solely the province of publicly funded academics. "The big companies aren't working on broccoli or carrots—there's just not enough profit in that," she says. "And they don't work on rice. It feeds half the world, but not the wealthy half."

Rice could be the ideal proving ground for genetic engineering to improve the environment while preparing for a warmer world, she says.

Take flooding, for instance. No one knows for certain how much flooding will increase as the planet warms, but scientists believe it will become more frequent and last longer in places such as Southeast Asia, where it already causes around $1 billion in annual damage to rice crops.

That's why Ronald's lab teamed up with colleague Dave Mackill in the late 1990s to create a species of rice that could be submerged for weeks and survive. Unlike many crops, rice has a dizzying number of varieties (as many as 140,000), all with distinct genetic codes. Mackill found one variety from eastern India with an unusual ability to live underwater for long spans. Ronald's team undertook the painstaking task of sorting through the genome until they found a single gene that seemed to act as a "master switch" for flood tolerance.

It was a neat trick, but the researchers wanted something that could be used easily by poor rice farmers. One method would have been to slice the gene out and simply slide it into a commercial crop, making it "genetically modified." However, they finally decided to simply breed the old with the new while targeting that specific place in the gene that held the precious submergence trait. This so-called marker-assisted breeding blends genetic work with old school, dirty-finger-nails farming. Because the actual genetic transfer was done in rice fields, the new strain is not considered modified and is thus under less scrutiny from government agencies than lab-modified strains are.

In a 2006 paper in *Nature,* the team announced a new strain of rice that could survive two weeks totally underwater. And it was easy to grow. By the end of 2010, the floodproof rice was expected to cover 125,000 acres in four countries. That's projected to jump tenfold this year.

This is just the beginning, Ronald says. Flooding is one of climate change's three key threats to agriculture. Drought and pest outbreaks are the other two, and Ronald believes lab-aided rice can be designed to resist them all. She is just beginning to work on drought-tolerant rice, and she believes a bug- and weed-resistant rice could slash the amount of pesticides used by rice farmers.

It's an example of how genetic engineering has accomplished exactly what many environmentalists and organic farmers want, Ronald says. Genetically modified cotton is a prime example. Little more than a decade ago, farmers in China started using "Bt cotton," a genetically engineered variety containing a protein that kills pests but is not toxic to mammals. (The Bt protein is a favorite insecticide among organic farmers.) Within four years, the Chinese cotton farmers reduced their annual use of poisonous insecticides by 70,000 metric tons—almost as much as is used in all of California each year.

The line between "genetically engineered" and "traditional" crops exists only in the media and politics. For scientists, it's more of a continuum.

Opponents worry that GM food carries some still-undiscovered health risks or that it's just a tool that helps big corporations sell more pesticides. And Doug Gurian-Sherman of the Union of Concerned Scientists worries that expensive GM research siphons money from less-sexy techniques. He likes marker-led breeding, he says, but he wants to see more money spent on organic techniques that reduce sprawling monocultures.

The danger of pesticides far outweighs that of switching a few base pairs in the DNA, Ronald says. She frequently notes that there's no record of anyone ever becoming sick from a GM crop.

Ronald also points out that the debate revolves around several false dichotomies. While naysayers declare genetic modification to be a new and evil practice, Ronald says the line between "genetically engineered" and "traditional" crops really exists only in the media and politics. For scientists, she says, it's more of a continuum—with traditional breeding on one end and crops with genes borrowed from vastly different creatures on the other.

Another false tradeoff is the idea that embracing genetic engineering means doing away with other environmentally friendly agriculture practices. If we are to feed the world without destroying the planet, Ronald believes, we must incorporate not just genetic modification but also crop rotations, crop diversity, and other ideas promoted by organic farmers.

To explain what might finally tip the scales, Ronald points to the developing world. As global warming intensifies, poor subsistence farmers will be devastated by food insecurity far more than the wealthy West.

"If farmers don't change the seed they're planting now, in 25 years they're going to be getting half the yield," Ronald says. She believes altering rice and other crops—such as strains of bananas—could help prevent future famine, much in the way that Borlaug's wheat spared millions of people from starvation. If we're going to accomplish that, environmentalists need to think more broadly. "You don't have to choose between productivity and sustainability," she says. "You can have both."

Critical Thinking

1. Evaluate the benefit of the initial work of Norman Borlaug.
2. Explain why agriculture research on rice is primarily conducted by academics, whereas wheat, corn, and soy are heavily researched by agriculture companies.
3. Justify the need for the current research on flood-resistant rice.
4. Critique the following statement: "The line between 'genetically engineered' and 'traditional' crops exists only in the media and politics."

Plant geneticist Pamela Ronald blogs about agriculture and genetics issues at scienceblogs.com/tomorrowstable. Reprinted from *Conservation* (July–Sept. 2010), "the magazine for environmental intelligence" published by the Society for Conservation Biology. www.conservationmagazine.org.

Engineering the Future of Food

Tomorrow's genetically modified food and farmed fish will be more sustainable and far healthier than much of what we eat today—if we can overcome our fears and embrace it. Here's how one foodie learned to stop worrying and love "Frankenfood."

JOSH SCHONWALD

The Plant Transformation Facility at the University of California, Davis, has been the scene of more than 15,000 "transgenic events," which is the term molecular biologists use when they blast DNA from one life form into another. In room 192 of Robbins Hall, a brick building not far from the student union, thousands of microscopic plantlets grow in Petri dishes bathed in pink and fluorescent blue light.

Here, molecular biologists can mix what were previously sexually incompatible species together using a gas-pump-like tool called the Helium Particle Delivery System. Using bullets (literally) made out of gold, they fire genes from one species into another in a bombardment chamber. The Davis lab has given birth to grapes spiked with jellyfish, tomatoes spiked with carp, transgenic squash, transgenic carrots, transgenic tomatoes.

Another important site in genetic engineering history, an innocuous office building about a ten-minute drive from Robbins Hall, is the birthplace of the most audacious plant in the history of high-tech plants. Among biotech people and anti-bio-tech people, this plant, a tomato, needs no introduction. The so-called Flavr Savr was supposed to be the game changer—longer shelf life, better yield, better taste. Calgene, the company that created the Flavr Savr, claimed it could bring "backyard flavor" to the supermarket tomato.

Achieving "backyard flavor" in an industrial-scale, California-grown tomato has long been one of the holy grails of the $4 billion-plus tomato industry. During the pre-tomato launch hype-a-thon, the president of Calgene claimed that genetic engineering could not only bring us the tomato of our childhood dreams, but also remake the taste of the tomato, tailored to our every desire: "Eventually we're going to design acidic tomatoes for the New Jersey palate and sweet tomatoes for the Chicago palate."

The Flavr Savr turned out to be the Edsel of the produce world, a spectacular failure not just for Calgene, but for the whole biotech industry. This purportedly longer-shelf-life tomato became the lightning rod for much of the anti-genetically modified organism (GMO) movement. People learned about other transgenic crops—a potato with a chicken gene, tobacco with a firefly gene, and, perhaps most notoriously, a tomato with an Arctic flounder gene, which provided an image for a Greenpeace anti-GMO campaign. Nongovernmental organizations cried foul. Consumers were alarmed. It was an op-ed about the Flavr Savr where the term *Frankenfood* first appeared. As for the tomato's taste, most reports said that, far from achieving backyard flavor, it was not that great.

By 1997, supermarkets stopped stocking the bioengineered tomato. The Flavr Savr was a financial disaster for Calgene.

But that was almost fifteen years ago.

One fall day, across campus from the Helium Particle Delivery System, I went to visit Kent Bradford, the director of UC Davis's Seed Biotechnology Center and presumably among the best-positioned people at Davis to answer my burning question: Whatever happened *after* the Flavr Savr?

The Culinary Potential of Frankenfood

Genetic engineering obviously didn't stop with the Flavr Savr debacle; the use of GMOs has exploded. Many genetically engineered foods can be found throughout our food supply. Genetically modified soybeans and canola dominate the market, which means that most processed food—everything from your spaghetti to your Snickers bar—has GM ingredients. More than 90 percent of American cotton and 80 percent of corn crops come from GM seed. All of these crops, though, are what are called "commodity crops." They're not what you pick up at your local greengrocer. They're industrial crops, secondary ingredients. Not what interested me.

What I wanted to know is what was happening with the quest to achieve "backyard flavor"? And what I couldn't get out of my head was this claim that tomatoes could be engineered for precise tastes—"acidic tomatoes for the New Jersey palate and sweet tomatoes for the Chicago palate."

> ## "The process is costly and time-consuming, which partly explains why biotech crop development is largely in the hands of the agribusiness giants."

What was going on? Did they just stop working on "sweet tomatoes for the Chicago palate"? Wouldn't the Flavr Savr creators be intent on redemption, going back to the bench to try again? Or did everything just stop?

Strangely, Bradford, a plant geneticist who has been at UC Davis since the early 1980s, shared my curiosity about the post–Flavr Savr world—he just had a different way of explaining it.

"Yes. Where are all these output traits?" he said. (Input traits are breederspeak for what's so often critical to agriculture—disease resistance, insect resistance, adaptability to particular environments. An output trait is breeder parlance for what I was looking for—traits that improve taste and texture, traits that could change the dining experience of the future.)

Bradford had observed that, almost twenty years after the biotech revolution began, there were few signs of any "Second Generation" crops. The First Generation was the commodity crops: soybean, maize, cotton, canola, sugar beets. Most expected that, after the first wave of crops proved their worth, the next wave would be more consumer focused—better tomatoes, tastier lettuce. But biotech specialty crops (that's the crop scientist term for produce) hadn't appeared. In fact, a GMO specialty crop hadn't been commercialized since 1998. Even Bradford, a longtime biotech believer, considered, "Maybe the genes weren't working?"

A few years ago, Bradford and his collaborator Jamie Miller set out to find out "what was going on" with bioengineered specialty crops. They surveyed the leading plant science journals and tracked GM crop field trials—all subject to government regulation—from 2003 to 2008. Searching for citations related to specialty crops, they found that research not only had never stopped but was thriving.

"There was research on 46 different species," says Bradford. "More than 300 traits were being tested." A lot of it was on input traits (disease, weed resistance), but breeders had also experimented with output traits. "It was happening at the research level, but it just didn't move to the next step. It just stopped there."

There was an obvious explanation, Bradford says, sighing. "It was regulatory."

Post Flavr Savr, in response to growing consumer concerns about transgenic breeding, a regulatory process was created that treated genetically modified foods differently from conventionally bred crops. If you have iceberg lettuce, using classic plant-breeding techniques (crossing, back-crossing), the assumption is that the resulting lettuce is safe. There's no requirement for pretesting. You just introduce the product into the market. But with GMOs, Bradford says, the attitude was that "it's guilty until proven innocent."

A genetically engineered crop must pass review by the U.S. Department of Agriculture, the Environmental Protection Agency, and the Food and Drug Administration before it is commercialized. The cost could range from $50,000 to tens of millions of dollars to win regulatory approval. For every "transgenic event," the genetic engineer must show exactly what genes went into the plant and how they function, and then prove how the plant makeup has been altered. That research is costly. So is plant storage. Once a transgenic creation is spawned at the Plant Transformation Facility, it is whisked to the UC Davis Controlled Environment Facility, where it will stay in a tightly secured warehouse. Or it will be airmailed to some other place, where it'll live out its life in another intensely biosecure environment.

The process is costly and time-consuming, which partly explains why biotech crop development is largely in the hands of the agribusiness giants—the Monsantos, Syngentas, and Bayer CropSciences of the world—who have the resources to undertake the process. With such high approval costs, big companies have favored commodity crops with market potential for hundreds of millions of dollars in sales, not tens of millions.

We talked about the reasons for what Bradford calls "the bottleneck" for the biotech specialty crops. It was NGOs such as Greenpeace and the Union of Concerned Scientists that were the bogeymen, in his view. Big Organic, a $20 billion industry, had a vested interested in stopping GMOs. Back in 2000, when the USDA was developing the National Organic Program standards, the first draft did not prohibit genetically modified foods, but then activists launched an anti-GMO campaign, flooding the USDA with a tidal wave of letters—275,026, to be exact. The USDA then determined that genetically modified organisms would not be included under the standard for organic produce. Being deemed un-kosher in the organic world is a hard stigma to overcome.

The anti-GMO movement hasn't lost momentum; the Non-GMO Project has become the fastest-growing food eco-label in North America, with sales eclipsing $1 billion in 2011. As for Europe: After a 12-year moratorium on GMO crops, the European Union greenlighted a GMO potato—but not for human consumption. It would be used to produce higher levels of starch, which is helpful for industries like paper manufacturing. In short, the European market is still overwhelmingly closed for genetically modified foodstuffs.

What If the World Embraced Agricultural Biotechnology?

According to the World Health Organization, 250 million children worldwide, mostly in the developing world, have diets lacking in vitamin A. Between 250,000 and 500,000 of these children go blind every year. Yet, there is a crop, developed more than 13 years ago, that is fortified with vitamin A compounds. If children unable to get vitamin A from other protein sources simply eat this crop, they will not go blind and die. It is named "golden rice" because of its yellowish hue, and every health organization in the world has declared it to be safe to eat.

But golden rice was not bred through traditional means; it was bred in a lab. So golden rice is, by its opponents' definition, Frankenfood, and therefore, like many other GMO crops, it's been ferociously opposed.

Now let's say that golden rice does get approved (as some predict it will in 2013), and let's say it saves millions of children from starvation and blindness in Asia. Or let's say bioengineered crops slow down the creation of algal dead zones in the Gulf of Mexico. Or a low-fat, anti-cancer potato becomes a smash hit at McDonald's. Consumer worries about GMOs evaporate, becoming as anachronistic as fears of microwave ovens causing cancer. The regulatory barriers are gone; transgenic plants are treated the same as any other. The Monsanto juggernaut is over; small, boutique companies and open-source plant breeders in the comfort of a Brooklyn loft have a chance to contribute to the vegetable economy. Then what happens?

- **Food will look different.** There will almost surely be more varieties. Austrian heirloom lettuce varieties like Forellenschluss and heirloom tomatoes like the Brandywines and Cherokee Purples could become readily available. So many vegetables today aren't commercially viable because of disease vulnerabilities or production inefficiencies. But in a genetically engineered future, all the flaws that make them ill-suited for commercialization become mere speed bumps.

  "You could have disease immunity almost immediately." says Bradford. "And it would be very easy to take care of these other variables. Instead of taking a decade to ready a crop for commercialization, it will take a matter of months."

  It's possible that colors would change. You could find pink lettuce and blue arugula—maybe with a green orange slice for St. Patrick's Day. Color becomes malleable because it's often a single trait.

- **Food will taste different.** It is also likely, some geneticists say, that in 2035 some lettuces won't taste anything like lettuce. The notion of tomatoes with customized flavor was a reckless ambition in the 1990s when the Flavr Savr debuted; modifying taste is among the most challenging tasks for plant geneticists. You can silence a gene in the potato genome, tuning down the bitterness or acidic quality, but it's still a fractional impact on taste.

> "With a few mouse clicks, geneticists say, they could choose from a range of flavors, textures, and colors."

  Taste is complex. A tomato, for instance, has between five and twenty compounds that influence flavor. Changing flavor requires not one gene, but packages of genes, and the genes must be placed precisely. Then there is texture, inextricably linked to flavor. Modifying taste eludes technologists today, but in the next ten years, that could change, as bioengineers will be able to choose from a genetic cassette—stacks of genes that together confer desired traits. With a few mouse clicks, geneticists say, they could choose from a range of flavors, textures, and colors.

"Think of it like Photoshop," says C. S. Prakash, director of the Center for Plant Biotechnology Research at Tuskegee University. "At some point that won't be a far-fetched metaphor." It will be technologically possible, therefore, to create a Caesar salad without the Caesar dressing; the flavor of the Caesar could be bred into the lettuce.

Textures would also be far easier to change. You could bite into an apple that has the consistency of a banana. In a biotech-friendly future, fruits and vegetables would merely be another frontier for adventurous and often mind-bending culinary pioneers.

- **We'll see produce that doesn't spoil.** In a biotech future, the sell-by dates will be different; instead of rushing to eat your lettuce in a week, loose leaf lettuce could languish, unsealed, for a month or more. One of the huge problems in the produce industry is perishability, with close to one-third of all fresh fruits and vegetables produced lost to over ripening or damage during shipment. But bioengineers are already making progress in changing the post-harvest behavior of plants. By having an enzyme shut off, an apple has been modified so that it won't turn brown after it is sliced, and a banana has been engineered to ripen more slowly.

  Although small organic farmers are often the most hostile to technologized solutions and may be the least likely group to adopt high-tech crops, it's possible that GMOs could change the farmers' markets in places like Chicago or Buffalo.

  "In New York and Illinois, it's pretty hard to grow a lot of crops because they're going to freeze," explains Dennis Miller, a food scientist at Cornell University. "But you could engineer in frost tolerance. You could extend the growing season and bring in more exotic crops into new regions. I don't know if we'll be growing bananas in upstate New York, but it would expand the options for locally grown fruits and vegetables."

How Frankenfood Will Improve Health

Most breeders expect that the biggest change for consumers would be something that's already familiar to any Whole Foods shopper. We already have calcium-fortified orange juice and herbal tea enhanced with antioxidants, but in an agbiotech-friendly world, the produce section would likely be overflowing with health enhancements. Orange potatoes enhanced with beta-carotene, calcium-enhanced carrots, and crops with enhanced antioxidants are already in the pipeline. By the 2030s, vegetables and fruits will be vitamin, nutrient, and beneficial-gene-delivery vehicles.

To illustrate how this would play out, Prakash points to the work of Cynthia Kenyon, a University of California—San Francisco molecular biologist, who extended the life span of a ground worm by six times by changing a gene called "def 2."

While this is in the realm of basic science, Prakash also suggests that, if something like a "fountain of youth" gene is found to benefit humans, it could be bred into vegetables. By combining genetics and plant science, a whole new realm of products would likely appear.

Some geneticists envision a future in which crop development would become a highly collaborative process: Nutritionists, geneticists, physicians, chefs, and marketers would work to develop new fruits and vegetables aimed at various consumer wants.

Another Kind of Foodie Hero

A scientist in a white lab coat doesn't conjure the same feelings as a micro-farmer in a straw hat. Growing fish in a warehouse isn't quite as stirring as pulling them out of a choppy Alaskan sea. A meat-spawning bioreactor doesn't have the same allure as a dew-covered Virginia pasture.

But it's time to broaden the foodie pantheon.

Let's continue to celebrate our heirloom-fava-bean growers and our grass-fed-goat herders. Let's carefully scrutinize the claims of nutritional science and keep a wary eye on new technologies, especially those with panacea-like claims from multinational corporations with monopolistic aims and a history of DDT and Agent Orange production. But let's not be so black-and-white; let's not be reflexively and categorically opposed to any and all technological solutions. Savoring the slowest food and foraging for wild asparagus shouldn't be viewed as at odds with championing lab-engineered vitamin A–enhanced rice that could save children from blindness.

Pairing a locally grown, seasonal mesclun mix from an organic micro-farm with cobia, a saltwater fish grown in an industrial-sized warehouse, is not an incompatible, ethically confused choice.

I make this point because of the rising tide of food-specific neo-Luddism in America. While well intentioned and often beneficial in its impact, this foodie fundamentalism is unfortunately often associated with a dangerous antiscientism. If we're going to meet the enormous challenges of feeding the world's still-growing population, we are going to need all the ingenuity we can bring to bear.

My modest hope: Let's keep an open mind. Let's consider even the fringy, sometimes yucky, maybe kooky ideas. Let's not miss opportunities to build a long-term sustainable future for our planet.

Critical Thinking

1. Define the potential "input traits" and "output traits" of genetically modified foods.

2. Outline the history of GM foods.

3. Explain why biotech crop development occurs primarily in large agribusiness corporations. Evaluate why opponents of large agribusiness corporations view this as negative.

4. Evaluate the potential benefits of GM foods.

Josh Schonwald is the author of *The Taste of Tomorrow: Dispatches From the Future of Food* (Harper, 2012). He will be speaking at World-Future 2012, the World Future Society's annual conference, to be held in Toronto, Ontario, Canada.

Food Fight

Genetically modified crops, says agro-research czar Roger Beachy, receive an unjustified shellacking from environmentalists.

BRENDAN BORRELL

Roger Beachy grew up in a traditional Amish family on a small farm in Ohio that produced food "in the old ways," he says, with few insecticides, herbicides or other agro-chemicals. He went on to become a renowned expert in plant viruses and sowed the world's first genetically modified food crop—a tomato plant with a gene that conferred resistance to the devastating tomato mosaic virus. Beachy sees no irony between his rustic, low-tech boyhood and a career spent developing new types of agricultural technologies. For him, genetic manipulation of food plants is a way of helping preserve the traditions of small farms by reducing the amount of chemicals farmers have to apply to their crops.

In 2009 Beachy took the helm of the National Institute of Food and Agriculture, a new research arm of the U.S. Department of Agriculture, where he controls a $1.5-billion budget for pursuing his vision of the future of agriculture. In the past year Beachy's institute has funded ambitious agricultural research, such as a massive genomic study of 5,000 lines of wheat and barley, alongside unexpected projects: a $15-million behavioral study on childhood obesity in rural states, for one.

Beachy's appointment sparked controversy among environmentalists because his work helped to kick-start the $11-billion global agricultural biotechnology industry. Seed companies never commercialized his virus-resistant plants, but their success—tomato plants that showed near-complete resistance to multiple virus strains—underlined the potential for a technology that was ultimately widely embraced by U.S. farmers. Today in the U.S. more than 90 percent of soybean and cotton crops and more than 80 percent of corn plants are genetically engineered to resist herbicides and insects using methods similar to the ones developed by Beachy. Organic farmers and locavores worry about Beachy's ties to big agriculture—much of his tomato work received funding from Monsanto—and his advocacy of genetic modification of food crops. Beachy, though, remains unrepentant. Although he believes seed companies can do more to improve food security in the developing world, he insists that genetic manipulation is essential to feed the earth's growing population

In Brief

A pioneer in developing genetically modified foods has assumed an influential role as head of the U.S. Department of Agriculture's research agency.

Roger Beachy continues to advocate for a prominent place for genetic engineering of crops, which he claims provides a basis for chemical-free, sustainable agriculture that will prove more of a boon for the environment than have conventional weed and pest control.

Detractors of GM foods, meanwhile, have expressed their chagrin at Beachy's appointment.

Without GM crops, Beachy contends that farmers would need to return to older practices that would produce lower crop yields, higher prices and an increase in the use of agrochemicals inimical to health.

sustainably. Edited excerpts of a phone conversation with Beachy follow.

SCIENTIFIC AMERICAN: *Did you actually get to see the first GM tomatoes when they were planted in the field in Illinois in 1987?*
BEACHY: Oh, my goodness, I planted them. I went out and hoed them. I was out there once a week looking at everything in the field, and my daughter K. C. even helped me weed the tomato patch one time. I really wanted to observe the patch and see how it was progressing.

Were you surprised by how effective the virus-resistance gene was?
Absolutely. As the parental plants without the resistance gene were getting sicker and sicker, the ones that had the gene looked just dynamite. I still have the original photos from 25 years ago, and it's pretty remarkable even now to look at them and say, "By George, our stuff really works!" Other people have seen the same kind of technology work in cucumbers and papaya and squash and green peppers; many are surprised at

how relatively simple the concept was and yet how much of an impact it can have.

That effectiveness does not last forever, of course. Today we are seeing the resistance these technologies provide against pests and disease being overcome. Do you think the industry has relied too much on GM as a "silver bullet"?

No, these things happen in plant breeding of all kinds, whether it's traditional breeding or molecular breeding like we're doing now. In the 1960s and 1970s new types of wheat rust spread up from Mexico on the wind, and the plant breeders would hustle and hustle to find resistance to one strain of rust, and then, several years later, another strain would come, so they would have to be looking ahead to find any new resistance.

Durable, permanent resistance is almost unheard of, which brings up the question of why did we create GM crops in the first place? What we've gotten over the past 15 to 20 years is a considerable amount of insecticides not being used in the environment. That's remarkable. What we're wondering now is if we will go back to using only chemicals or if we will be able to find new genes that will capture the diversity of pests that we're seeing around the world.

Unlike in the U.S., tropical regions of the world, including parts of China, face constant pressure from multiple insects. To control the variety of crop-damaging insects, scientists will need a variety of different genetic technologies, or it may be necessary to apply nongenetic technologies, such as different proven insecticides to control them. Overall, we'll find the kinds of genes that will protect against white flies in one country and aphids in another country. If we manage this right, we'll have the genetic solutions to these questions and not chemical solutions and will therefore, in my opinion, be more sustainable.

Critics of the agricultural biotechnology industry complain that it has focused on providing benefits to farmers rather than improving foods for consumers. What do you say to them?

In the early years many of us in the university community were looking at using genetic engineering to enhance vitamin content of foods, improve the quality of seed proteins and develop crops that don't require use of pesticides—all things we thought would benefit agriculture and consumers. The process for approval of a biotechnology product was onerous, expensive and unknown for academics. It would take the private sector to make the new technologies successful and find an opportunity to give farmers crops with higher productivity. But the food companies that purchased these crops—General Mills, Kellogg's—were not used to paying more for wheat or oats that had more nutritional content or for vegetables that were higher in minerals.

Why not?

Because the American public would not be willing to pay more for those products.

Today consumers are willing to pay more for crops that are labeled "organic" or even "GM-free" because they view them as more sustainable. How do you think GM crops can help make agriculture more sustainable?

In my opinion, the GM crops we have today already contributed to sustainable agriculture. They have reduced the use of harmful pesticides and herbicides and the loss of soils because they promote the use of no-till methods of farming. Nevertheless, there is much more that can be done. As you know, agriculture and forestry account for approximately 31 percent of global greenhouse gas emissions, larger than the 26 percent from the energy sector. Agriculture is a major source of emissions of methane and nitrous oxides and is responsible for some of the pollution of waterways because of fertilizer run-off from fields. Agriculture needs to do better.

We haven't reached the plateau of global population and may not until 2050 or 2060. In the interim, we must increase food production while reducing greenhouse gas emissions and soil erosion and decrease pollution of waterways. That's a formidable challenge. With new technologies in seeds and in crop production, it will be possible to reduce the use of chemical fertilizers and the amount of irrigation while maintaining high yields. Better seeds will help, as will improvements in agricultural practices.

Environmentalists have been reluctant to embrace GM crops because of concerns about genes flowing to non-GM crops and also to wild native plants. That's one reason a federal judge in California recently ordered genetically modified sugar beets to be destroyed.

You are correct. Nevertheless, it is important to note that the court ruling is not about the safety of the sugar beets or the plants that result from cross-pollination. The farmers who brought suit charge a premium for their crops because they are branded as organic—a definition that does not include genetic engineering. They are worried that their non-GM crops will be pollinated by pollen from GM crops, reducing their value. In this case, it is not an issue of food safety but of product marketing.

On the other hand, it's true that there are reasons why we want to preserve wild populations of crop plants: they act as a reservoir for genetic diversity. Here in the U.S., we are not, for instance, planting GM corn alongside wild maize, which is from Mexico. There are some native species for which there is a cross-pollination possibility, for example, squashes and melons, where there are some wild progenitors out in the field. It will be important to ensure that such germplasm is preserved.

In some quarters it might actually be seen as positive if a trait for disease or pest resistance, whether or not it was of GM origin, was transferred to weedy relatives, because it will reduce pests or pathogens in the area.

It may be a positive thing for agriculture, but not necessarily for wild ecosystems. What are the consequences if you create a vitamin A–rich rice and that gene spreads into an environment where vitamin A is scarce?

Most scientists do not predict any negative consequences if the genes used to develop Golden Rice [vitamin A–rich rice] are transferred to other varieties or to wild relatives. In contrast, the payoff for making Golden Rice widely available to those with vitamin A–poor diets is enormous. Imagine if we further delayed the release of such improved foods, leaving many hundreds of thousands of children with blindness and impaired vision and early deaths because of deficiency of vitamin A. What is the value of sight in children? What is the potential damage should the genetic trait be transferred to wild or feral rice? You're right—you can't say that every place in the country or every place in the world or every environment, hot or cold, that it won't have an impact, but we need to weigh the risks and benefits.

Some scientists have complained that biotech companies have stymied research on GM crops. Aren't these studies needed to get accurate answers about the risks of these crops?

That's a complex question with many different factors at play. In my opinion, the field would be more advanced if more academic scientists were involved in testing and other types of experimentation. We've had too little involvement of the academic sector in some of these cases. Many of us urged early on that there be more sharing, and I can understand the concerns of the academics.

On the other hand, I've asked companies why seed isn't made readily available for academic scientists' use. Some point out that there have been a number of academic studies in the past 20 years about using GM crops that were incomplete or poorly designed. And as a result, there was a lot of wasted effort by many other scientists that follow up on such studies.

Take the case of the report that pollen from insect-resistant corn harms larvae of Monarch and other butterflies, which led many to conclude that GM corn would have a devastating effect on Monarch populations. This finding was widely quoted in the media, and the USDA spent a great deal of energy and investment on follow-up research, which in the end showed that Monarch larvae were likely to be affected under very restricted conditions: for example, if the pollination of a crop occurs at the same time and place as the larval growth of the butterfly—a very, very rare occasion.

Furthermore, because the use of insect-resistant corn reduced the use of chemical pesticides, the outcome increased the population of butterflies and other insects. From this and other examples, companies were justifiably concerned about the quality of some academic studies and felt that they had more to lose than to gain in such cases. Yet there is much to be gained from academic scientists conducting well-designed studies with GM crops, and I hope that the future brings greater collaboration and less suspicion between public-sector and private-sector scientists in agriculture biotechnology.

What would be the consequence if GM crops were suddenly removed from the market?

Here in the U.S., there would likely be a modest increase in food prices because the efficiency of food production is currently high as a consequence of using GM traits, resulting in low food prices. We would have to go back to older types of production that would result in lower density of planting and likely lower per-acre outputs. We would likely see an increase in acreage planted, including the use of some marginal lands to increase total output. In the U.S. and other countries, there would be a significant increase in the use of agrochemicals, and the related health issues associated with such use would increase. Although there have been great advances in plant breeding during the past 20 years, the yields of the major commodity crops, such as maize, soybeans and cotton, would be less in the absence of biotechnology than with it. If total global crop production drops, the impacts would, of course, be greater on poorer nations than on those that are wealthier. The agriculturally poor countries would certainly suffer more than those that have a strong foundation of food agriculture production.

More to Explore

Genetically Modified Foods: Debating Biotechnology. Edited by Michael Ruse and David Castle. Prometheus Books, 2002.

Safe Food: The Politics of Food Safety. Marion Nestle. University of California Press, 2010.

Critical Thinking

1. Describe the first genetically modified crop. Who designed it and why?
2. Explain why Roger Beachy's appointment as the head of the National Institute of Food and Agriculture is controversial.
3. What percentage of corn, cotton, and soybeans grown in the United States are genetically modified?
4. Discuss the advantages and disadvantages of genetically modified crops.

BRENDAN BORRELL is based in New York City and frequently writes about science and the environment for *Scientific American* and *Nature*.

Food That Lasts Forever

Want to shop once a month? New techniques can keep meals fresh longer—much longer

Deborah Blum

In his basement office at the University of Wisconsin, Rich Hartel lines up the failures. The 10-year-old jar of marshmallow crème in which the corn syrup settled into a thick amber pool at the bottom. The two-year-old petrified Peeps. "I have some one-year-old Twinkies at the back of my cabinet," offers Hartel, a professor of food science. Contrary to popular belief that they're immortal, Twinkies are designed for no more than a four-week shelf life, and they tend to become more chewy than soft after the first week. The fact is that most desserts—barring, famously (or infamously), fruitcake—devolve into a sticky wad of starch in a depressingly short time.

At least for now. Scientists like Hartel are working to change that, with some startling recent success. A new generation of food-preservation technologies is starting to transform how long we can keep food tasting fresh, exponentially increasing its life span. NASA recently reported that it has come up with bread pudding that can last a solid four years. Over at the Pentagon, there's pound cake that stays springy for up to five years. And that's just the desserts. Long-lasting entrées and side dishes are being concocted, with enormous implications: in the future we may have to go to the grocery store only once a month and will rarely, if ever, need to throw out food because it has gone bad. Further, if fruits and vegetables can be better preserved, food scientists hope they will become less expensive and more available for people on limited budgets.

Without new and more sophisticated methods of preservation, we could fall short of feeding a global population expected to top 7 billion this year

Consumers are already taking advantage. Tuna in those vacuum-sealed pouches that started popping up in stores a few years ago tastes fresher than canned tuna and has a similar shelf life, about 2 ½ years. Foodmakers had conquered one part of the equation. Spam is famously imperishable—but palate-wise, it's practically in a category of its own and not a likely standard bearer for fresh-tasting, everyday meals. Though Spam is sold with an expiration date two years in the future, Phil Minerich, vice president of research at Hormel, says that actually underestimates its durability. "We really put that on there to help the consumer move

it through," he says. "We don't want it to be sitting on the shelf for 12, 15 years." But, he adds, a well-sealed can of Spam would remain edible that long, if not longer.

The new food preservationists aren't just after longevity; they're reaching for a different standard of edibility. "In the last decade, there's been an evolution in the way we think of long-lasting foods," says Lauren Oleksyk, leader of the food-processing, engineering and technology team at the U.S. Department of Defense Combat Feeding Directorate.

"We're not just talking about long-term space missions," says John Floros of Penn State. "We're talking about survival here on earth."

Much of the new technology stems from the military's need for long-lasting food for troops, packaged as MREs (meals, ready to eat)—rations that have never been famous for tasting good. In 2002, Oleksyk and her colleagues introduced their first alternative option, an "indestructible" sandwich: a bread envelope stuffed with pepperoni or barbecued chicken, designed to last three to five years without refrigeration at standard room temperature.

There are three big challenges to making food with a long life span, and a sandwich presents all of them: controlling moisture, controlling atmosphere and controlling microorganisms, from bacteria to mold. (Many traditional food-preservation techniques, such as drying and salting, work because they kill microorganisms or limit their growth.) Oleksyk's team members needed to keep liquids from the sandwich filling from seeping into the bread, so they mixed water-absorbing ingredients including glycerol and sorbitol into the filling. They also increased the use of fine, edible polymer films, which are undetectable in the mouth. (Hartel notes that in desserts, chocolate is often used as a moisture barrier. His favorite example is the Twix, designed so that chocolate separates the dry cookie from the moist peanut butter or caramel inside.)

The supersandwich also limits exposure to oxygen, which accelerates chemical changes in food, by tucking packets of oxygen-scavenging chemicals in the outer wrapping. And the packaging is as impervious as possible, with layers of heat-resistant polypropylene and metal foil.

But the most important advance may be innovative ways of controlling bacteria, like a newly refined method of high-pressure processing (HPP), which greatly improves taste. The old method of sterilization requires 30 minutes of 250°F (121°C) heat, and as any cook knows, every hot minute changes the food. With HPP, food is sealed in a plastic pouch, placed in a chamber and subjected to 87,000 lb. of pressure per sq. in., effectively killing any bacteria. The makers of some commercially available lunch meats, like Hormel's Natural Choice line, already rely on high-pressure processing rather than chemical preservatives. Companies that handle delicate seafood products like raw oysters are also adopting the approach. Oleksyk says the technique may soon allow the military to offer sandwiches stuffed with ingredients like tuna salad and mayonnaise.

Will consumers bite? Better taste and texture are critical for makers to change the way people think about preserved foods

"It's night and day compared to the old heating process," Oleksyk says. "The foods taste like they're freshly prepared." The Defense Department hopes to introduce packaged HPP fruit that will retain its crispness for at least three years in a way that cannot be achieved by canning. Oleksyk's goal is to eventually create meals that can last up to 10 years. That would mean—especially if combat rations continue to be delivered on the standard three-to-five-year schedule—that there would never be a point when the food didn't taste fresh, she says. "They wouldn't have any idea how old it actually was."

Oleksyk admits that these are still mostly dreams of the future, but researchers at NASA have also been pushing the boundaries of old-time heat treatment. A report published in December in the *Journal of Food Science* offered a detailed portrait of the outer limits of shelf stability for heat-treated, or thermostabilized, foods. The report was based on a three-year study of 13 foods, including vegetable side dishes (carrot coins, three-bean salad), pork chops, vegetable omelettes and apricot cobbler. Once processed and packaged, the foods were stored at Johnson Space Center and

taste-tested on a regular basis over the three years. They remained edible for a surprising length of time, although they had clearly aged, turning darker and changing in texture. "We tested a tuna-fish casserole," says lead author Michele Perchonok, a food scientist at the center's Habitability and Environmental Factors Division. "The pasta got soft, but the tuna held up very well."

"It's night and day compared to the old heating process. The foods taste like they're freshly prepared," says the U.S. Defense Department's Lauren Oleksyk

The best results consistently came from meat products, she says. For instance, extrapolating from its three-year study, the agency calculated that grilled pork chops could remain edible for nearly seven years and tuna or salmon for close to eight years (far longer than desserts, which had shelf lives of 1¼ to five years). She attributes the durability of meats mostly to their tough protein fibers.

Ultimately, long-lasting foods could have global impact. We rely on shelf-stable foods after disasters and when electricity fails. After Hurricane Katrina in 2005, many Gulf Coast residents subsisted on MREs provided by the military; these and similar products feed victims of everything from earthquakes and blizzards to drought. What's more, frozen- and chilled-food sections are expensive for grocers. In a future when energy supplies may be increasingly limited, researchers suggest, investment in food preservation looks like a smart move.

That's one of the main messages in a recent analysis titled "Feeding the World Today and Tomorrow" from the Chicago-based Institute of Food Technologists. The lead author, John Floros, head of the food-science department at Penn State University, says that without good food preservation, we could fall short of meeting the needs of a global population expected to top 7 billion this year. The problem, he says, is that we lose too much food to rot and decay. In developing countries without sophisticated food-distribution and cooling systems, the loss is consistently 30 percent a year and in some places as high as 70 percent. He expects such challenges to increase, along with uncertainties in food production related to projected global climate change. Floros works with NASA on its food-stability projects, but "we're not just talking about long-term space missions," he says flatly. "We're talking about survival here on earth."

Critical Thinking

1. Identify the three big challenges of producing food with a long shelf life.
2. Describe methods used as moisture barriers in food processing
3. Define high pressure processing (HHP). List three examples of foods preserved by (HHP).

BLUM is a science writer and the author of *The Poisoner's Handbook*

Shelf Lives in the Balance

- **Bread:** Fresh bread quickly gets moldy when unrefrigerated
- **Twinkies:** Rumors of their immortality are greatly exaggerated
- **Canned Peas:** It's best to throw out canned goods after about a year
- **Tuna:** Vacuum packaging means even more salad days
- **Pork Chops:** Thermostabilizing grilled chops gives a boost to longevity
- **Spam:** No everyday food lasts longer than this icon (yet)

Inside the Meat Lab

A handful of scientists aim to satisfy the world's growing appetite for steak without wrecking the planet. The first step: grab a petri dish.

JEFFREY BARTHOLET

It is not unusual for visionaries to be impassioned, if not fanatical, and Willem van Eelen is no exception. At 87, van Eelen can look back on an extraordinary life. He was born in Indonesia when it was under Dutch control, the son of a doctor who ran a leper colony. As a teenager, he fought the Japanese in World War II and spent several years in prisoner-of-war camps. The Japanese guards used prisoners as slave labor and starved them. "If one of the stray dogs was stupid enough to go over the wire, the prisoners would jump on it, tear it apart and eat it raw," van Eelen recalls. "If you looked at my stomach then, you saw my spine. I was already dead." The experience triggered a lifelong obsession with food, nutrition and the science of survival.

One obsession led to another. After the Allies liberated Indonesia, van Eelen studied medicine at the University of Amsterdam. A professor showed the students how he had been able to get a piece of muscle tissue to grow in the laboratory. This demonstration inspired van Eelen to consider the possibility of growing edible meat without having to raise or slaughter animals. Imagine, he thought, protein-rich food that could be grown like crops, no matter what the climate or other environmental conditions, without killing any living creatures.

If anything, the idea is more potent now. The world population was just more than two billion in 1940, and global warming was not a concern. Today the planet is home to three times as many people. According to a 2006 report by the Food and Agriculture Organization, the livestock business accounts for about 18 percent of all anthropogenic greenhouse gas emissions—an even larger contribution than the global transportation sector. The organization expects worldwide meat consumption to nearly double between 2002 and 2050.

Under normal conditions, 10 cells could grow into 50,000 metric tons of meat in just two months. One such cell line would be sufficient to feed the world.

Meat grown in bioreactors—instead of raised on farms— could help alleviate planetary stress. Hanna Tuomisto, a Ph.D. candidate at the University of Oxford, co-authored a study last year on the potential environmental impacts of cultured meat. The study found that such production, if scientists grew the muscle cells in a culture of cyanobacteria hydrolysate (a bacterium cultivated in ponds), would involve "approximately 35 to 60 percent lower energy use, 80 to 95 percent lower greenhouse gas emissions and 98 percent lower land use compared to conventionally produced meat products in Europe."

As it is, 30 percent of the earth's ice-free land is used for grazing livestock and growing animal feed. If cultured meat were to become viable and widely consumed, much of that land could be used for other purposes, including new forests that would pull carbon out of the air. Meat would no longer have to be shipped around the globe, because production sites could be located close to consumers. Some proponents imagine small urban meat labs selling their products at street markets that cater to locavores.

The Only Choice Left

Even Winston Churchill thought in vitro meat was a good idea. "Fifty years hence, we shall escape the absurdity of growing a whole chicken in order to eat the breast or wing by growing these parts separately under suitable medium," he predicted in a 1932 book, *Thoughts and Adventures*. For most of the 20th century, however, few took the idea seriously. Van Eelen did not let it go. He worked all kinds of jobs—selling newspapers, driving a taxi, making dollhouses. He established an organization to help underprivileged kids and owned art galleries and cafes. He wrote proposals for in vitro meat production and eventually plowed much of his earnings into applying for patents. Together with two partners, he won a Dutch patent in 1999, then other European patents and, eventually, two U.S. patents. In 2005 he and others finally convinced the Dutch Ministry of Economic Affairs to pledge €2 million to support in vitro meat research in the Netherlands—the largest government grant for such research to date.

By that time, an American scientist had already succeeded in growing a piece of fish filet in a lab. Using a small grant from NASA, which was interested in developing food sources for deep-space voyages, Morris Benjaminson removed skeletal muscle from a common goldfish and grew it outside the fish's body. Then an associate briefly marinated the explants in olive oil, chopped garlic, lemon and pepper, covered them in bread crumbs and deep-fried them. "A panel of female colleagues gave it a visual and sniff test," says Benjaminson, now an emeritus professor at Touro College in Bay Shore, N.Y. "It looked and smelled pretty much the same as any fish you could buy at the supermarket." But NASA, apparently convinced there were easier ways to provide protein to astronauts on long deep-space voyages, declined to further fund Benjaminson's research.

The Dutch money was used by van Eelen and H. P. Haagsman, a scientist at Utrecht University, to fund a consortium that would aim to show that stem cells could be taken from farm animals, cultured and induced to become

GLOBAL TRENDS

Meaty Problems

The rich world already eats a lot of meat; the developing world is catching up. One reason is that as more people move to cities, improved infrastructure means that meat can be kept cold throughout its journey from the slaughterhouse to the kitchen. Yet as demand for meat increases, so will the environmental consequences. Livestock farming already accounts for 17.8 percent of all anthropogenic greenhouse gas emissions.

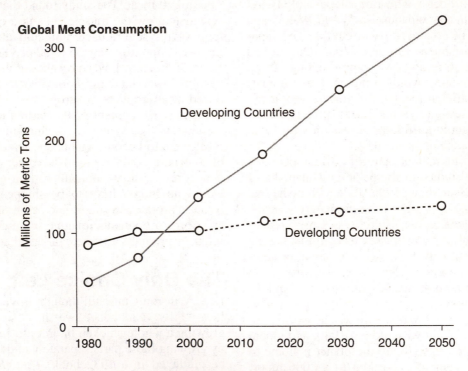

Global Meat Consumption

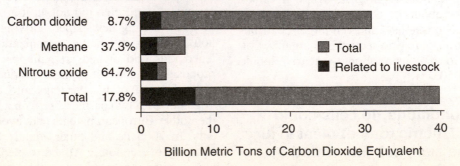

Livestock's Current Contribution to Greenhouse Gas Emissions

skeletal muscle cells. The team included a representative from meat company Meester Stegeman BV, then part of Sara Lee Corporation in Europe, and top scientists at three Dutch universities. Each university studied different aspects of in vitro meat production. Scientists at the University of Amsterdam focused on producing efficient growth media; a group at Utrecht worked on isolating stem cells, making them proliferate and coaxing them into muscle cells; and those at Eindhoven University of Technology attempted to "train" the muscle cells to grow larger.

The scientists made some progress. They were able to grow small, thin strips of muscle tissue in the lab—stuff that looked like bits of scallop and had the chewy texture of calamari—but several obstacles remained to commercial-scale production. "We gained knowledge; we knew a lot more, but we still didn't have [something that tasted like] a T-bone steak that came from a petri dish," says Peter Verstrate, who represented Meester Stegeman in the consortium and now works as a consultant. In time, the Dutch money ran out.

Van Eelen now fumes that one scientist involved was "stupid" and others just milked him and the Dutch government for money. "I don't know what they did in four years—talking, talking, talking—every year taking more of the money," he says. For their part, the scientists say that van Eelen never understood the scale of the challenge. "He had a naive idea that you could put muscle cells in a petri dish and they would just grow, and if you put money into a project, you'd have meat in a couple of years," says Bernard Roelen, a cell biologist who worked on the project at Utrecht.

Van Eelen was not the only one who imagined a revolution. In 2005 an article in *The New York Times* concluded that "in a few years' time there may be a lab-grown meat ready to market as sausages or patties." A couple of months before the story appeared, researchers had published the first peer-reviewed article on cultured meat in the journal *Tissue Engineering*. The authors included Jason G. Matheny, co-founder of the lab-produced meat advocacy group New Harvest. He understands the challenges better than most. "Tissue engineering is really hard and extremely expensive right now," he says. "To enjoy market adoption, we mainly need to solve the technical problems that increase the cost of engineered meat." That will take money, he notes, and few governments or organizations have been willing to commit necessary funding.

To the scientists involved, that failure seems short-sighted. "I think [in vitro meat] will be the only choice left," says Mark J. Post, head of the physiology department at Maastricht University. "I'm very bold about this. I don't see any way you could still rely on old-fashioned livestock in the coming decades."

Assembly Required

In theory, an in vitro meat factory would work something like this: First, technicians would isolate embryonic or adult stem cells from a pig, cow, chicken or other animal. Then they would grow those cells in bioreactors, using a culture derived from plants. The stem cells would divide and redivide for months on end. Technicians would next instruct the cells to differentiate into muscle (rather than, say, bone or brain cells). Finally, the muscle cells would need to be "bulked up" in a fashion similar to the way in which animals build their strength by exercising.

For now there are challenges at every stage of this process. One difficulty is developing stem cell lines that can proliferate for long periods without suddenly deciding they want to differentiate on their own. Another challenge is to be sure that when stem cells are prompted to differentiate, the overwhelming majority of them turn into muscle as instructed. "If 10 cells differentiate, you want at least seven or eight to turn into muscle cells, not three or four," Roelen says. "We can achieve 50 percent now."

The Utrecht scientists tried to extract and develop embryonic stem cell lines from pigs. Such cells would, in normal conditions, be able to duplicate every day for long periods, meaning 10 cells could grow into a staggering amount of potential meat in just two months—more than 50,000 metric tons. "Culturing embryonic stem cells would be ideal for this purpose since these cells have an (almost) infinite self-renewal capacity," according to a 2009 report by the Utrecht team. "In theory, one such cell line would be sufficient to literally feed the world."

Until now, however, such cell lines have been developed only from mice, rats, rhesus monkeys and humans. Embryonic cells from farm animals have had a tendency to differentiate quickly—and of their own accord—into specialized cells. In the report, Utrecht team's porcine cells often veered toward "a neural lineage"—brains, not bacon.

The Utrecht group also worked with adult stem cells, which have the advantage of being largely preprogrammed. These cells exist within skeletal muscle (as well as other parts of the body) with a specific mission: to do repair work when tissue is injured or dies off. So if you are making in vitro meat and want stem cells that will almost surely turn into muscle tissue, adult stem cells from skeletal muscle tissue should work very well. Until now, however, scientists have not been able to get these cells to proliferate as readily as they can embryonic cells.

Cost is another barrier. The culture used to grow stem cells of any kind is very expensive. With currently available media, it might cost $50,000 to produce a pound of meat, according to Roelen, and the most efficient nutrient bath is derived from fetal calf or horse serum taken from slaughtered animals. In recent years scientists have developed their own recipes for "chemically defined media" that include no animal products. By using recombinant-DNA technology, they have also been able to get plant cells to produce animal proteins that could be used to grow the meat. But both these types of media are, for now, prohibitively expensive. An algae-based medium may eventually work best because algae can produce the proteins and amino acids necessary to sustain cell life, but that, too, is costly—at least for now.

Once the researchers get a big supply of muscle cells, they will need to keep them alive and bulk them up. It is possible now to engineer a thin strip of tissue, but if it gets thicker than a few cell layers, parts of it start to die off. The cells need a constant flow of fresh nutrients to stay alive. In the body, these nutrients are delivered by the bloodstream, which also removes waste. Post is working on how to develop a three-dimensional system that delivers such nutrients.

He is also exploring bulking up the muscle cells. "If you take your cast off after a bone break, it scares you: the muscles are gone," he says. "But within a couple of weeks they're back. We need to replicate that process." The body achieves this in several ways, including exercise. In a lab setting, scientists can stimulate the tissue with electrical pulses. But that is costly and inefficient, bulking up the cells by only about 10 percent. Another method is simply to provide anchor points: once the cells are able to attach to different anchors, they develop tension on their own. Post has made anchors available by providing a scaffold of sugar polymers, which degrades over time. But at this stage, he says, "We're not looking at Schwarzenegger muscle cells."

He has one more method in mind, one he thinks might work best. But it is also more complex. The body naturally stimulates muscle growth with tiny micropulses of chemicals such as acetylcholine. These chemicals are cheap, which is part of what makes this approach appealing. "The trick is to do it in very, very short pulses," Post says. The hurdles to that are technological, not scientific.

Breakthroughs in all these areas will take money, of course. In 2008 People for the Ethical Treatment of Animals (PETA) offered $1 million to the first person or persons who could grow commercially viable chicken in a lab by 2012. But that was mainly a publicity stunt and no help to scientists who need money to get research done now. More seriously, the Dutch government recently pledged roughly €800,000 toward a new four-year project that would continue the stem cell research at Utrecht—and also initiate a study on the social and moral questions related to in vitro meat.

The Ick Factor

Some see social acceptance as the biggest barrier of all to producing in vitro meat on a commercial scale. "I've mentioned cultured meat to scientists, and they all think, 'great idea,'" says Oxford's Tuomisto. "When I talk to nonscientists, they are more afraid of it. It sounds scary. Yet it's basically the same stuff: muscle cells. It's just produced differently."

Cor van der Weele of Wageningen University is heading up the philosophical aspects of the new Dutch study (for example, is cultured meat a moral imperative or morally repugnant, or some combination of the two?). She has been intrigued by the emotional reactions that some people have toward the idea. "We call it the 'yuck response,'" she says. "People initially think that it might be something contaminated or disgusting."

But that perception can change quickly, van der Weele observes. She notes that people often associate cultured meat with two other ideas: genetically modified foods—which are often seen, particularly in Europe, as a dangerous corporate scheme to dominate or control the food supply—and negative perceptions of the meat industry in general, with its factory farms, disease and mistreatment of animals. Once people realize that cultured meat is not genetically modified and could be a clean, animal-friendly alternative to factory farms, she says, "the scared, very negative response is often very fleeting."

Such observations are only anecdotal, of course. The study will assess popular responses to in vitro meat in detail—comparing reactions across different regions and cultures—and will determine ways to frame the issue that might enhance consumer interest. Proponents imagine a day when governments will levy special environmental taxes on meat produced from livestock or when consumers will be able to opt for in vitro meat that is labeled "cruelty-free."

"I don't think you want to know about the hygienic conditions in the majority of slaughterhouses in the U.S. or the efficiency of euthanasia," says Post, who spent six years at Harvard University and Dartmouth College before returning home to the Netherlands in 2002. Another outbreak of disease—like mad cow or bird flu—could make cultured meat seem all the more appetizing. "We are far from what we eat," Roelen says. "When we're eating a hamburger, we don't think, 'I'm eating a dead cow.' And when people are already so far from what they eat, it's not too hard to see them accepting cultured meat."

Post has a bold scheme to attract new funding: he aims to create an in vitro sausage just to demonstrate that it is possible. He estimates that it will cost €300,000 and take six months of work by two doctoral students using three incubators. "We'll take two or three biopsies of a pig—say, 10,000 stem cells," Post says. "After 20 population doublings, we'll have 10 billion cells." The students will use 3,000 petri dishes to produce many tiny bits of porcine muscle tissue, which then will be packed into a casing with some spices and other nonmeat ingredients to give it taste and texture. In the end, scientists will be able to display the sausage next to the living pig from which it was grown.

"It's basically a stunt to generate more funds," Post says. "We're trying to prove to the world we can make a product out of this." But will it taste like a sausage? "I think so," Roelen says. "Most of the taste in a chicken nugget or a sausage is artificially made. Salt and all kinds of other things are added to give it taste."

Van Eelen, who regards himself as "the godfather of in vitro meat," is not a fan of the sausage proposal. He is a diehard idealist and thinks it is important to launch the in vitro revolution with meat that looks, smells and tastes just like anything you would buy off the farm. Van Eelen probably also realizes that time is running out to realize a dream that he has pursued nearly his entire life. "Every time you talk to him, he's speaking about someone else he's found who will be the top scientist who will solve his problems," Roelen says. "I can understand his point of view. But I can't change the laws of the universe."

More to Explore

Production of Animal Proteins by Cell Systems. H. P. Haagsman, K. J. Hellingwerf and B. A. J. Roelen. University of Utrecht, October 2009.

Livestock Production: Recent Trends, Future Prospects. Philip K. Thornton in *Philosophical Transactions of the Royal Society B*, vol. 365, no. 1554, pages 2853–2867; September 27, 2010.

Food: A Taste of Things to Come? Nicola Jones in *Nature,* vol. 468, pages 752–753; 2010.

Animal-Free Meat Biofabrication. B. F. Bhat and Z. Bhat in *American Journal of Food Technology,* vol. 6, no. 6, pages 441–459; 2011.

New Harvest: www.new-harvest.org.

Critical Thinking

1. What life events led Willem van Eelen to pursue a career of producing meat in a lab?

2. Discuss the advantages and disadvantages to growing meat in a lab.

3. Critique the concept of meat grown in a petri dish going mainstream.

4. Explain how the world's food supply and agriculture change if we could harvest meat in a petri dish

Jeffrey Bartholet is a veteran foreign correspondent and former Washington bureau chief for *Newsweek* magazine.

H₂ Uh–Oh

Do You Need to Filter Your Water?

NUTRITION ACTION NEWSLETTER

"For years, people said that America has the cleanest drinking water in the world," William K. Reilly, the Environmental Protection Agency's administrator under President George H. W. Bush, told *The New York Times* last year.

"That was true 20 years ago. But people don't realize how many new chemicals have emerged and how much more pollution has occurred. If they did, we would see very different attitudes."

Part of the problem: "The regulatory system is, frankly, slow to respond to emeriging threats to water safety," says Shane Snyder, a water-contaminant expert and professor of environmental engineering at the University of Arizona.

Here's some of what may be lurking in your tap water . . . and why you may not be able to rely on your local water utility to keep you safe.

Germs

"We estimate that 19.5 million illnesses occur each year in the United States that are caused by microorganisms in drinking water," says University of Arizona microbiologist Kelly Reynolds. Particularly vulnerable are older adults, young children, and people with weakened immune systems.

The culprits: viruses (primarily Norovirus), bacteria (like *Campylobacter, E. coli,* and *Shigella*), and cysts that are produced by protozoa like *Cryptosporidium* and *Giardia.* They can cause diarrhea, headaches, and, in rare cases, chronic conditions like reactive arthritis.

How do germs get into drinking water?

- **Contaminated surface water.** About two-thirds of Americans get their water from surface water sources like reservoirs, lakes, and rivers. "And all surface waters, no matter how pristine, contain water-borne pathogens from birds and animals, such as *Campylobacter* and *Salmonella,*" notes Reynolds.

  Surface water can also harbor gastrointestinal germs that are flushed down the toilet by humans when they're sick. How do they get into waterways? Blame it, at least in part, or the weather.

  The water systems that serve some 40 million Americans—often older systems in the Northeast, the Great Lakes region, and the Pacific Northwest—carry sewage and storm water in the same pipes. When water from heavy or sustained rains overloads a system, the overflow—wastewater along with rainwater—is discharged into rivers and creeks to prevent it from backing up.

  At least 40,000 sewage overflows occur each year in the United States. And that wastewater could become your drinking water after it's been treated by your local water utility. Since treatment plants can't eliminate 100 percent of the germs, some can get through to your tap.

  Climate change will likely add to the stress on water utilities in the Northeast and Midwest if, as predicted, it results in more and heavier precipitation there. Researchers at Johns Hopkins University in Baltimore found that heavy downpours preceded half of the 548 reported water-borne disease outbreaks in the United States from 1948 to 1994.[1]

- **Contaminated groundwater.** "Historically, groundwater supplies were thought to be free of disease-causing microorganisms because the soil naturally filters them out," says Reynolds. But viruses and other microbes from contaminated septic tanks, landfill leaks, or inadequate disposal of animal waste or wastewater can end up in water beneath the surface.

  The Environmental Protection Agency now requires utilities to disinfect ground-water that has a history of contamination.

- **Leaks in the distribution pipes.** Disease-causing microorganisms can also get into drinking water after it leaves the treatment plant. About a quarter of the nation's water distribution pipes are in poor condition, with leaks, cracks, and corrosion. On average, a city loses 18 to 44 percent of its water from leaking pipes, notes Yale University microbiologist Stephen Edberg.

Those pipes are often buried in the same trenches as sewer pipes. Changes in water pressure can allow contaminants in the soil to be sucked into the water pipes, fouling the drinking water.

"The proportion of disease outbreaks linked to breaches in the water distribution has increased over the past decade," says Reynolds, "and it's going to be a continuing problem."

- **Plumbing.** In 2004, University of Arizona researchers measured bacteria in the tap water of seven Tucson homes. The EPA limits the amount of these bacteria—which in most cases are harmless—to no more than 500 per milliliter of drinking water. Tucson's public water averaged only about 50, so it was relatively clean.

Not so most of the homes. Water from kitchen and bathroom faucets in the seven houses averaged more than 3,000 bacteria per milliliter. Levels varied among homes (one had virtually none, while another had 13,000 bacteria), and from day to day within the same house. Bathroom tap water in two homes averaged 2,400 bacteria first thing in the morning, then dropped to 140 after running the water for 30 seconds.[2]

Where do the bacteria come from?

"If you have pets that lick the faucet, or children with dirty hands who play with the faucet, or if you handle raw meats and then touch the faucet, bacteria can enter the pipes and grow," says Reynolds. "They get backwashed into the pipes, where they can form a layer, or biofilm."

Another potential source of bacteria is stagnant water sitting in pipes. "Maybe you're on vacation or maybe you have a second home," says Reynolds. "Bacteria can grow in pipes while you're gone, and then you can get a big dose when the water is turned back on again."

The antidote: "Flush out the system by letting the water run until it's as cold as it gets," suggests Reynolds. "That will certainly rinse out bacteria that haven't established a biofilm on the inside of the pipes."

If a bacteria biofilm has developed, it could loosen over time as the water faucet is used, says Reynolds, "and a chunk can break off and you can suddenly get exposed to a big dose of bacteria. It could be a significant health risk."

What to Do

Use a filter that has been certified for microbiological purification by the Water Quality Association (WQA), NSF International, or Underwriters Laboratories (UL).

Lead

It's clear that lead can damage the brains and nervous systems of children. But it may also cause high blood pressure, cataracts, decline in mental abilities, and kidney problems in adults. (See *Nutrition Action,* March 2005, cover story.)

"We're learning that older adults should also be concerned about lead poisoning," says researcher Marc Edwards, a professor of civil and environmental engineering at Virginia Tech University in Blacksburg.

"Recent studies have shown that low levels of lead in the blood that we once considered safe are causing health problems in adults. No one thinks to ever look for it in older people." (The most common symptoms are abdominal pain, headache, fatigue, muscular weakness, and pain, numbness, or tingling in the extremities.)

The evidence that lead affects the brain is troubling. In one study of nearly 600 women aged 47 to 74, those with higher levels of lead in their bones scored worse on memory and other cognitive tests than those with lower levels.[3] The women with higher lead had scores comparable to women who were three years older.

Where does lead in water come from?

"The lead or brass service lines that connect the community water supply from streets to homes in older cities can leach lead," says Edwards. So can the lead solder or brass and lead plumbing fixtures inside many buildings.

"Sometimes just one tap in a house might be providing water loaded with lead," notes Edwards. "It could be because some plumber had a bad day and did some sloppy soldering 40 years ago when your house was being built."

A case in point: The ex-mayor of a North Carolina town had suffered from chronic fatigue for years. "The kitchen tap in her apartment was perfectly clean," Edwards reports. "It was her bathroom faucet that had just outrageously high amounts of lead." All it took was an occasional drink of water from the bathroom tap.

Another potential source: hot tap water, which can contain high levels of dissolved lead.

"We're finding that there's quite a heavy use of hot tap water by the elderly to make tea, coffee, soup, and other foods," says Edwards. "And some devices that are used to heat water—like coffeemakers and those electric heating coils that are submerged directly into a cup of water—can dissolve high levels of lead into the water. It's safer to take cold water and heat it in a teapot on the stove."

What to Do

"People shouldn't panic, because the vast majority of taps in this country are safe," says Edwards. "Maybe only one out of 100 faucets is dispensing hazardous levels of lead into the water." That may not seem like many, says Edwards, "but if that's your family and that's your house, it's not good."

For about $20 per sample, you can have your water tested for lead. But testing isn't 100 percent reliable.

"We're discovering that little pieces of lead particles or solder, or lead rust that has corroded, can flake off the insides of pipes," says Edwards. "And that can deliver very, very high doses of lead" that a one-time test can miss.

The solution: a filter that removes lead at the faucet for all the water you use for cooking and drinking. "If there's a lead problem; it's probably coming from your plumbing, so you've got to treat it right at the end of the system," says Edwards.

Disinfection Byproducts

"Chlorine is an extremely good disinfectant for killing disease-causing bacteria and viruses in drinking water," says Paul Westerhoff director of Arizona State University's School of Sustainable Engineering and the Built Environment. "Plus, it's cheap."

That's why more than half the country's water treatment plants use chlorine. Another 30 percent use chloramine, a combination of chlorine and ammonia. Others use ozone. But there's a downside to those disinfectants.

"Chlorine combines with organic matter that is naturally found in water to form hundreds of compounds called disinfection byproducts, or DBPs," says Westerhoff. Chloramine and ozone produce smaller amounts of DBPs.

The EPA regulates the 11 most common and best-studied DBPs. Nine of the 11 cause cancer in laboratory animals.[4]

"This is an absolutely clear-cut case of humans' being exposed to chemicals that are known to be toxic in high doses," says David Savitz of the Mount Sinai School of Medicine in New York. "We all drink this water." (The EPA estimates that 94 percent of Americans consume foods and beverages that are made with chlorinated water.)

"The question is whether the DBPs are present at high enough levels to have measurable adverse effects on our health," Savitz explains. Researchers have focused on bladder cancer and pregnancy.

- **Bladder cancer.** "Using water with elevated levels of DBPs over years or decades does appear to be associated with a small increased risk of bladder cancer," says Savitz.

A 2004 meta-analysis of studies pooled from the United States, Canada, France, Italy, and Finland found that men—but not women—whose tap water contained an average of more than 1 part per billion of DBPs (the legal limit is 80 ppb) had a 24 percent greater risk of being diagnosed with bladder cancer than men who had no more than 1 ppb in their water.[5]

The EPA estimates that from 2 to 17 percent of the 56,000 new cases of bladder cancer each year in the United States may be caused by DBPs in

Is Bottled Water Better?

Is bottled water safer than tap water?

"There are not a lot of outbreaks associated with bottled water," notes the University of Arizona's Kelly Reynolds. But it's not clear whether that's because bottled water is less contaminated, or because it's harder to pin outbreaks on it.

"Bottled water gets distributed all over the country," says Reynolds. "If it caused an outbreak, that might be hard to identify."

In theory, *purified* bottled water should be safer. "Many bottled water companies start with tap water that has met all federal standards," notes Reynolds. "And the companies often add an additional treatment"—something like ultraviolet light or ozone to further disinfect the water or reverse osmosis to remove chemicals. "So you do sometimes get a higher standard of treatment."

The two big differences between tap and bottled water:

- The EPA, which regulates tap water, requires utilities to notify consumers when their water fails to meet legal standards. The FDA, which regulates bottled water, doesn't require bottlers to do the same. (The EPA's and FEA's standards are essentially the same.) So bottled-water drinkers are unlikely to know about any violations.
- Tap water doesn't come in plastic bottles that can end up in landfills.

BOTTLE BASICS

Purified Water: Most likely municipal tap water that has been distilled or treated with a process like deionization or reverse osmosis to remove impurities. The two major bottled drinking waters, Dasani and Aquafina, are purified water.

Spring Water: Comes from an underground formation from which water flows naturally to the surface of the earth. May be collected only at the spring or through a borehole tapping the underground formation that feeds the spring.

Mineral Water: Contains not less than 250 parts per million total dissolved mineral solids when it emerges from its source. No minerals can be added.

Sparkling Bottled Water: Contains the same amount of carbon dioxide that it had as it emerged from its source. (Companies sometimes add CO_2 to replace what's lost during bottling.) Depending on the source, it may be labeled something like "sparkling drinking water," "sparkling mineral water," or "sparkling spring water."

Source: Adapted from the International Bottled Water Association (bottledwater.org/content/labeling-0).

drinking water. When the agency slightly lowered the maximum levels of some DBPs permitted in water in 2006, it estimated that the move would prevent about 275 cancer cases a year.

New research suggests that breathing in some DBPs and absorbing them through the skin could be more harmful than swallowing DBPs. Roughly half of our exposure to chlorinated water comes from washing with it and being near running water and flushing toilets, notes Savitz.

- **Pregnancy.** "Tap Water can Increase Risk of Miscarriages During First Trimester," warned the Associated Press headline in 1998. In a study of roughly 5,000 pregnant women in northern California, those who lived where the tap water contained more than 75 parts per billion of disinfection byproducts were nearly twice as likely to miscarry, but only if they drank at least five glasses of water a day.[6]

But a later study by Savitz found no link between DBPs and miscarriage in 2,400 pregnant women in Texas, Tennessee, and North Carolina.[7] "It was a pretty sophisticated study and it didn't corroborate the California research," says Savitz, then at the University of North Carolina in Chapel Hill.

Levels of the 11 regulated DBPs in drinking water have dropped by 60 to 90 percent since the early 1970s. "Their regulation has led to a huge improvement in drinking water quality," notes Westerhoff.

But there are more than 600 DBPs in water, and "new research over the last decade suggests that some of the unregulated ones that occur at very low concentrations are actually more genotoxic than the 11 regulated ones," he adds.

Genotoxic compounds damage DNA and can cause cancer. Among the metropolitan areas with the highest levels of the 11 regulated DBPs: Baltimore, Boston, Little Rock, Phoenix, and Washington, DC.

What to Do

Use a water filter that's certified to reduce volatile organic compounds (VOCs), which include DBPs.

Other Chemicals

"There's growing evidence that numerous chemicals in water are more dangerous than previously thought, but the EPA still gives them a clean bill of health," Linda Birnbaum, director of the government's National Institute of Environmental Health Sciences, told *The New York Times* in December 2009.

"These chemicals accumulate in body tissue. They affect developmental and hormonal systems in ways we don't understand." Some examples:

- **Atrazine.** It's the pesticide most often found in drinking water, especially in the Midwest, where it's applied to cornfields to kill weeds. It's also widely used on lawns, in parks, and on golf courses.

All of the watersheds monitored by the EPA, and some 40 percent of groundwater samples from agricultural areas, test positive for atrazine, according to the Natural Resources Defense Council.

In some studies, women living in areas with higher levels of atrazine in the drinking water were more likely to have lower-birth-weight babies. And in two studies, women in those areas were at higher risk of having babies with gastroschisis, a birth defect in which the intestines, stomach, or liver push through a hole in the abdominal wall.[8]

The EPA limits atrazine in drinking water to 3 parts per billion when averaged over an entire year. But people in agricultural areas may be exposed to much higher levels when use of the pesticide spikes during the growing season. The EPA says that it is reevaluating the safety of atrazine, and will decide "whether new restrictions are necessary to better protect health and the environment."

- **Perchlorate.** It's an ingredient in solid fuels used for explosives, fireworks, road flares, and rocket motors. It also occurs naturally and is a byproduct that forms in bleach. And it can be detected in drinking water and groundwater in 35 states and in the urine of just about every American.[9]

In large amounts, perchlorate blocks iodine from reaching the thyroid gland, which can make it harder to produce thyroid hormone. Perchlorate may also block the transfer of iodine from mother to fetus, which can hinder normal growth.

California, Massachusetts, and New Jersey limit perchlorate levels in drinking water. In 2008, the EPA concluded that national perchlorate regulations wouldn't produce a great enough public health benefit. The agency now says that it's reevaluating its decision.

"It's extremely difficult for water utilities to remove perchlorate," says University of Arizona water expert Shane Snyder. "The only technologies available are ion exchange, which is extremely rare in water treatment systems, or a reverse osmosis system that's also rarely used because it is energy-intensive."

How to Choose a Water Filter

Point-of-use filters remove contaminants at the faucet, so they protect you from lead and other pollutants that may have gotten into your water after it left the treatment plant.

How do you go about choosing one for your home? "There's no one technology that takes everything out of water," says Joseph Harrison, former technical director at the Water Quality Association, a trade group of water filter manufacturers. Your choice generally narrows down to one or a combination of these basic types of filters:

Activated carbon: When water passes over the granular activated carbon or powdered carbon block, the negative ions of the contaminants are attracted to the slight positive charge of the carbon.

Reverse osmosis: A semipermeable membrane traps contaminants that activated carbon can't. Chlorine degrades the membranes, so most units contain activated carbon pre-filters. Reverse osmosis is inefficient; it typically wastes three to five gallons of water for every gallon filtered. And it filters out good minerals like calcium and fluoride along with the contaminants.

Ion exchange: As water percolates through bead-like resins, ions in the water are swapped for ions on the beads. The system is used mostly to soften water.

Which filtration system is for you? That depends on what kind of protection you want and how much you're willing to spend:

1. **For basic protection.** Get an activated carbon filter that's certified to reduce lead, cysts, and volatile organic compounds (VOCs). Filtering VOCs should help protect you from disinfection byproducts (DBPs), atrazine and some other pesticides, and several dozen other contaminants. The filter should also be certified to eliminate the taste and smell of chlorine.

   Check the filter's box or literature to make sure that the claims for lead, VOCs, and any other contaminants have been certified using NSF/ANSI Standard 53. Claims that the filter eliminates "aesthetic" contaminants (like taste, odor, or chlorine) should be certified using NSF/ANSI Standard 42. The non-profit NSF International establishes standards for consumer goods and certifies products.

2. **To filter out bacteria and viruses.** Get a system that has been certified for micro-biological purification by the Water Quality Association (WQA), NSF International, or Underwriters Laboratories (UL). It could consist of an ultraviolet light to disinfect the water or a filter with pores so fine that microorganisms can't get through them.

3. **To target contaminants you know are in your water.** Have your tap water tested. Or get a copy of the Consumer Confidence Report that most water utilities are required to mail out by July 1 of every year, Many utilities also post the reports on their website. If your water has elevated levels of any contaminants, look for a filter that has been certified to reduce them.

4. **For the cleanest water on your block.** "Get a reverse osmosis system plus an activated carbon system," says Harrison. Then add a filter that has been certified for microbiological purification.

Before You Buy Any Filter

Check the website of the California Department of Public Health (cdph.ca.gov/certlic/device/Pages/WTD2009Directory.aspx). If the filter you're looking at is sold in California, the website will tell you whether its claims have been verified by independent, state-approved laboratories.

The website lists all approved models and what they are certified to remove, and has separate lists of filters that have been certified to remove arsenic, *Cryptosporidium* and *Giardia* cysts, fluoride, chromium, lead, bacteria and viruses, MTBE (a gasoline additive), nitrates, perchlorate, radium, and volatile organic compounds (VOCs) like disinfection byproducts (DBPs) and atrazine.

For basic information on the water supply and the effectiveness of different kinds of filters, see the EPA's booklet "Water on Tap" (www.epa.gov/safewater/wot/pdfs/book_waterontap_full.pdf). For questions about your drinking water, you can call the EPA's Safe Drinking Water Hotline (800-426-4791).

- **Drugs.** When you take an aspirin, or birth control pills, or Lipitor, or another drug, tiny amounts end up in the toilet bowl, where they're flushed into the sewage system and, eventually, into a wastewater treatment plant.

  "Conventional wastewater plants typically remove more than 90 percent of these compounds," explains Snyder. "But even if you have 99.99 percent removal, that still leaves parts per trillion in the water which is subsequently discharged into rivers and streams." And that water, with its drug residues, can eventually end up coming out of your tap.

While the traces of drugs in drinking water are one-ten-thousandth to one-hundred-thousandth the amount in any therapeutic dose, "I don't know that we can completely dismiss the impact on human health," says Snyder, "because we don't know much about the toxicity of mixtures of drugs. But based on the concentrations of the individual compounds, harm to humans doesn't appear to be likely."

What to Do

- **Atrazine.** Use a filter that's certified to reduce levels of volatile organic compounds (VOCs), which include atrazine.

- **Perchlorate.** Only reverse osmosis and ion exchange filters reduce perchlorate.
- **Drugs.** Claims that filters reduce drug residues are based on the manufacturers' own tests. Official standards to verify the tests are in the works, though.

Notes

1. *Am. J. Public Health 91:* 1194, 2001
2. *Int. J. Food Microbiol. 92:* 289, 2004.
3. *Environ. Health Perspect. 117:* 574, 2009.
4. *Mutation Research 636:* 178, 2007.
5. *Epidemiology 15:* 357, 2004.
6. *Epidemiology 9:* 134, 1998.
7. *Epidemiology 19:* 729 and 738, 2008.
8. *Am. J. Obstet. Gynecol. 202:* 241, 2010.
9. *J. Expo. Sci. Environ. Epidemiol. 17:* 400, 2007.

Critical Thinking

1. What are the four most common biological contaminants (bacteria and viruses) found in our water supply?

2. How can water from household faucets be contaminated with bacteria by humans or pets?

3. What are the detrimental effects of consuming lead, other than the well-known effects on the brain and nervous system?

Arsenic in Your Juice

How much is too much? Federal limits don't exist.

Arsenic has long been recognized as a poison and a contaminant in drinking water, but now concerns are growing about arsenic in foods, especially in fruit juices that are a mainstay for children.

Controversy over arsenic in apple juice made headlines as the school year began when Mehmet Oz, M.D., host of "The Dr. Oz Show," told viewers that tests he'd commissioned found 10 of three dozen apple-juice samples with total arsenic levels exceeding 10 parts per billion (ppb). There's no federal arsenic threshold for juice or most foods, though the limit for bottled and public water is 10 ppb. The Food and Drug Administration, trying to reassure consumers about the safety of apple juice, claimed that most arsenic in juices and other foods is of the organic type that is "essentially harmless."

But an investigation by Consumer Reports shows otherwise. Our study, including tests of apple and grape juice, a scientific analysis of federal health data, a consumer poll, and interviews with doctors and other experts, finds the following:

- Roughly 10 percent of our juice samples, from five brands, had total arsenic levels that exceeded federal drinking-water standards. Most of that arsenic was inorganic arsenic, a known carcinogen.

In our tests, apple and grape juice had arsenic and lead at varying levels.

- One in four samples had lead levels higher than the FDA's bottled-water limit of 5 ppb. As with arsenic, no federal limit exists for lead in juice.
- Apple and grape juice constitute a significant source of dietary exposure to arsenic, according to our analysis of federal health data from 2003 through 2008.
- Children drink a lot of juice. Thirty-five percent of children 5 and younger drink juice in quantities exceeding pediatricians' recommendations, our poll of parents shows.
- Mounting scientific evidence suggests that chronic exposure to arsenic and lead even at levels below water standards can result in serious health problems.

- Inorganic arsenic has been detected at disturbing levels in other foods, too, which suggests that more must be done to reduce overall dietary exposure.

Our findings have prompted Consumers Union, the advocacy arm of Consumer Reports, to urge the FDA to set arsenic and lead standards for apple and grape juice. Our scientists believe that juice should at least meet the 5 ppb lead limit for bottled water. They recommend an even lower arsenic limit for juice: 3 ppb.

"People sometimes say, 'If arsenic exposure is so bad, why don't you see more people sick or dying from it?' But the many diseases likely to be increased by exposure even at relatively low levels are so common already that its effects are overlooked simply because no one has looked carefully for the connection," says Joshua Hamilton, Ph.D., a toxicologist specializing in arsenic research and the chief academic and scientific officer at the Marine Biological Laboratory in Woods Hole, Mass.

As our investigation found, when scientists and doctors do look, the connections they've found underscore the need to protect public health by reducing Americans' exposure to this potent toxin.

Many Sources of Exposure

Arsenic is a naturally occurring element that can contaminate groundwater used for drinking and irrigation in areas where it's abundant, such as parts of New England, the Midwest, and the Southwest.

But the public's exposure to arsenic extends beyond those areas because since 1910, the United States has used roughly 1.6 million tons of it for agricultural and other industrial uses. About half of that cumulative total has been used since only the mid-1960s. Lead-arsenate insecticides were widely used in cotton fields, orchards, and vineyards until their use was banned in the 1980s. But residues in the soil can still contaminate crops.

For decades, arsenic was also used in a preservative for pressure-treated lumber commonly used for decks and playground equipment. In 2003 that use was banned, (as was most residential use) but the wood can contribute to arsenic in groundwater when it's recycled as mulch.

Other sources of exposure include coal-fired power plants and smelters that heat arsenic-containing ores to process copper or lead. Today the quantity of arsenic released into the environment in the U.S. by human activities is three times more than that released from natural sources, says the federal Agency for Toxic Substances and Disease Registry.

The form of arsenic in the examples above is inorganic arsenic. It's a carcinogen known to cause bladder, lung, and skin cancer in people and to increase risks of cardiovascular disease, immunodeficiencies, and type 2 diabetes.

The other form that arsenic takes is organic arsenic, created when arsenic binds to molecules containing carbon. Fish can contain an organic form of arsenic called arsenobetaine, generally considered nontoxic to humans. But questions have been raised about the human health effects of other types of organic arsenic in foods, including juice.

Use of organic arsenic in agricultural products has also caused concern. For instance, the EPA in 2006 took steps to stop the use of herbicides containing organic arsenic because of their potential to turn into inorganic arsenic in soil and contaminate drinking water. And in 2011, working with the FDA, drug company Alpharma agreed to suspend the sale of Roxarsone, a poultry-feed additive, because it contained an organic form of arsenic that could convert into inorganic arsenic inside the bird, potentially contaminating the meat. Or it could contaminate soil when chicken droppings are used as fertilizer. Other arsenic feed additives are still being used.

What Our Tests Found

We went shopping in Connecticut, New Jersey, and New York in August and September, buying 28 apple juices and three grape juices. Our samples came from ready-to-drink bottles, juice boxes, and cans of concentrate. For most juices, we bought three different lot numbers to assess variability. (For some juices, we couldn't find three lots, so we tested one or two.) In all, we tested 88 samples.

Five samples of apple juice and four of grape juice had total arsenic levels exceeding the 10 ppb federal limit for bottled and drinking water. Levels in the apple juices ranged from 1.1 to 13.9 ppb, and grape-juice levels were even higher, 5.9 to 24.7 ppb. Most of the total arsenic in our samples was inorganic, our tests showed.

As for lead, about one fourth of all juice samples had levels at or above the 5-ppb limit for bottled water. The top lead level for apple juice was 13.6 ppb; for grape juice, 15.9 ppb.

The following brands had at least one sample of apple juice that exceeded 10 ppb: Apple & Eve, Great Value (Walmart), and Mott's. For grape juice, at least one sample from Walgreens and Welch's exceeded that threshold. And these brands had one or more samples of apple juice that exceeded 5 ppb of lead: America's Choice (A&P), Gerber, Gold Emblem (CVS), Great Value, Joe's Kids (Trader Joe's), Minute Maid, Seneca, and Walgreens. At least one sample of grape juice exceeding 5 ppb of lead came from Gold Emblem, Walgreens, and Welch's. Our findings provide a spot check of a number of local juice aisles, but they can't be used to draw general conclusions about arsenic or lead levels in any particular brand. Even within a single tested brand, levels of arsenic and lead sometimes varied widely.

Arsenic-tainted soil in U.S. orchards is a likely source of contamination for apples, and finding lead with arsenic in juices that we tested is not surprising. Even with a ban on lead-arsenate insecticides, "we are finding problems with some Washington state apples, not because of irresponsible farming practices now but because lead-arsenate pesticides that were used here decades ago remain in the soil," says Denise Wilson, Ph.D., an associate professor at the University of Washington who has tested apple juices and discovered elevated arsenic levels even in brands labeled organic.

Over the years, a shift has occurred in how juice sold in America is produced. To make apple juice, manufacturers often blend water with apple-juice concentrate from multiple sources. For the past decade, most concentrate has come from China. Concerns have been raised about the possible continuing use of arsenical pesticides there, and several Chinese provinces that are primary apple-growing regions are known to have high arsenic concentrations in groundwater.

How to Reduce Your Family's Risk

Test your water. If your home or a home you're considering buying isn't on a public water system, have the home's water tested for arsenic and lead. To find a certified lab, contact your local health department or call the federal Safe Drinking Water Hotline at 800-426-4791. To find contact information for your public water system, go to cfpub.epo.gov/safewater/ccr/index.cfm.

Limit children's juice consumption. Nutrition guidelines set by the American Academy of Pediatrics can help. The academy recommends that infants younger than 6 months shouldn't drink juice; children up to 6 years old should consume no more than four to six ounces a day and older children, no more than 8 to 12 ounces a day. Diluting juice with water can help meet those goals.

Consider your food. Buying certified organic chicken makes sense because organic standards don't allow the use of chicken feed containing arsenic. But for juice and other foods, it's not so certain. Organic standards prohibit the use of synthetic fertilizers and most pesticides, but organic juices still may contain arsenic if they're made from fruit grown in soil where arsenical insecticides were used.

Need a home-treatment system? Contact NSF International at www.nsf.org/certified/DwTu or 800-673-8010 for info on systems certified to lower arsenic levels to no more than 10 ppb. The University of Georgia Cooperative Extension discusses treatment technologies at aesl.ces.uga.edu/publications/watercirc. (Click on "Removal of Arsenic from Household Water.")

If you're concerned, get tested. Ask your doctor for a urine test for you or your child to determine arsenic levels. Don't eat seafood for 48 to 72 hours before being tested to avoid misleadingly high levels from "fish arsenic." For a medical toxicologist in your area who can interpret results, call the American Association of Poison Control Centers at 800-222-1222.

A much bigger test than ours would be needed to establish any correlation between elevated arsenic or lead levels and the juice concentrate's country of origin. Samples we tested included some made from concentrate from multiple countries including Argentina, China, New Zealand, South Africa, and Turkey; others came from a single country. A few samples solely from the United States had elevated levels of lead or arsenic, and others did not. The same was true for samples containing only Chinese concentrate.

The FDA has been collecting its own data to see whether it should set guidelines to continue to ensure the safety of apple juice, a spokeswoman told us.

The Juice Products Association said, "We are committed to providing nutritious and safe fruit juices to consumers and will comply with limits established by the agency."

Answering a Crucial Question

We also wanted to know whether people who drink juice end up being exposed to more arsenic than those who don't.

So we commissioned an analysis of data from the National Health and Nutrition Examination Survey (NHANES), conducted annually by the National Center for Health Statistics. Information is collected on the health and nutrition of a nationally representative sample of the U.S. population, based on interviews and physical exams that may include a blood or urine test. Officials and researchers often use the data to determine risk factors for major diseases and develop public health policy. In fact, data on lead in the blood of NHANES participants were instrumental in developing policies that have successfully resulted in lead being removed from gasoline.

Our analysis was led by Richard Stahlhut, M.D., M.P.H., an environmental health researcher at the University of Rochester with expertise in NHANES data, working with Consumer Reports statisticians. Ana Navas-Acien, M.D., Ph.D., a physician—epidemiologist at Johns Hopkins University's Bloomberg School of Public Health, also provided guidance. She was the lead author of a 2008 study in the Journal of the American Medical Association that first linked low-level arsenic exposure with the prevalence of type 2 diabetes in the U.S.

Over time, people who ingest even low arsenic levels can become sick.

Stahlhut reviewed NHANES data from 2003 through 2008 from participants tested for total urinary arsenic who reported their food and drink consumption for 24 hours the day before their NHANES visit. Because most ingested arsenic is excreted in urine, the best measure of recent exposure is a urine test.

Following Navas-Acien's advice, we excluded from our NHANES analysis anyone with results showing detectable levels of arsenobetaine, the organic arsenic in seafood. That made the results we analyzed more likely to represent inorganic arsenic, of greatest concern in terms of potential health risks.

The resulting analysis of almost 3,000 study participants found that those reporting apple-juice consumption had on average 19 percent greater levels of total urinary arsenic than those subjects who did not, and those who reported drinking grape juice had 20 percent higher levels. The results might understate the correlation between juice consumption and urinary arsenic levels because NHANES urinary data exclude children younger than 6, who tend to be big juice drinkers.

"The current analysis suggests that these juices may be an important contributor to dietary arsenic exposure," says Keeve Nachman, Ph.D., a risk scientist at the Center for a Livable Future and the Bloomberg School of Public Health, both at Johns Hopkins University. "It would be prudent to pursue measures to understand and limit young children's exposures to arsenic in juice."

Robert Wright, M.D., M.P.H., associate professor of pediatrics and environmental health at Harvard University who specializes in research on the effect of heavy-metals exposure in children, says that findings from our juice tests and database analysis concern him: "Because of their small size, a child drinking a box of juice would consume a larger per-body-weight dose of arsenic than an adult drinking the exact same box of juice. Those brands with elevated arsenic should investigate the source and eliminate it."

A Chronic Problem

Arsenic has been notoriously used as a poison since ancient times. A fatal poisoning would require a single dose of inorganic arsenic about the weight of a postage stamp. But chronic toxicity can result from long-term exposure to much lower levels in food, and even to water that meets the 10-ppb drinking-water limit.

A 2004 study of children in Bangladesh suggested diminished intelligence based on test scores in children exposed to arsenic in drinking water at levels above 5 ppb, says study author Joseph Graziano, Ph.D., a professor of environmental health sciences and pharmacology at Columbia University. He's now conducting similar research with children living in New Hampshire and Maine, where arsenic levels of 10 to 100 ppb are commonly found in well water, to determine whether better nutrition in the United States affects the results.

People with private wells may face greater risks than those on public systems because they're responsible for testing and treating their own water. In Maine, where almost half the population relies on private wells, the USGS found arsenic levels in well water as high as 3,100 ppb.

And a study published in 2011 in the International Journal of Environmental Research and Public Health examined the long-term effects of low-level exposure on more than 300 rural Texans whose groundwater was estimated to have arsenic at median levels below the federal drinking-water standard. It found that exposure was related to poor scores in language, memory, and other brain functions.

Warning Signs

Chronic arsenic exposure can initially cause gastrointestinal problems and skin discoloration or lesions. Exposure over time, which the World Health Organization says could be five to

20 years, could increase the risk of various cancers and high blood pressure, diabetes, and reproductive problems.

Signs of chronic low-level arsenic exposure can be mistaken for other ailments such as chronic fatigue syndrome. Usually the connection to arsenic exposure is not made immediately, as Sharyn Duffy of Geneseo, N.Y., discovered. She visited a doctor in 2007 about pain and skin changes on the sole of her left foot. She was referred to a podiatrist and eventually received a diagnosis of hyperkeratosis, in which lesions develop or thick skin forms on the palms or soles of the feet. It can be among the earliest symptoms of chronic arsenic poisoning. But she says it was roughly two years before she was finally referred to a neurologist, who suggested testing for arsenic. She had double the typical levels.

"Testing for arsenic isn't part of a routine checkup," says Duffy, a retiree. "When you come in with symptoms like I had, ordering that kind of test probably wouldn't even occur to most doctors."

Michael Harbut, M.D., chief of the environmental cancer program at Karmanos Institute in Detroit, says, "Given what we know about the wide range of arsenic exposure sources we have in this country, I suspect there is an awful lot of chronic, low-level arsenic poisoning going on that's never properly diagnosed."

Our Test Findings of Apple and Grape Juice

There's no federal limit for arsenic or lead in juice. In our tests, 25 percent of samples exceeded the 5-ppb lead limit for bottled water, and 10 percent exceeded the 10-ppb limit for arsenic in drinking water. Most arsenic we detected was inorganic. Our tests don't offer conclusions about overall levels in any juice type or brand. We tested three lots of most juices. Smaller containers are noted. For more details see www.ConsumerReports.org/juicebox.

Juice (in alphabetical order)	Total arsenic[1] (ppb)	Lead (ppb)
365 Everyday Value Organic 100 percent Apple Juice (Whole Foods)[2]	7.0 to 7.1	3.5 to 3.8
America's Choice 100 percent Apple Juice (A&P)	1.4 to 4.4	0.5 to 5.6
Apple & Eve 100 percent Apple Juice (6.75-ounce juice boxes)	5.0 to 10.5	1.9 to 3.4
Gerber 100 percent Apple Juice (4-ounce bottles)	5.8 to 9.7	3.4 to 13.6
Gerber Organic 100 percent Apple Juice (4-ounce bottles)	5.5 to 5.7	2.2 to 2.3
Gold Emblem 100 percent Apple Juice (CVS)	3.1 to 9.4	2.9 to 5.6
Gold Emblem 100 percent Grape Juice (CVS)	5.9 to 7.5	6.5 to 8.6

Juice (in alphabetical order)	Total arsenic[1] (ppb)	Lead (ppb)
Great Value 100 percent Apple Juice (Walmart)	10.1 to 13.9	3.7 to 5.1
Great Value 100 percent Apple Juice (Walmart, 10-ounce bottles)[3]	5.5	3.4
Great Value 100 percent Apple Juice with fiber Not from Concentrate (Walmart)	2.9 to 3.9	0.1 to 0.2
Joe's Kids 100 percent Apple Juice (Trader Joe's, 6.75-ounce Juice boxes)	4.1 to 5.7	5.3 to 9.7
Juicy Juice 100 percent Apple Juice Non Frozen Concentrate[4]	1.9 to 4.2	1.4 to 2.2
Juicy Juice 100 percent Apple Juice	1.7 to 3.0	0.8 to 2.3
Juicy Juice 100 percent Apple Juice (10-ounce bottles)	1.7 to 1.9	1.1 to 3.5
Juicy Juice 100 percent Apple Juice (6.75-ounce juice boxes)	1.3 to 2.8	1.4 to 2.8
Lucky Leaf 100 percent Apple Juice[2]	2.3 to 3.2	0.8 to 1.2
Minute Maid 100 percent Apple Juice (10-ounce bottles)	6.2 to 6.7	4.2 to 6.5
Minute Maid 100 percent Apple Juice (juice box packaged for McDonald's)	2.0 to 5.6	0.8 to 5.3
Mott's Original 100 percent Apple Juice	4.0 to 7.9	2.1 to 3.8
Mott's Original 100 percent Apple Juice (4.23-ounce juice boxes)	4.0 to 10.2	0.6 to 0.7
Mott's Original 100 percent Apple Juice (6.75-ounce juice boxes)	2.1 to 2.8	0.6 to 1.3
Nature's Own 100 percent Apple Juice[2]	2.3 to 2.4	0.9 each
Old Orchard 100 percent Apple Juice Frozen Concentrate[4]	1.6 to 4.8	0.6 to 1.3
Red Jacket Orchards 100 percent Fuji Apple Juice	1.3 to 1.8	0.1 to 0.2
Rite Aid Pantry 100 percent Apple Juice	1.1 to 6.4	0.4 to 2.6
Seneca 100 percent Apple Juice Frozen Concentrate[4]	2.3 to 4.4	0.9 to 5.5
Tropicana 100 percent Apple Juice (15.2-ounce bottles)	1.5 to 2.1	0.5 to 1.0
Walgreens 100 percent Apple Juice	4.0 to 6.8	2.3 to 6.9
Walgreens 100 percent Grape Juice	9.7 to 24.7	10.1 to 15.9
Welch's 100 percent Apple Juice Pourable Concentrate[4]	1.1 to 4.1	0.6 to 1.3
Welch's 100 percent Grape Juice	7.1 to 12.4	3.5 to 9.2

[1] Includes organic and inorganic arsenic.
[2] Two lots tested.
[3] One lot tested.
[4] Reconstituted; assumes no arsenic or lead from added water.

Emerging research suggests that when arsenic exposure occurs in the womb or in early childhood, it not only increases cancer risks later in life but also can cause lasting harm to children's developing brains and endocrine and immune systems, leading to other diseases, too.

Case in point: From 1958 through 1970, residents of Antofagasta, Chile, were exposed to naturally occurring arsenic in drinking water that peaked at almost 1,000 ppb before an arsenic removal plant was installed. Studies led by researchers at the University of California at Berkeley found that people born during that period who had probable exposure in the womb and during early childhood had a lung-cancer death rate six times higher than those in their age group elsewhere in Chile. Their rate of death in their 30s and 40s from another form of lung disease was almost 50 times higher than for people without that arsenic exposure.

"Recent studies have shown that early-childhood exposure to arsenic carries the most serious long-term risk," says Joshua Hamilton of the Marine Biological Laboratory. "So even though reducing arsenic exposure is important for everyone, we need to pay special attention to protecting pregnant moms, babies, and young kids."

Other Dietary Exposures

In addition to juice, foods including chicken, rice, and even baby food have been found to contain arsenic—sometimes at higher levels than the amounts found in juice. Brian Jackson,

Ph.D., an analytical chemist and research associate professor at Dartmouth College, presented his findings at a June 2011 scientific conference in Aberdeen, Scotland. He reported finding up to 23 ppb of arsenic in lab tests of name-brand jars of baby food, with inorganic arsenic representing 70 to 90 percent of those total amounts.

Similar results turned up in a 2004 study conducted by FDA scientists in Cincinnati, who found arsenic levels of up to 24 ppb in baby food, with sweet potatoes, carrots, green beans, and peaches containing only the inorganic form. A United Kingdom study published in 2008 found that the levels of inorganic arsenic in 20-ounce packets of dried infant rice cereals ranged from 60 to 160 ppb. Rice-based infant cereals are often the first solid food that babies eat.

Consumers Union wants federal limits for arsenic and lead in juice.

Rice frequently contains high levels of inorganic arsenic because it is among plants that are unusually efficient at taking up arsenic from the soil and incorporating it in the grains people eat. Moreover, much of the rice produced in the U.S. is grown in Arkansas, Louisiana, Mississippi, Missouri, and Texas, on land formerly used to grow cotton, where arsenical pesticides were used for decades.

"Initially, in some regions rice planted there produced little grain due to these arsenical pesticides, but farmers then bred a type of rice specifically designed to produce high yields on the contaminated soil," says Andrew Meharg, professor of biogeochemistry at the University of Aberdeen, in Scotland. Meharg studies human exposures to arsenic in the environment. His research over the past six years has shown that U.S. rice has among the highest average inorganic arsenic levels in the world—almost three times higher than levels in Basmati rice imported from low-arsenic areas of Nepal, India, and Pakistan. Rice from Egypt has the lowest levels of all.

Infant rice cereal for the U.S. market is generally made from U.S. rice, Meharg says, but labeling usually doesn't specify country of origin. He says exposure to arsenic through infant rice cereals could be reduced greatly if cereal makers used techniques that don't require growing rice in water-flooded paddies or if they obtained rice from low-arsenic areas. His 2007 study found that median arsenic levels in California rice were 41 percent lower than levels in rice from the south-central U.S.

Setting a Standard

Evidence of arsenic's ability to cause cancer and other life-threatening illnesses has surged because some of the diseases linked to it have latency periods of several decades. Only recently have scientists been able to more fully measure the effects in populations that were exposed to elevated levels of arsenic in drinking water many years ago.

The Environmental Protection Agency periodically revises its assessment of the toxicity of various chemicals to offer

---

How Much Juice Do Children Drink?

Too many children drink too much juice, according to our poll of parents. One in four toddlers 2 and younger and 45 percent of children ages 3 to 5 drink 7 or more ounces of juice a day.

The American Academy of Pediatrics cautions that to help prevent obesity and tooth decay, children younger than 6 should drink no more than 6 ounces a day, about the size of a juice box. (Infants younger than 6 months shouldn't drink any.) The possible presence of arsenic or lead in juices is all the more reason to stick with those nutrition-based limits.

Our findings are from 555 telephone interviews in October with parents, who were asked about children's juice consumption the previous day. Totals don't equal 100 percent because some said they didn't know how much juice their kids drank.

Amount of juice consumed	Children 2 and under	Children 3 to 5	Total children 5 or younger
None	40 percent	22 percent	31 percent
1 to 6 oz.	28	26	27
7 to 12 oz.	18	29	23
16 oz. or more	8	16	12

---

guidance on drinking-water standards. Based on such a review, the agency changed the water standard for arsenic to 10 ppb, effective in 2006, from the 50-ppb limit it set in 1975. The EPA had proposed a 5-ppb limit in 2000, so the current limit is a compromise that came only after years of haggling over the costs of removing arsenic. Since 2006, New Jersey has had a 5-ppb threshold, advising residents that water with arsenic levels above that shouldn't be used for drinking or cooking.

For known human carcinogens such as inorganic arsenic, the EPA assumes there's actually no "safe" level of exposure, so it normally sets exposure limits that include a margin of safety to ideally allow for only one additional case of cancer in a million people, or at worst, no more than one in 10,000. For water with 10 ppb of arsenic, the excess cancer risk is one in 500.

Debate over that standard is likely to begin anew. The agency's latest draft report, from February 2010, proposes that the number used to calculate the cancer risk posed by ingesting inorganic arsenic be increased 17-fold to reflect arsenic's role in causing bladder and lung cancer. The proposal "suggests that arsenic's carcinogenic properties have been underestimated for a long time and that the federal drinking-water standard is underprotective based on current science," says Keeve Nachman, the Johns Hopkins scientist.

Each year the FDA tests a variety of foods and beverages for arsenic and other contaminants. It also started a program in 2005 to test for specific toxins such as arsenic and lead in domestic and imported products. As of late November, that program had published results for 160 samples of apple juice and concentrate. And the agency can alert inspectors at U.S. ports to conduct increased surveillance for products suspected to pose risks. Currently there's an alert for increased surveillance of apple concentrate from China and six other countries "where we have a suspicion there may be high levels of arsenic in their products," says FDA spokeswoman Stephanie Yao. But

in fiscal 2010, the agency conducted physical inspections of only 2 percent of imported food shipments.

Consumers Union urges federal officials to set a standard for total arsenic in apple and grape juice. Our research suggests that the standard should be 3 ppb. Concerning lead, juice should at least meet the bottled-water standard of 5 ppb. Such standards would better protect children, who are most vulnerable to the effects of arsenic and lead. And they're achievable levels: 41 percent of the samples we tested met both thresholds.

Moreover, the EPA should impose stricter drinking-water standards for arsenic, Consumers Union believes. (The drinking-water threshold for lead is 15 ppb, which acknowledges that many older homes have water pipes or solder with lead.) Officials should also ban arsenic in pesticides, animal-feed additives, and fertilizers.

As our tests show, sources of lead haven't been eliminated, but dramatic progress has been made: Since the 1970s, average blood lead levels in children younger than 6 have dropped by about 90 percent, thanks to a federal ban on lead in house paint and gas. The U.S. should be equally aggressive with arsenic, suggests Joseph Graziano at Columbia University. "We tackled every source, from gasoline to paint to solder in food cans," he says, "and we should be just as vigilant in preventing arsenic from entering our food and water because the consequences of exposure are enormous for adults as well as children."

Critical Thinking

1. Identify the natural and man-made sources of exposure to lead and arsenic.
2. Differentiate between organic and inorganic arsenic.
3. Describe how the FDA regulates arsenic and lead in US food and beverages.
4. Identify potential signs of chronic low-level exposure to arsenic.

UNIT 8

Hunger, Nutrition, and Sustainability

Unit Selections

Learning Outcomes

After reading this unit, you will be able to:

- Summarize the impact of weather, oil prices, the expansion of agrofuels, the financial crisis of 2008–2009, increases in meat consumption, and population growth on global food prices.

- Describe how the U.S. policies to manage its food supply has impacted world food trade and prices.

- Evaluate the effectiveness of the price premium on production of fair-trade agriculture.

- Summarize how price competition from large retail stores impacts the laborers on plantations where organic and fair trade products are grown.

- Define food insecurity.

- List the factors that impact the price of the global food supply.

- Identify the barriers to international food assistance and education programs.

- Evaluate the causes of the nutrition and health disparities among native people.

- Evaluate the advantages and disadvantages of using synthetic fertilizers.

- Explain why a plant-based diet will lead to less destruction of the atmosphere and pollutants of our water supplies.

- Define perennial grain crops and explain how perennial grain crops differ from annual grain crops.

- Identify the three grain crops that provide 70 percent of the calories for human consumption worldwide.

Student Website
www.mhhe.com/cls

Internet References

Food and Agriculture Organization of the United Nations (FAO)
www.fao.org

Population Reference Bureau
www.prb.org

International Food Information Council Foundation (IFIC)
www.FoodInsight.org

U.S. Sustainable Agriculture Research and Education Program, University of California-Davis
www.sarep.ucdavis.edu/concept.htm

World Health Organization (WHO)
www.who.int/en

Considering the economic instability of the past few years, more Americans are living at or below the poverty level. The changes in our economy and employment rates have caused many Americans to spend less money on food for themselves and their families. It is possible to consume fresh and nutritious foods on a tight budget, but it is challenging in our current food culture. Several articles in this unit describe some of the challenges that low-income populations face in obtaining nutritious foods and what can be done to improve the accessibility of nutritious foods for those who struggle to feed their families.

The international food supply is a complex global process that is impacted by natural and secular phenomena. Unpredictable weather, climate change, government regulation of agriculture, tariffs on trade, trading and speculation of commodity crops, and increased meat consumption have all impacted the world's food supply. Global food prices are directly linked to changes in supply and the price of food around the world has increased because of changes in the food supply. Over the past eight years food prices have increased at dramatic rates, with prices of grains increasing at the highest rates. The sharp increases in food prices lead to political protests in African, South American, and Asian countries. The food crisis has culminated in greater political instability in developing countries that rely on rice and wheat as their main source of calories.

The regulations that helped to stabilize agriculture prices and production after the Great Depression and World War II have diminished or been eliminated. As a result of this deregulation, the price of food has increased and has experienced much great volatility in prices. The populations that feel the most effect of rising food costs are the poorer areas of developing countries.

Nutrient deficiencies magnify the effect of disease, resulting in more severe symptoms and greater complications in countries with developing economies. For example, vitamin A deficiency leads to blindness in about 250,000–300,000 children annually and exacerbates the symptoms of measles. Iron deficiency, which is widespread among pregnant women and those in the child-bearing years in developing countries, increases the risk of death from hemorrhage in their offspring and reduces physical productivity and learning capacity. Finally, iodine deficiency causes brain damage and mental retardation. It is estimated that 1.5 billion people are at risk for iodine deficiency disorders.

Malnutrition is the main culprit for lowered resistance to disease, infection, and death, especially in children in developing countries. The malnutrition infection combination results in stunted growth, lowered mental development in children, lowered productivity, and higher incidence of degenerative disease in adulthood. This directly affects the economies of developing countries. Over 1 billion people globally suffer from micronutrient malnutrition frequently called "hidden hunger." In addition, partnerships between the public and private sectors may prove valuable in combating malnutrition. Solutions to these problems such as building sustainable systems through indigenous knowledge and practices that are community based and environmentally friendly with emphasis on biofortification and dietary diversification may combat hunger and nutrient deficiencies in the future.

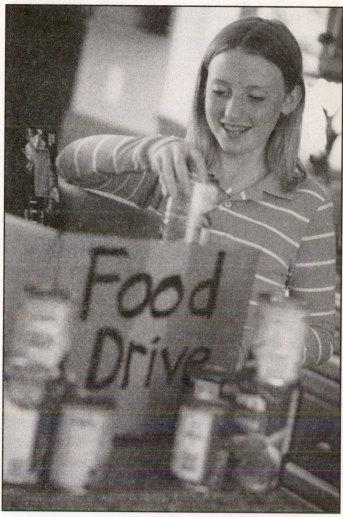

© Design Pics/SW Productions

Malnutrition not only affects children and adults in developing countries, but it is also prevalent in the United States. Thirty million Americans (including 11 million children), experience food insecurity and hunger. In a country where one-fifth of the food is wasted and 130 pounds of food per person is disposed of, it is unacceptable that Americans go hungry. Food security is now critical to consumers worldwide.

The final two articles are about sustainable agriculture versus conventional agricultural practices. Current conventional agricultural techniques depend on nitrogen-based fertilizers for crop production; however, as the use of these chemical fertilizers spreads to other countries, it is posing threats to our health and the health of our ecosystems. The article by Townsend and Howarth describes the history of nitrogen-based fertilizers and the damage that results from too much nitrogen in our atmosphere. The other agriculture article addresses food security through genetically modifying grain crops to be perennial crops rather than annual crops. Our agricultural grain crops are annuals, meaning the plants must be planted each year from seed and the plants are cleared from the fields at the end of the growing season. Plant geneticists are now able to develop perennial grain plants that could have significant ecological, environmental, and health benefits to the world's food supply.

Many of the articles in this unit focus on food insecurity, hunger, and food/health disparities. This topic was emphasized in this unit because of the growing number of food-insecure households in the United States as a result of the economy. The topic of hunger has always been a central focus in international nutrition; however, more people in the United States are affected by food insecurity, even with the abundant amount of food that is wasted here. Food assistance programs are needed domestically as well as for the millions of undernourished people living in developing countries.

The Food Crisis and the Deregulation of Agriculture

BILL WINDERS

Food prices began to climb throughout the world in 2007. World wheat prices climbed from an average of $127 per ton in 2004–2005 to $397 per ton in the spring of 2008—an increase of more than 200 percent—and rice prices rose by more than 250 percent to $962 per ton in 2008.[1] Prices for corn, meat, oils, and dairy products saw similar though less dramatic increases at this time as well.[2] Not surprisingly, world hunger and malnutrition rose along with food prices. The Food and Agriculture Organization (FAO) estimates that more than one billion people were undernourished in 2009, representing a dramatic increase from 15 years before when fewer than 800 million people were hungry.[3]

As food prices rose and the threat of hunger spread in 2007 and 2008, protests struck dozens of countries, including Argentina, Mexico, India, Italy, Bangladesh, Egypt, Somalia, and Morocco. These protests contributed to political instability in a number of countries. In Haiti, for example, the prime minister was removed after a week of food riots in April 2008.[4] Although rising food prices did not lead to disruptive protests in every nation, reduced access to food was undoubtedly a destabilizing political force in many.

Though food prices declined in 2009 and protests faded, prices began to increase again in 2010 and continued rising in early 2011. In fact, the FAO's food price index (a composite look at real food prices) was higher in February, March, and April of 2011 than at any other point in the previous 20 years. Wheat prices, for example, rose to $336 per ton in April.[5] Also, of course, protests rocked the Middle East in the first three months of 2011. This "Arab Spring" began in January with food riots in Tunisia, which were soon followed by protests in Algeria, in which rising food prices also played a role.

The food crisis, then, has entailed not only rising food prices and increasing world hunger, but also greater political instability and change. Food crises hold the potential to destabilize existing political alliances, mobilize masses against regimes, and prompt some people to begin questioning economic systems. Given the possibility of such significant scenarios, how can we explain this food crisis in the world economy? Why did it come about? We might start by putting the factors behind this crisis into two categories: immediate (or proximate) causes

and secular (or systemic) causes.[6] The immediate or proximate factors are those current elements and conditions surrounding the rise in food prices, while the secular or systemic causes are more long-term trends and changes that are not as immediately visible.

While most public attention is paid to the immediate context of the food crisis—issues such as weather conditions and ethanol production—I argue that deregulation in agriculture in both national policies and the level of the world economy set the stage for the crisis. Over the past 40 years, regulations that had helped stabilize agricultural prices and production were eroded or eliminated altogether. Recognizing the role of long-term deregulation also reveals an important insight about the recent food crisis: the instability and volatility of prices is as important as the existence of high prices. Before we explore this point, however, I will first turn briefly to the factors commonly cited as contributing to the food crisis.

Immediate Causes of Rising Food Prices

Observers tend to point to several factors in explaining recent increases in food prices: inhospitable weather and climate, the proliferation of agrofuels, rising oil prices, commodity speculation, greater meat consumption, and population growth. There should be little doubt that most of these factors played a role in rising food prices in the past four years, and certainly these factors receive the most public attention. While this immediate context is not my central focus, acknowledging the part that these factors played in the food crisis is important nonetheless.

First, harsh or inhospitable weather clearly affects crop harvests and result in higher prices due to unexpected decreases in the supply of food. Leading up to the 2007–2008 food crisis, Australia suffered from a drought, which affected wheat and rice production, and a cyclone hurt rice production in Thailand—the world's leading rice exporter.[7] Then in the summer of 2010, Russia and parts of Europe experienced a severe drought that reduced wheat harvests and pushed the Russian government to ban wheat exports. A *New York Times* article on the drought noted, "Wheat prices have soared by about 90 percent since June because of the drought in Russia and parts of the European Union, as well as floods in Canada, and the ban pushed prices even higher."[8] Food prices are likely to rise if weather patterns depress agricultural production.

Second, the shift from food grains to agrofuels undermined food supply and drove prices up. In particular, observers have highlighted the increased use of corn for ethanol production in 2006–2008, especially in the United States and European Union. As Fred Magdoff and Brian Tokar note, "Close to one-third of the entire 2008 United States corn crop was used to produce ethanol to blend with gasoline to fuel cars."[9] In 2007, Congress tried to encourage the use of corn for ethanol production by passing the Energy Independence and Security Act, which "mandates the increase of agro-fuels production [...] from 4.7 billion gallons in 2007 to at least 36 billion gallons in 2022."[10] To encourage agrofuel production, the United States has also created a number of subsidies.[11] This push to increase agrofuel production reduced the supply of food in the world economy.

This push to increase agrofuel production reduced the supply of food in the world economy.

Third, rising oil prices can contribute to higher food prices. Agricultural production, especially grain production, in developed countries relies heavily on oil as industrial agriculture employs heavy machinery as well as petroleum-based chemical fertilizers. The food crisis of 1973, for example, was exacerbated by the historic rise in oil prices. Oil prices began to rise in 2007 and peaked in 2008 (when gasoline in the United States rose above $4 per gallon).[12]

Fourth, the financial crisis of 2008–2009 contributed to rising food prices. As real estate markets began to falter, investors sought alternative outlets such as commodities futures markets. Farmers and others use futures markets to lock in a price for a commodity, allowing them "some protection from price fluctuations and allow[ing] them to plan their business effectively."[13] The financial crisis, however, increased the level of speculation, which is basically a "bet on the probability that the price of a commodity will rise or fall in order to profit from changes in prices."[14] This influx of money into the futures market drove up commodity prices, increasing the price of food.[15]

Fifth, rising meat consumption in the world contributed to higher food prices. Though meat consumption has increased in the past 20 years in the United States and Europe, it has risen much more in countries such as China and India. In the latter, growth in the middle class and rising per capita income have helped to fuel increased per capita meat consumption. And as meat consumption increases, more land is used for pasture or to grow feed grains, such as corn and soybeans. This reduces the land devoted to food crops to be consumed directly by people. In addition, meat production is a less efficient way to feed people since it "takes seven to eight kilos of grain to produce one kilo of beef."[16]

Though it was cited as an important factor in the 1970s, population growth has rarely been singled out as a significant contributor to the recent food crisis. Nonetheless, *The Economist* recently published a special report titled, "The 9 billion-people question," which focused on the implications of population growth. The world's population is projected to reach 9 billion by 2050. This report asked: Will there be enough food?[17]

This immediate context undoubtedly contributed in varying degrees to recent increases in food prices. Yet focusing on these factors really remains at the surface and leaves fundamental trends and processes unexplored. The broader political-economic context was such that these trends could come together. Understanding how this context came about is central to understanding the fundamental processes leading to this crisis.

Secular Causes of Rising Food Prices

The commonly cited factors are not the only forces contributing to rising food prices, nor are high food prices the only concern. Greater instability in agricultural prices and production is also an important problem. In the past five years, food prices have fluctuated dramatically. For example, wheat prices rose by about 200 percent, then fell by 55 percent, then rose again by almost 100 percent—all within the span of a few years. This volatility is linked to policies of deregulation in the United States and elsewhere over the past 40 years. This instability in prices and production was central to rising food prices and the food crisis.

Importantly, food prices have historically been a function of international food regimes—the institutions, rules, and norms that shape food and agricultural production, trade, and consumption in the world economy. Therefore, the ebb and flow of food prices and the degree to which prices are volatile are functions of the changes in food regimes, which are shaped by national policies and agrarian politics.[18]

To put this process into proper context, we need to begin with the mid-twentieth century, when the United States created global institutions to support its position as the dominant economic and political power in the world economy. At that time, the United States food regime came to stress regulation in agriculture with the aim of stabilizing prices and production.

Regulating Food and Agriculture, 1945–1970

Following the Great Depression and World War II, the United States set out to liberalize the world economy. In particular, the United States sought to tear down many of the trade barriers and regulations created during the Depression. The General Agreement on Tariffs and Trade (GATT) was the primary vehicle for trade liberalization. Coming into effect in 1948, GATT set forth rules for trade and aimed to reduce trade barriers in the world economy through multilateral trade agreements. It was effective at reducing trade barriers, as the average tariff rate on dutiable imports fell from about 40 percent when GATT was formed to five percent by 1990. GATT had one important caveat, however: it exempted agriculture from liberalization. As a result, nations could still regulate agricultural production, prices, and trade.

The exemption of agriculture from GATT was, of course, due to the United States' desire to protect its policy of supply management, which rested on three programs: price supports, production controls, and export subsidies. Price supports provided a minimum price for agricultural goods, thereby protecting farmers from severe downturns in the market. Production controls restricted the amount of acreage that farmers could devote to particular commodities (e.g., corn, wheat, cotton), but also regulated production in a manner that helped to guarantee a steady production of these commodities.[19] Export subsidies, including international food aid, were created to help lower the price of agricultural exports, which had been artificially inflated because of price supports. Together, these programs aimed to stabilize the market for agriculture.

In part because agricultural regulations were exempt from GATT, many other nations adopted similar agricultural policies including France, Canada, Mexico, Germany, Australia, and Japan. These nations adopted supply management not simply because GATT allowed it, but also because they faced competition from United States agriculture concerns, which were subsidized and extensively regulated. This competition prompted many farmers around the world to push their respective governments for protections from United States agriculture. United States agricultural policy, then, encouraged other nations to extensively regulate agriculture. Thus, supply management was a widespread national policy in the world economy.[20]

Just as importantly, the regulation of agriculture existed at the level of the world economy beyond GATT. Indeed, while GATT merely allowed—and encouraged—the national regulation of agriculture, a variety of international organizations and agreements were created to oversee extensive regulations of agriculture, in effect instituting supply management policy at the international economic level.

For example, the International Wheat Agreement (IWA) brought wheat-exporting and wheat-importing nations together to coordinate the market to ensure supply and prices. The first IWA went into effect in 1949 and was "a long-term, multilateral commodity contract, which specifies the basic maximum and minimum prices at which 'guaranteed quantities' of wheat will be offered by designated exporting countries or purchased by designated importing countries."[21] IWA-exporting countries included the United States, Canada, and Australia, which combined accounted for more than 75 percent of world wheat exports at the time. The International Wheat Council oversaw the terms of the IWA, which was renegotiated seven times over the next two decades. While not all world wheat exports went through the IWA, the agreement nonetheless offered significant stability in terms of world wheat prices and production between 1949 and 1970.[22]

Other commodities had similar institutions and agreements. The International Coffee Agreement (ICA) set export quotas and prices, overseen by the International Coffee Organization. Created in 1962, the ICA governed the international coffee market until 1989, when the agreement broke down. Like the IWA, the ICA had a significant stabilizing effect on world coffee prices, which fluctuated between $1.00 and $1.50 per pound during this period.[23] Sugar, cocoa, wool, cotton, and rubber also had international agreements and organizations that helped to stabilize prices, production, and trade.

Of course, not all agricultural commodities had international agreements regulating trade, production, and prices. The world corn market, for instance, did not have such regulation. This was in part because market stability existed without regulation since the United States dominated world corn exports and regulated corn prices and production domestically. Between 1957 and 1970, for example, the United States accounted for roughly 57 percent of world corn exports.[24] This dominance helped to stabilize the market for corn.

Did these national policies and international agreements regulating prices and production help to stabilize agriculture? Yes and no. We should first recognize that because agricultural production is so dependent on the weather, some fluctuations in production and, hence, prices are bound to occur. Some years bring good weather and large harvests, while other years see bad weather and crop shortfalls. Also, of course, prices and farm income do not necessarily vary with production; when good harvests abound, prices and income may drop. When crops fall short of expectations, prices may rise but farmers may not have the crop to take advantage of high prices. Such fluctuations in fortunes occur in agriculture with or without state intervention.

Nonetheless, national agricultural policies that rested on supply management policies used price supports to help prevent market collapses by instituting a minimum price. Furthermore, price supports generally involved buying excess commodities with the aim of eliminating oversupply and low prices. The government-held stocks could then be released during periods of unexpected crop shortfalls. Such price support programs helped to stabilize production, as well as prices, by removing excess commodities during times of surplus and adding previously purchased and stored commodities during shortages. Thus, national policies of supply management helped to smooth out the vagaries of the market on prices and of nature on production, thereby creating greater stability in agriculture.

Fluctuations in fortunes occur in agriculture with or without state intervention.

In addition, international commodity agreements had similar effects: they helped to reduce market instability by setting a minimum price, or at least a range in which prices could vary. These agreements also worked to regulate production, trade, or both. This kind of coordination helped to prevent some of the steep fluctuations in prices that we have seen recently.

During the mid-twentieth century, agriculture was regulated at both the level of national policy and world economy. These policies helped to stabilize agriculture prices and production. In the 1970s, however, deregulation began and marked a significant shift in agriculture.

Deregulating Agriculture, 1970s-Present

The United States food regime, with its extensive economic regulation, was gradually dismantled during the last quarter of the twentieth century. This process of deregulation was apparent at three levels: the breakdown of international commodity agreements, the incorporation of agriculture into GATT, and the retrenchment of national agricultural policies emphasizing supply management.

First, international agreements such as the IWA and ICA began to weaken during this period, resulting in greater instability in commodity markets. The last wheat agreement was approved in 1967 and lasted only three years. Though there were two subsequent attempts to establish another agreement in 1970 and 1971, no deals regulating prices or exports were approved.[25] The ICA lasted until 1989, when the United States withdrew from the International Coffee Organization. Disagreements between producing and consuming nations about quotas and prices were generally at the core of these collapses. After the failure of these international agreements, the markets for these commodities demonstrated much more price volatility.

Second, the Uruguay Round of GATT talks began in 1986 and included agriculture for the first time, thus starting the process of incorporating that sector in GATT's general push toward liberalization. This same round of GATT talks led to the creation of the World Trade Organization (WTO) in 1995. The WTO replaced GATT as the locus of trade rule negotiations, implementation, and dispute settlement, including agriculture. Consequently, international pressure increased on nations to reduce regulations in agriculture. This pressure was central enough to the WTO's trade policies that it led several ministerial meetings to collapse as many nations resisted liberalizing agriculture.[26]

Other international organizations, including the International Monetary Fund (IMF) and World Bank also pushed nations to liberalize their agricultural policies. The IMF and World Bank often made agricultural liberalization a condition of loans.

Third, individual nations—most notably the United States—began to weaken their policies of agriculture supply management. This tended to happen after the elements of supply management at the level of the world economy had been washed away. For example, although the IWA effectively ended in 1970, the national regulation of wheat prices and production remained (at least in the United States) until the 1990s. In this way, the end of the international commodity agreements was the first phase of liberalization in agriculture, followed later by the retrenchment of national policies of supply management.

In 1996, the United States passed the Federal Agriculture Improvement and Reform (FAIR) Act, which eliminated production controls and decoupled farm subsidies from market prices. By removing production controls, in particular, it essentially ended supply management policy after almost 60 years. While the United States eliminated production controls, it reinstituted income supports for farmers in response to the decline in prices precipitated by the passage of the FAIR Act.[27]

Not all nations, however, were in a position to continue subsidizing farmers. Some simply did not have the national budget resources to do so, while others were limited by IMF or World Bank restructuring agreements. With the creation of NAFTA, for example, Mexico agreed to end its long-standing policy protections of corn and open its market to corn from the United States. Consequently, Mexican imports of corn increased substantially, depressing prices and flooding the Mexican market.

The elimination of stabilizing policies signaled fundamental shifts in agricultural and food production, trade, and prices. The safeguards against market volatility were weakened or eliminated beginning in the 1970s. What were the effects of this deregulation? How exactly did this contribute to the food crisis?

The Consequences of Liberalization

The elimination of price supports and production controls made agriculture more vulnerable to market vagaries. First, this deregulation destabilized production and prices. Consequently, the supplies of grains and other foods that poorer countries had come to depend on between 1945 and 1975 were no longer reliable. Following the passage of the FAIR Act, between 1996 and 2005, United States corn production increased by about 20 percent. By contrast, wheat production fell slightly by about five percent. Without regulations on production, farmers could more easily shift between crops, resulting in less stable supply of various commodities.

The collapse of international agreements had similar effects on agricultural production in the Global South. When the ICA broke down in 1989, for example, coffee production shifted dramatically. Vietnam went from being a small producer of Robusta coffee (about 400,000 60-kilogram bags annually) in the mid-1980s to being the dominant producer (almost 11 million bags) by 2000. Consequently, Vietnam alone increased total world production of Robusta coffee by about 50 percent in less than ten years.[28] This dramatic shift in production would not have been possible under the stricter arrangements of the mid-twentieth-century ICA. With the collapse of the coffee agreement, however, a nation could emerge as a top coffee producer and add enough coffee to flood the market.

Second, this deregulation made markets for commodities originating from the Global South less stable. Fluctuating commodity prices, especially price collapses, can endanger the incomes of producers and raise the poverty level in developing countries. Falling incomes inevitably reduce access to food and food insecurity rises.

Returning to the example of coffee, a crisis plagued the world coffee market for about two decades. When the ICA broke down in 1989, coffee production and prices became much less stable. The ICO's composite price fell from $1.15 per pound in 1988 to $0.63 in 1993. After rising again between 1994 and 1998, the composite price fell further to $0.47 per pound in 2002. While coffee prices rose between 2003 and 2008, the peak in this was still below the average price of $1.31 for 1982–1988.[29] As the gourmet coffee market (e.g., Starbucks) took off and American consumers paid more for their daily cup of coffee, world production increased and prices to producers fell. As Daniel Jaffee notes, "The share of the purchase price kept by coffee-producing nations, then, plunged from between 30 and 33 percent to less than 8 percent in a little more than a decade."[30] Higher prices paid by American coffee drinkers have not necessarily meant higher incomes for coffee farmers around the world.

Higher prices paid by American coffee drinkers have not necessarily meant higher incomes for coffee farmers around the world.

Instability in the price of a central commodity produced in the Global South, such as coffee, has important implications for income and poverty in that part of the world.[31] These commodities are important sources of income for nations and individuals, and the prices of the commodities do not necessarily vary with prices for commodities that are imported, such as rice, wheat, or other grains. Therefore, the collapse in the price of coffee had the effect of increasing poverty in coffee-producing nations such as Brazil, Kenya, Ethiopia, India, and Vietnam. Increasing poverty contributes to the likelihood of a food crisis because food is a commodity that must be purchased. When incomes fall while the prices for basic foodstuffs rise, people lose adequate access to food. The deregulation in agriculture over the past 40 years contributed to the food crisis by undermining incomes around the world and contributing to spikes in food prices. The food crisis, then, is merely exacerbated poverty and hunger.

Conclusion

The immediate context certainly helped to create the recent food crisis. Bad weather, the diversion of crops to biofuel and livestock feed, oil prices, and financial speculation all played a role in increasing prices. But to focus on these short-term trends at the expense of understanding the secular effects of liberalization over the past 40 years is a mistake. The shift toward deregulated agriculture between 1970 and the 1990s played a fundamental role in creating the context that allowed for the recent extreme volatility seen in food prices.

From the 1940s to the 1970s, agricultural production, prices, and trade were regulated at the level of national policy and the world economy. These regulations attempted to manage the supply of various commodities, and in doing so they also worked to stabilize prices. This food system was by no means perfect, but it nonetheless helped to eliminate some of the worst excesses of the market economy, smoothing out the sharp fluctuations in prices and shifts in production. The push for deregulation beginning in the 1970s removes these stabilizing policies.

The current food crisis has revealed how precarious the underlying system has become. The food regime is increasingly susceptible to sharp changes in prices as the buffers that had been in place for decades are now either severely weakened or eliminated. This change has left many people and nations throughout the world more vulnerable to extreme market swings in prices and production. The food crisis occurred at least in part because of that vulnerability.

What does such a food crisis mean? What are the implications of being more susceptible to sharp fluctuations in prices? First, such crises affect individuals, and those most vulnerable are the poor in developing countries. A high proportion of their budget is devoted to food, and they generally have few resources to absorb sudden and sharp increases in food prices.[32] This is, at its root, a very personal side of food crises as food is a basic need that every one of us has. When food is a commodity that becomes swept up in a wave of economic crisis, it often means even tougher times for those who are already struggling.

Second, food crises bring the possibility of political and economic instability. Food riots, political shifts, economic downturns, increased debt and financial problems, and other potential troubles can accompany food crises—particularly for food-importing and developing countries. As with individuals, food crises can exacerbate the financial, economic, or political difficulties that countries may face, especially in a global context in which buffers against extreme volatility have been significantly weakened.

Nonetheless, we should remember that political decisions construct the market and build the parameters of international regimes. The long-term movement between regulation and deregulation in food regimes is an ongoing process that can be traced back to the mid-1800s, when Britain established a food regime based primarily on free trade. The ebb and flow of regulations will continue. The question now is: How can we move toward a food regime that offers more food security to people around the world?

Notes

1. Based on monthly world prices from FAOSTAT. See: Food and Agriculture Organization of the UN, *International Commodity Prices Database,* www.fao.org/es/esc/prices/PricesServlet .jsp?lang=en.
2. Food and Agriculture Organization of the UN, *FAO Food Price Index,* August 2011, www.fao.org/worldfoodsituation/ wfs-home/foodpricesindex/en/.
3. Food and Agriculture Organization of the UN, *The State of Food Insecurity in the World: Addressing Food Insecurity in Protracted Crises,* 2009.
4. Joseph Guyler Delva and Jim Loney, "Haiti's Government Falls after Food Riots," *Reuters,* April 12, 2008.
5. While the food price index was higher in early 2011 than in 2008, the prices of rice and wheat were not. Wheat and rice prices in 2011 were still notably higher than the average for 2004–2005, but they did not reach the heights of 2008. This, of course, means that other food prices are higher than in 2008 See: FAO, *Food Price Index.*
6. Others use this or a similar distinction. For example, see: Eric Holt-Gimenez and Raj Patel, *Food Rebellions! Crisis and the Hunger for Justice* (Oakland, CA: Food First Books, 2008); Walden Bello, *The Food Wars* (London: Verso Books, 2009).
7. Keith Bradsher, "A Drought in Australia, a Global Shortage of Rice," *New York Times,* April 17, 2008; "Cyclone fuels rice price increase," *BBC News,* May 7, 2008.

8. Andrew E. Kramer, "Russia, Crippled by Drought, Bans Grain Exports," *New York Times,* August 5, 2010.

9. Fred Magdoff and Brian Tokar, "Agriculture and Food in Crisis: An Overview," in *Agriculture and Food in Crisis,* edited by Fred Magdoff and Brian Tokar (New York: Monthly Review Press, 2010), 9–30, 11.

10. Walden F. Bello, *The Food Wars* (New York: Verso Books, 2009), 107.

11. Saturnino M. Borras, Jr., Philip McMichael, and Ian Scoones, "The Politics of Biofuels, Land and Agrarian Change," *Journal of Peasant Studies* 37, no. 4 (2010): 575–92.

12. From June 9 to July 24, average retail gas prices were above $4 per gallon. United States Energy Information Administration, *Weekly Retail Gasoline and Diesel Prices (Dollars per Gallon, Including Taxes),* www.eia.gov/dnav/pet/pet_pri_gnd_dcus_nus_w.htm.

13. Holt-Gimenez and Patel, *Food Rebellions,* 16.

14. Ibid.

15. Jayati Ghosh, "The Unnatural Coupling: Food and Global Finance," *Journal of Agrarian Change* 10, no. 1 (2010): 72–86.

16. Holt-Gimenez and Patel, *Food Rebellions,* 14.

17. "The 9 billion-people question," *The Economist,* February 26, 2011.

18. For food regimes, see: Harriet Friedmann, "The Political Economy of Food: A Global Crisis," *New Left Review* 197 (1993): 29–57.

19. In the United States, production controls and price supports rested on "base acreage," which restricted eligibility for subsidies and acreage allotments for particular commodities based on the farm's historical production patterns. To maintain a steady base acreage for wheat, for example, a farm generally had to continue growing wheat. This helped to ensure fairly stable production levels.

20. For a more extensive discussion of agriculture in GATT, see: Bill Winders, "The Vanishing Free Market: The Formation and Spread of the British and US Food Regimes," *Journal of Agrarian Change* 9, no. 3 (2009): 315–44.

21. Helen C. Farnsworth, "International Wheat Agreements and Problems, 1949–56," *The Quarterly Journal of Economics* 70, no. 2 (1956): 217–48.

22. C. D. Harbury, "An Experiment in Commodity Control—The International Wheat Agreement, 1949–1953," *Oxford Economic Papers* 6, no. 1 (1953): 82–97. See also: Ian McCreary, "Protecting the Food Insecure in Volatile International Markets: Food Reserves and Other Policy Options," *Canadian Foodgrains Bank Occasional Paper,* March 2009, Figure 4.

23. Daniel Jaffee, *Brewing Justice: Fair Trade Coffee, Sustainability, and Survival* (Berkeley, CA: University of California Press, 2007): 42.

24. Bill Winders, *The Politics of Food Supply: U. S. Agricultural Policy in the World Economy* (New Haven: Yale University Press, 2009), Figure 6.4, 152.

25. There have since been several wheat agreements, but they have not entailed the kind of regulations seen before 1970.

26. This was most apparent in the ministerial meeting in Cancun, Mexico, in 2003. See: Gimenez and Patel, *Food Rebellions,* 50–52.

27. For an extensive discussion of the history and politics of US agricultural policy, including the FAIR Act, see: Winders, *Politics of Food Supply.*

28. United States Department of Agriculture: Foreign Agricultural Service, *Production, Supply and Distribution Online Database,* www.fas.usda.gov/psdonline/.

29. International Coffee Organization, ICO Indicator Prices, www.ico.org/.

30. Jaffee, *Brewing Justice,* 45.

31. For example, see: Jaffee, *Brewing Justice.*

32. Food and Agriculture Organization of the UN, *The State of Food Insecurity in the World* (Rome: FAO, 2011): 13–20.

Critical Thinking

1. Differentiate between the immediate (short-term) and secular (long-term) causes of increases in global food prices.

2. Explain how unpredictable weather, oil prices, the expansion of agrofuels, the financial crisis of 2008–2009, increased meat consumption, and population growth impact global food prices.

3. Summarize the methods by which the United States controls its food supply.

BILL WINDERS is an associate professor of sociology in the School of History, Technology, and Society at the Georgia Institute of Technology. His publications include *The Politics of Food Supply: United States. Agricultural Policy in the World Economy.* He would like to thank Rick Rubinson for his comments and encouragement on this article.

Behind the Label: How Fair Are Organic and Fairtrade Bananas?

The Dominican Republic's organic and Fairtrade boom has helped banana growers, but what about the slum-dwelling Haitian migrant workers? Tom Levitt reports on the plight of the forgotten people in the banana trade.

TOM LEVITT

Like many young Dominicans, Federico left for the United States when he finished school to look for work, ending up in a Spanish store in New York. After 20 years working seven days a week he grew tired of the long hours and yearned for his homeland and the tropical climate of the Caribbean.

He had heard about the booming banana trade with the export market growing fast, a cheap and plentiful workforce, and land and water in abundance. It seemed like an ideal opportunity, with money to be made for entrepreneurs willing to set up a plantation. Today he is half way towards his dream, 35 hectares of indigenous forest have been cleared with half already planted with banana trees. The other half will be up and running later this year, together with a new building to wash and pack the harvested bananas.

Not far away Jan Luis Moneta is still waiting for his dream: a work visa. He migrated from Haiti, one of the poorest countries in the world, when he was 14 years old. After 30 years working on banana plantations he is still classed as an illegal worker. With his daily wage he cannot afford to live in anything more than a corrugated iron hut, with no water, toilet facilities or electricity.

Jan Luis is just one of many thousands of 'invisible' Haitian migrants working in the banana sector, where they make up an estimated 90 per cent of the total workforce [the government says the figure is 66 per cent]. Union activists told the *Ecologist* that 90–95 per cent of them are working in the country illegally.

Although their stories are wildly different, both Federico and Jan Luis have together helped fuel the Dominican Republic's banana boom. The country is the UK's biggest supplier in value terms, with more than half of all their bananas exported to our shores. The majority of these are Fairtrade and/or organic. Despite the economic downturn, overall Fairtrade sales in the UK grew by 12 per cent in 2011.

But by buying organic and Fairtrade bananas, are consumers in the UK helping to improve conditions for workers and the environment on the ground? And is the switch to organic and Fairtrade providing a template for other banana-producing countries to replicate?

A favourite at breakfast and in packed lunches, the banana's unrivalled popularity has seen major supermarkets such as Tesco and Asda vying to offer the best deal. Between 2002 and 2008, a price war between major supermarkets saw the price of bananas plummet by up to 41 per cent. The price cuts are almost invariably kicked off by Walmart (owner of Asda in the UK) and have continued to this day. At one point in 2009, German discounter Aldi led others down to the UK's lowest price ever, at 37p per kilo, one third the price at the beginning of the decade.

A decision by Sainsburys and Waitrose to only source Fairtrade bananas from 2007 seemed to signal a change or at least a part change. In 2012 the Co-op followed suit. These decisions have contributed to creating a £150 million Fairtrade banana market, accounting for one in every three bananas sold.

The Dominican Republic has been one the main beneficiaries of this boom. Its Fairtrade and organic banana industry has been growing rapidly over the past decade with an estimated 60 per cent of banana production certified organic and a quarter certified Fairtrade.

The principles of organic farming insist on fairness to all workers, while Fairtrade standards are meant to ensure fair payments to banana plantation owners and their workers, with the additional Fairtrade premium being spent on projects to help small producers and plantation workers.

While the health problems normally associated with banana plantations and daily contact with toxic pesticides and fungacides were not apparent in the Dominican Republic, the industry the *Ecologist* saw in the country was still one reliant on a migrant workforce paid poverty wages, living in slums and with no legal status. What's more, in an effort to tackle criticism of its treatment of illegal workers, the Dominican Republic government is now planning to force many of these migrants underpinning the banana industry to leave the country.

The Organic and Fairtrade Boom

The seeds of an organic, and latterly, Fairtrade industry in the Dominican Republic were sown in the 1980s when private foundations from Germany encouraged organic cocoa production. Producers later switched to bananas. Growing consumer demand, together with technical support from multinational marketing companies, helped the banana sector grow considerably from the 1990s onwards.

The organic farms we visited had managed to replace often dangerous chemicals used to protect banana trees with a natural pesticide, a mixture of garlic and rotting vegetables. But the prevalence of black sigatoka (or 'leaf streak'), the fungal disease that wreaks havoc in banana growing countries across the world, is becoming a major problem, with farms regularly reporting losses of up to 30 per cent of their crop. The disease attacks the tree and can cut fruit production by half.

A particularly devastating outbreak in late 2011 wiped out an estimated 40 per cent of production in the main banana growing region. For smaller producers in particular, the growing prevalence of diseases like black sigatoka make it a struggle to meet the low and non-chemical requirement in Fairtrade and organic standards. Larger conventional and organic farms in the country can afford to operate aerial spraying every 20 to 30 days to protect their crops.

Federico runs an organic plantation in the north-west of the Dominican Republic in the province of Monte Cristi. Like many organic farms he hopes to get Fairtrade certification soon too. Along with the neighbouring province of Valverde, this is the heart of the banana-growing industry in the country. One government official we spoke to estimated 90 per cent of employment here is related to bananas.

On his farm, Federico is proud of his chemical-free plantation, even as it expands onto more former forested land. The irony is that forested land can be converted straight into organic production whereas former conventional agricultural land would have to go through a two-year conversion period to remove traces of chemicals in the soils.

He uses a mixture of roots and chicken manure to fertilise the plants, which means he loses out on the unnaturally large bananas of conventional farms. 'My smaller bananas are much healthier and stronger', says Federico. Like all other plantations, every bunch of bananas is protected by a plastic bag, although in his case dipped in a mixture of hot pepper, garlic and soap rather than chemicals.

The use of plastic bags in particular is one of the most wasteful parts of banana production. On both conventional and organic farms, they are used to protect the bananas from over-exposure to the sun and thrown out after three months. Disposal of the bags is badly regulated and local roads and rivers throughout the banana growing regions are strewn with plastic waste, white bags from organic plantations and blue chemical coated bags from the conventional ones.

Ironically, if it wasn't for the colour coded plastic bags covering the bunches of bananas, it would be impossible to spot the difference between the organic and conventional farms. They often lie just metres apart (sometimes even on the same farm) and look identical in terms of layout, stretching for tens of acres with no attempt at mixed cropping or diversity to encourage natural wildlife. The monoculture landscape is little different to the oil palm plantations of south-east Asia which have devastated the once biodiversity-rich tropical rainforests of countries like Malaysia and Indonesia.

'This region has lost its biodiversity,' says Fasto Pena, director of Naturaleza, a local environmental group. 'It's equally bad on organic and conventional farms. Plantation owners need to look after the natural environment better so it is still there for us in the future.'

The Forgotten Banana Workers

There is also a less visible side to banana production. As with the majority of banana growing countries, a key component of the growth in the Dominican Republic has been a cheap migrant workforce. When the Haiti earthquake struck in 2010, thousands fled across the border, ending up in the north-west banana-growing states. However, the supply of migrant workers has actually been constant for the past 20 to 30 years. But a better life is unlikely to be found on a banana plantation.

Lying hidden off a main road, around 1,000 Haitian migrants live crowded together in a community of corrugated iron shacks. Most of them are young and male, some have families but no-one has water, toilets or electricity. Some of them have jobs. Some don't. Of the ones that do, nearly all work on banana plantations, including some for a well-known organic plantation.

Most of the workers get 250 to 300 pesos a day when they work (about £4). 'It is barely enough to eat,' a group of young men tell us. 'It allows us one meal a day of beans and rice but is not enough to rent a house or look after a family.'

Nearby, off a main road near the town of Mao in Valverde, in another community of mainly wooden huts, live around 130 Haitian migrants. One of them, a 34-year-old Haitian Sabin James, told us he works on an organic plantation and after 15 years in the country is still trying to get legal status. Even though he gets paid 300 pesos, Sabin can't afford to buy a US$225 (8,800 pesos) passport that would give him access to social security. His company offers help to apply for one but won't help him pay for it. 'They say they are helping us but they know it's no help at all,' says Sabin.

'The companies don't want to know about workers or bother themselves with how much they earn, where they live or what they eat,' says Padre Regino Martinez, co-founder of Asomilin.

His organisation has been helping migrants get passports at a reduced cost of US$140 and overcoming their fears of being deported if they try and apply.

Padre says Dominican workers don't get paid more but were given fixed contracts and the opportunity for promotion to higher paid positions, which Haitians never occupied, leaving them trapped in poverty.

'They don't have enough to cover the costs of living. And have no way of getting a higher salary to rent a home or buy a visa or passport. No power to negotiate with plantation owners. There are plenty of workers who need a job, so they are all too scared to stand up to employers,' says Padre.

Another migrant, Emmantel Audige, was one of a number of workers we met living near the Haitian border and is employed on a Fairtrade certified banana plantation. He told us that he and other migrants had signed a contract for eight hours a day but actually worked six am to five pm without rest or overtime and for wages of no more than the average 250 pesos reported by non-Fairtrade workers. He said he had been in the country for 11 years but was still an illegal worker, with no rights to social security. All migrants can use state hospitals but we were told care was very poor, with long waiting times.

According to the Fairtrade Foundation the premium consumers pay for Fairtrade bananas has been used to help migrants get passports and working visas, however, Emmantel says he has no idea what the premium gets spent on. He and other migrants would like to have access to a healthcare centre to deal with work injuries and for use by their families. After one year workers should also get 14 days paid holiday but Emmantel says he gets none.

Even migrants like Jean Baptiste who has been working in the country in the banana sector for over 30 years—currently six days a week for an organic and Fairtrade certified plantation—are still forced to live in the community of wooden huts with no electricity, water or toilet facilities. Jan gets 280 pesos a day but says a fair wage would be 500 pesos (£8), something that would allow him to continue to live comfortably in the wooden huts with fellow migrants, but not enough to rent a home with water and electricity.

Back on his organic farm, Federico, who hopes to be certified Fairtrade, admits that some of his workers are illegal migrants with no work permits. He uses around 40 workers on day-to-day contracts, although he is not sure about where they live or their living conditions. He says his farm does not have enough money yet to help workers get visas or passports.

The Fairtrade Foundation in the UK acknowledges that migrant workers in Dominican Republic's banana industry need help in getting better housing, access to healthcare and legal status. It says many of the small-scale producers are often disadvantaged themselves and it takes time for them to assume more responsibility for the living conditions of migrant workers.

Trade union groups in the Dominican Republic say Fairtrade standards do not do enough to help migrant workers. 'There is no doubt that they are improving international trade but it isn't helping migrant workers to earn a fair salary,' says Luciano Robles, from the Trade Union Autonomous Federation (CASC). 'International standards need to be adapted to local situations.'

Supermarket Price Wars

The Fairtrade Foundation says calls for using the Fairtrade premium to subsidise migrant workers' wages may undermine the responsibility of farm owners and employers to tackle the 'living wage' issue. It points the blame, in part, at the continual use of bananas in price wars between supermarkets, saying it has devalued the fruit in the eyes of the consumer and left producers with low returns, even in the Fairtrade sector, which has to remain competitive against conventional alternatives. Although the minimum price for Fairtrade bananas has risen slightly in the past two years, the price wars make it harder than ever to improve the conditions of slum-dwelling Haitian migrants.

Campaigners are hoping the new supermarket watchdog, the Groceries Code Adjudicator, will help stop supermarkets pressurising their suppliers. 'Supermarkets are the most powerful actors along supply chains and make vast profits however the unsustainably low prices they pay to suppliers can leave the workers who plant, harvest and pack our food in poverty,' says Banana Link campaigner Anna Cooper.

While campaigners fight for a better standard of living for banana workers, there are fears many of the illegal Haitian migrants could soon be expelled. Tough new rules, which union groups say are politically motivated, state that at least 80 per cent of a firm's employees must be Dominican—a figure at odds with the reality of the migrant-dominated banana industry. Government officials told the *Ecologist* this was to 'regularise' the workforce and ensure Haitians were legal citizens in the country. But it puts the plight of thousands of other illegal migrants in peril.

'Until now the Dominican Republic government has allowed the existence of illegal Haitian workers, knowing the extreme difficulties they face in their own country and which can be partly solved by work here,' says Marike de Pena, from Banelino, a well-known Fairtrade producer group that sells bananas to many UK supermarkets.

She admits some of their small-scale producers may be using illegal workers but says the group wants more Haitian migrants to be able to stay in the country and get better wages and legal status. To that end, the Fairtrade Foundation, together with banana producers, have been lobbying the government to resolve the issue.

For now though, the difficulties for many migrants persist. 'The network of migration, exploitation and violation of rights is mutually beneficial for Haiti and Dominican Republic. There is even money to be made on the border from trafficking people. The institutions issuing visas, the Dominican economy and the banana industry getting cheap labour. Everyone benefits,' union organiser Luciano Robles told the *Ecologist*.

Critical Thinking

1. Describe the working conditions of organic and Fairtrade banana plantations in the Dominican Republic.

2. Evaluate the effectiveness of the price premium on production of fair trade agriculture.

3. Summarize how price competition from large retail stores impacts the laborers on plantations where organic and Fairtrade agriculture is grown.

Rising Prices on the Menu

Higher Food Prices May Be Here to Stay

THOMAS HELBLING AND SHAUN ROACHE

Around the world, poor weather has reduced harvests and driven up food prices, fueling inflation risks and hitting the most vulnerable. Floods in Australia, Pakistan, and parts of India have helped push up the cost of food, as have droughts in China, Argentina, and Eastern Europe. Energy prices are again on the rise, with likely knock-on effects for food.

Many countries—especially developing and emerging economies—are struggling with the implications of high food prices, given their effects on poverty, inflation, and, for importing countries, the balance of payments. Higher food prices may also have contributed to social unrest in the Middle East and North Africa.

International food prices were broadly stable through the first half of 2010, but they surged in the second half of 2010, and have continued rising in 2011. The IMF's food price index (see box) is now close to the previous spike in June 2008.

The increase in food prices is, of course, bad news for all consumers. But the poor—as well as consumers in developing and emerging economies in general—are hit harder by higher food costs because food represents a much larger share of their overall spending (IMF, 2011). At the same time, rapidly rising food prices pose important macroeconomic policy challenges for decision makers in emerging and developing economies.

International Food Markets

Food, more than perhaps any other product, is laden with both symbolic and practical value. Concerns about food security, sufficient domestic production, and relative incomes in agriculture mean that food is not traded as readily as manufactured goods, because of protectionist agricultural policies. Despite these trade barriers, some major food items—especially major grains and oilseeds—are traded internationally. In this article we focus on the international prices of such products. Much food is not traded, so international food prices are only one determinant of domestic food inflation.

The world grew accustomed to relatively low international food prices in the 1980s and the 1990s, when prices adjusted for inflation were below those recorded during the Great Depression. But since the turn of the century, food prices have been rising steadily—except for declines during the global financial crisis in late 2008 and early 2009—and this suggests that these increases are a trend and don't just reflect temporary factors.

Expensive Tastes

Perhaps the most important explanation for the trend increase in food prices is that consumers in emerging and developing economies are becoming richer and changing their diet as a result. In particular, consumers in these economies are eating more high-protein foods such as meat, dairy products, edible oils, fruits and vegetables, and seafood. These products are more "income elastic" than staple grains. In other words, as people get richer, they demand more of these high-protein foods, whereas their consumption of grains may grow more slowly or even decline.

This increases the demand for scarce agricultural resources—for example, more land might be devoted to cattle grazing instead of crop planting, while more crops are used for animal feed. Reflecting these changes, emerging and developing economies have accounted for about three-quarters of the total growth in global demand for major crops since the early 2000s.

Food and Fuel

Another influence on the markets for food products over the past decade has been the boom in biofuels. High oil prices and policy support have boosted demand for biofuels, which are used as supplements in transportation fuels, particularly in the advanced economies and also in some emerging economies, including Brazil. This demand, in turn, has buoyed the demand for feedstock crops. In 2010, for example, the production of corn-based ethanol absorbed some 15 percent of the global corn crop. Other crops whose demand is correlated with that of biofuels are cane sugar, palm kernels, and rapeseed.

In addition to these indirect effects, high oil prices also have a direct effect on the cost of producing food because fuel—including natural gas—is used to produce inputs, such as fertilizers. Fuel is also used in all stages of the agricultural production cycle—from sowing to harvesting to distribution. Food prices are partly dependent on oil prices, and biofuels have likely strengthened this link.

Tracking Food

The IMF food price index tracks the spot prices of the 22 most commonly internationally traded agricultural food items.

These include major grains—wheat, rice, and corn; oil seeds—soybeans; edible oils—palm oil; basic meats—beef carcasses; some basic seafood items—fish meal; some tropical fruits—bananas; and sugar.

The index was created to facilitate assessment of food market developments and prospects for the IMF's *World Economic Outlook*. The commodities it follows are those with the largest shares in international trade, and those shares determine the weight of each commodity in the index. These items generally have an international reference price—for example, the price of U.S. corn exports at Gulf of Mexico ports.

Yielding Crops

With the structural increases in the demand for many crops and other foods, prices can only remain stable over the medium term if there is a matching structural increase in supply. In other words, average prices have to increase to provide the incentives for increased supply. While farmers have responded to the opportunities from rising demand, their response has only been gradual. The interplay between productivity and acreage growth is key to understanding the supply response. Traditionally, rapid productivity growth in agriculture helped drive down food prices. But over the past decade, global productivity growth—as measured by the amount of crop produced per hectare—has fallen for rice and wheat compared with the 1980s and 1990s and has been broadly stagnant for corn and soybeans. Less productivity growth means higher prices, everything else being equal.

With lower yield growth, production increases have had to be achieved by using more land. But increasing the amount of land devoted to producing more of a crop comes at a cost, which is reflected in higher prices. The higher cost is due to two main factors.

First, crops compete for land. Since there are geographical limits to where crops can be produced, higher acreage for one crop often means lower acreage for another. Farmers decide what to plant depending on crops' relative prices. Second, because demand for many crops has been rising at the same time, overall acreage also had to increase. To encourage farmers to plant and harvest more acreage, particularly on marginal land that is less productive, crop prices need to rise.

From a longer-term perspective, the recent decline in yield growth is worrying. It means that continued growth in demand for food will require further increases in acreage. But some of the additional land will be less productive than that now being used, whether due to lack of irrigation in arid areas, poor infrastructure, or simply lower soil fertility. In areas with rapid urbanization, fertile land is being used for purposes other than agriculture. And soil degradation and climate change have hampered yield growth.

Low yield growth and limited land availability amid rapid demand growth in an economy can lead to shifts in international trade patterns. In China, for example, rising demand for animal feed has turned that country into a net importer of corn and soybeans. Because international food markets are still relatively shallow—that is, only a small share of global production is exported, as most production is consumed locally—such developments can have large effects on world prices.

Weathering Production Cuts

The ongoing structural change in international food markets is clearly one factor behind the trend increase in food prices. But trends usually don't result in abrupt price movements. To really understand recent price surges, we have to look at other factors. Indeed, the catalyst of the food price surge since mid-2010 has been a series of weather-related supply shocks. The sequence of events is well known by now.

First, drought and wildfires caused a decline in wheat production in Russia, Ukraine, and Kazakhstan. As a result, the global wheat harvest for the current crop year is now estimated to have declined by over 5 percent. Then, a hot and wet summer led to a lower-than-expected corn harvest in the United States. Finally, starting in fall 2010, one of the strongest La Niña weather episodes in the past 50 years began to hit harvests—including rice—in Asia. The damage to harvests in Asia not only caused rises in the price of international food commodities but also affected local food markets, notably through the negative impact on local fruit and vegetable production.

The global price response to a supply shortfall depends not only on the size of the shortfall but also on other factors. One amplifying factor was the imposition of grain export restrictions in Russia and Ukraine. This helps to keep domestic prices low and stable but leads to higher world prices. A pattern of protectionist trade policy responses to supply shocks have also been observed during past price surges for food commodities, including in the 1973–74 and the 2006–08 booms (see Martin and Anderson, 2011).

Stocking Up

Food prices are also affected by the level of stocks. Many of the major food commodities—as opposed to perishable food—are storable and, when there are harvest shortfalls, stocks can add to supply. The lower stocks are relative to consumption—the so-called stock-use ratio—the more reluctant inventory holders will be to release parts of their stocks at any given price, assuming they are maintaining them partly to protect against future shortages. So the effect of supply shocks on prices goes up as stock-use ratios fall.

Low stock-use ratios have amplified the effects on prices of recent supply disappointments and have contributed to an uptick in food price volatility. Stock levels relative to consumption decreased substantially over the past decade. At the previous food price peak in 2008, they had reached a low comparable to that recorded during the 1973–74 commodity and food price boom. Favorable harvest outcomes in the second half of 2008 and early 2009 allowed for only minor rebuilding of stocks. So when supply shocks started to hit in mid-2010, food markets were still vulnerable.

The effects of supply shocks tend to be short lived. Crop production usually returns to trend quickly as weather normalizes. Indeed, periods with production shortfalls and large price spikes are usually bracketed by long periods of relative price stability (Deaton and Laroque, 1992, among others, have emphasized this pattern). In the absence of further weather disturbances, the recent food price surge can be expected to ease when the new Northern Hemisphere crop season begins later this year. But the upward trend in prices is unlikely to reverse soon because the supply adjustment to the structural increases in demand for major food commodities will take time.

Impact

The surge in international food prices has already caused higher domestic food inflation and headline consumer price inflation as of early 2011 in many economies. Such direct effects are referred to as "first-round," and are part of the normal pass-through of prices. As in 2007–08, these effects have been greater in emerging and developing economies, where the share of food items in the consumer basket is higher than in advanced economies (IMF, 2008).

Just as poorer countries and households spend a higher proportion of their budget on food, so too the actual cost of food makes up a larger proportion of the cost of food products in poor countries than in rich countries, where the cost of labor, transportation, marketing, and packaging add value that are not in the form of calories.

But if international food prices stabilize, the first-round effects fade unless underlying, or core, inflation is affected. Economists call these indirect or "second-round" effects and they occur if the food price increases affected expectations of future inflation. If people expect food to continue to go up in price, they begin to demand higher wages, leading to increased core inflation.

The experience of the past two decades has been that risks of a pass-through from rising food prices to core inflation are low for advanced economies, but are significant for emerging and developing economies.

The main reasons for this difference are twofold (IMF, 2008). First, with the much larger expenditure shares for food and larger cost shares of raw food in the latter group of countries, food price spikes are more likely to unhinge inflation expectations and trigger increases in wage demands. Second, monetary policy credibility in emerging and developing economies remains lower despite recent improvements, implying that economic actors will be less confident in a strong central bank response to emerging inflation pressures and will thus be more likely to adjust their medium-term inflation expectations.

The IMF has traditionally advised countries to accommodate the first-round, direct effects of rising commodity prices on inflation, but to be prepared to tighten monetary policy to avoid second-round effects. At the same time, such policies have to be complemented by measures that strengthen social safety nets and protect the poor from the ravages of rising grocery bills.

Higher Food Prices—Here to Stay?

The world may need to get used to higher food prices. A large part of the recent surge is related to temporary factors, such as the weather. Nevertheless, the main reasons for rising demand for food reflect structural changes in the global economy that will not be reversed.

Over time, supply growth can be expected to respond to higher prices, as it has in previous decades, easing pressures on food markets, but this will take time counted in years rather than months. There is also the prospect that the world may face increasing scarcity in inputs important for food production, including land, water, and energy. Technology and higher yield growth could compensate for such scarcity.

In the meantime, policymakers—particularly in emerging and developing economies—will likely have to continue confronting the challenges posed by food prices that are both higher and more volatile than the world has been used to.

References

Deaton, Angus, and Guy Laroque, 1992, *"On the Behavior of Commodity Prices," Review of Economic Studies,* vol. 59, no. 1, pp. 1–23.

Grilli, Enzo, and Maw Cheng Yang, 1988, *"Primary Commodity Prices, Manufactured Goods Prices, and the Terms of Trade of Developing Countries: What the Long Run Shows," The World Bank Economic Review,* vol. 2, no. 1, pp. 1–47.

International Monetary Fund, 2008, *World Economic Outlook,* Chapter 3, *"Is Inflation Back? Commodity Prices and Inflation"* (Washington, October).

_____, 2011, *World Economic Outlook* (Washington, April).

Martin, Will, and Kym Anderson, 2011, *"Export Restrictions and Price Insulation During Commodity Price Booms"* Revised version of a paper presented at the World Bank-UC Berkeley Conference on Agriculture for Development—Revisited, Berkeley, October 1–2, 2010.

Pfaffenzeller, Stephan, Paul Newbold, and Anthony Rayner, 2007, *"A Short Note on Updating the Grilli and Yang Commodity Price Index," The World Bank Economic Review,* vol. 21, no. 1, pp. 151–63.

Critical Thinking

1. List the factors that impact the price of the global food supply.

2. How has the economic growth in emerging and developing countries impacted the price and supply of food?

3. Explain why growing crops for biofuels impacts the supply and price of food crops.

THOMAS HELBLING is an Advisor and **SHAUN ROACHE** is an Economist, both in the IMF's Research Department.

Tackling Undernutrition the Right Way

GARY R. GLEASON, PhD

While many problems facing nutritionists in the United States today involve overnutrition, undernutrition affects more than 360 million undernourished children in more than 36 of the world's poorer countries. Undernutrition contributes to more than 3.5 million related child deaths each year.[1] Despite this tragic situation, improving nutrition is often neglected and given low priority among national development policies. Nutrition is rarely listed as one of the key elements of international assistance.

Neglect of nutrition may change if a recent major international effort by a broad coalition of the United Nations (UN) and multilateral organizations, bilateral agencies, civil society organizations, and developing country partners takes hold. The coalition is growing and strengthens a movement aimed at placing undernutrition toward a central position in international assistance and national planning in poorer countries. The main product of this broad and growing coalition is a powerful global "Policy Brief, Scaling Up Nutrition: A Framework for Action" released in March 2010 and posted on the World Bank Web site and published in the Food and Nutrition Bulletin.[2] The document was written by a team of experts targeting political and opinion leaders rather than nutrition specialists. It is being broadly disseminated and promoted by many large international donors, UN, and organizations in the international nutrition community. The policy brief is in the hands of leaders of the G8 group of countries including Canada, France, Germany, Italy, Japan, Russia, the United Kingdom, and the United States.

The policy brief on scaling up nutrition reflects a broad international consensus that a multisectoral approach with adoption and scale-up of high-impact nutrition interventions are needed to make UN's Millennium Development Goals a reality (see Box 1). Clear justification for moving nutrition into the central core of international assistance and national development strategies of sectors responsible for food security and agriculture, health, and social protection sectors has been well documented in the more detailed preliminary drafts of the policy brief (personal correspondence with Meera Shekar, lead health and nutrition specialist, Human Development Network, World Bank, November 2009) that draws substantially from a major position paper of the World Bank with the bold title "Repositioning Nutrition as Central to Development."[3]

The first of the 8 Millennium Development Goals calls for elimination of extreme poverty and hunger by 2015 (see Box 1). Despite global and national commitments to this goal, nutrition has been a neglected policy area in many of the poorer developing countries and also in the context of international aid. Management of malnutrition in children is clearly the responsibility of the health sectors in these countries, but the broader areas of nutritional improvement and the prevention of malnutrition usually lack a clear organizational home in governments structures. This is because multiple interventions are required to improve nutrition, and these are often spread across the responsibilities of several different sectors such as agriculture, education, social protection, health, light industry, and, in many cases, trade. Even within the UN organizations, the various factors that contribute to adequate nutrition for children are spread across the mandates of several agencies. Thus, the multisector policies needed to prevent undernutrition lack clear ownership, the necessary legislation to implement them, and coordination to make the programs realities.

In 2004, economists working with the Copenhagen Consensus Center, a world-renowned development aid think tank, concluded that poverty would not be easily addressed without concurrent interventions targeting malnutrition among the poor.[4] They also found that nutrition interventions such as vitamin and mineral supplementation, food fortification, and breast-feeding promotion were among the most cost-effective in terms of development assistance. The World Bank report noted above as calling for moving nutrition toward the center of international and national development agendas was complemented in 2008, by a special series in the *Lancet,* with 5 substantial papers focused on maternal and child nutrition. The *Lancet* series provided evidence supporting a set of potentially high-impact interventions that would improve child nutrition because of their effectiveness in improving health and development[5] and also showed their potential to improve nutrition to an extent where there would be positive impact on national economies.[6] These interventions mainly target pregnant women and young children and aim to ensure normal growth and development during fetal development and from birth to 24 months of age (see Box 2).

Box 1
Millennium Development Goals

The Millennium Development Goals are 8 international development goals set in 2001 that all 192 UN member states and at least 23 international organizations have agreed to achieve by the year 2015

1. Eradicate extreme poverty and hunger
2. Achieve universal primary education
3. Promote gender equality and empower women
4. Reduce child mortality
5. Improve maternal health
6. Combat HIV/AIDS, malaria, and other diseases
7. Ensure environmental sustainability
8. Develop a global partnership for development

Box 2
Major Intervention Areas and Key Interventions for Scale-up to Act Against Malnutrition

1. Prepregnancy and maternal nutrition
   a. Adequate maternal nutrition and prevention of low birth weight
      i. Maternal protein/calorie supplementation
      ii. Iron-folate supplementation
      iii. Multiple micronutrient supplements
      iv. Iodized salt and oil
      v. Food fortification; biofortification
   b. Prevention and management of infection
      i. Deworming during pregnancy
      ii. Use of insecticide-treated bed nets and intermittent preventive treatment of malaria
2. The infant and young child nutrition
   a. Adequate infant nutrition
      i. Promotion and protection of breast-feeding
      ii. Promotion of appropriate and safe complementary foods
3. Micronutrient investments
   a. Supplementation
      i. Vitamin A supplementation
      ii. Iron supplementation
      iii. Therapeutic zinc supplements
      iv. Multiple supplements for children
   b. Fortification
      i. Salt fortified with iodine
      ii. Fortification of different vehicles with multiple micronutrients (wheat flour, cooking oils, rice condiments)
4. Management and prevention of severe acute malnutrition
   a. Prevention of acute undernutrition in emergency situations
   b. Prevention of acute undernutrition in nonemergency situations
      i. Facility-based treatment of severe acute undernutrition
      ii. Community-based management of severe acute undernutrition
5. Prevention and management of infection
   a. Hygiene measures and hand washing
   b. Deworming
   c. Use of insecticide-treated bed nets

The harm, both acute and permanent to health and cognitive development from undernutrition during this critical "human development window" of −9 to 24 months continues well beyond those ages and has substantial adverse impacts across the full life cycle. This overall impact of poor nutrition during pregnancy and early childhood includes lost productivity, a massive burden on educational systems, and excess costs in the health services that will be needed to deal with the effects many years later.

On an organizational note, the *Lancet* series also concluded that the field of nutrition was fraught with problems, including a breakdown in international guidance, low organizational priorities, and lack of leadership.[7]

International agencies and other donors often provide assistance for a limited range and type of interventions, such as food fortification, improved crops, micronutrient supplements (food aid, etc), without requiring linkage to alternative or complementary interventions. They need to move nutrition toward a more central and integrated position on their development assistance agendas.

On the positive side, a number of potent new nutrition interventions have been developed during the past decade. For example, small, inexpensive packets of encapsulated micronutrients, often called "sprinkles" (see Sprinkles Global Health Initiative at www.sghi.org), can be safely and effectively added to all home-prepared complementary foods for young children. This type of product is an effective alternative to both commercially fortified complementary foods and to micronutrient supplement syrups. Another example is "Ready-to-Use Therapeutic Foods" (see www.fantaproject.org/downloads/pdfs/D3.S8Jarrett.pdf), which provide a specific dose of key nutrients in highly convenient packages that are easy to keep clean and can be squeezed directly into a young child's mouth. Ready-to-Use Therapeutic Food greatly curtails the need for hospital-based care for children with severe acute malnutrition and allows many to be managed by their families in their homes.

Multi-intervention, community-based nutrition programs are vital with multisectoral participation and coordination with community participation and ownership as key elements. Their number and quality are growing in several developing countries and that some international assistance agencies are helping to move such programs toward effective reality.

Positive signs of greater national commitment to eliminate malnutrition among young children are also evident in acceleration of efforts in some countries to complete national nutrition policies and work out cross-sector coordinating procedures. Rwanda, for example, launched a national "Emergency Plan to Eliminate Malnutrition" in May 2009. More than 1.4 million young children were screened in their villages and neighborhoods, and more than 84 000 were treated for moderate or severe acute malnutrition. The country held its first National Nutrition Summit in November 2009 and called for developing District Malnutrition Elimination Plans across the country that target children younger than 5 years. These plans are likely to be cross-sector strategies that involve collaboration among district officials in local government, health, agriculture, social protection, education, and a number of nongovernmental, private, and voluntary aid organizations. To be effective such plans will need to focus on both treatment and prevention of childhood undernutrition and the interventions will need to involve organizing communities to improve both food security at the household level and the nutrition security of children.

Community-organized growth monitoring systems can provide an early warning system on nutrition problems for families with children. Families in which acute malnourishment is found will need to be better linked into social safety net programs such as free health insurance, income generating activities, and household gardens and livestock.

Other counties including Namibia, Kenya, Malawi, Swaziland, and Zimbabwe have recently completed various stages in producing national nutrition policies, strategies, and plans of action. Some have phases that cover several years and include sections as diverse as micronutrient nutrition, land reform, and emergency nutrition in the case of natural disasters and civil disturbances. All of the newer nutrition policies in African countries include a substantial section on Nutrition and HIV/AIDS.

The "Food, Fuel and Finance" crisis that had such a great adverse effect on nutrition in 2008 was a wake-up call to nutrition planners in many countries.[8] It made them realize the need for much stronger linkage between agricultural policies, food security programs, and nutrition improvement. Efforts are now under way to link nutrition improvement more directly with the rapidly accelerating and well-resourced programs to improve agricultural productivity of small African farmers. The best plans also tackle household food security with interventions to better ensure nutrition security of the women and young children in farm families and in rapidly growing town and urban populations.

The new policy brief on Scaling Up Nutrition is a solid, evidence-based resource from which to advocate for greater and more focused international and national investments in nutrition interventions that protect the growth and development of young children. Critical information on costs is drawn from economic analysis of implementing the interventions. In late 2009, a World Bank meeting centered around discussions of "Scaling Up Nutrition: What Will It Take."[8] A detailed analysis of the costs and benefits of scaling up key interventions needed to eliminate undernutrition among young children estimated US $10.3 billion would be needed annually from international and national sources. A positive rate of return should result from lower needs of heath care, lower level of chronic disease during adulthood, and improved productivity across the life cycle.

Multiple interventions across multiple governmental sectors are needed.

Despite the progress on nutrition policy development, greater emphasis on multiple intervention packages, and cross-sectoral and community nutrition programs is needed in a number of African countries, powerful advocacy to catalyze major new international action and national commitments at the needed levels.

Scaling Up Nutrition provides an action framework supporting greater investment in scale-up of proven investments that can eliminate undernutrition in young children. The impact of effective scale-up goes beyond ameliorating the impact of undernutrition on individual lives to include national social and economic development and greater likelihood of achieving the Millennium Development Goals. Economic modeling has generated models that clearly demonstrate the national costs and benefits of young child nutrition.

There is a political window of opportunity for nutrition programs if they can attract key decision makers in governments.

These factors point to a powerful "political window of opportunity" for success with nutrition program advocacy that targets national leaders and heads of major donor organizations. Advocacy efforts for an increased focus and resources for nutrition of young children and pregnant women are bolstered by linkage of child nutrition to human rights. Thus, there is much promise for generating greater investment in effective interventions and promoting the capacity building needed to support their effective scale-up.

Advocacy at the level of senior political and opinion leaders requires targeting of experts as well. National experts and researchers must agree on the technical side and also come together to support cross-sectoral collaboration, community participation, and involvement of the private sector and civil society.

Box 3
Scale-Up Challenges for Nutrition Interventions

Despite growing acceptance of the high potential impact of key interventions affecting maternal and child nutrition, there are many challenges to their promotion, introduction, and, particularly, to their effective and sustainable scale-up to national levels. Constraints to sustainable, national scale-up success are common even with what seem to be simple and inexpensive child nutrition interventions. For example:

- Exclusive breast-feeding promotion can be constrained by private sector promotion of breast milk substitutes, by unsupportive peer pressure, work environment circumstances, or limited support from medical professionals.
- Micronutrient supplementation interventions, ranging from periodic vitamin A supplementation, to use of "packets" for in-home fortification of common complementary foods, can be constrained by logistics, commodity costs, regulations, health worker training, marketing, community awareness, and concern about potential adverse effects.
- Lack of donor-supplied commodities and "invisible symptoms" contribute to why few sub-Saharan African countries implement effective anemia prevention and control programs at national scale despite international guidelines.
- Decades of successful implementation in North America, powerful international advocacy, and availability of technical and funding support have brought salt iodization to universal production or access levels in many countries where iodine deficiency disease remains prevalent. However, major populations are still missed. In China, for example, despite major international and national investments and achieving universal salt iodization levels, more than 130 million Chinese citizens remain without access to iodized salt.
- Deworming, treated bed nets, hand washing, and other straightforward infection control interventions are synergistic with child nutrition but large-scale implementation and sustainability face many constraints.
- Community nutrition programs incorporating growth monitoring and other nutrition interventions, community ownership, and participation are known to be effective in principle and on a large sale in some countries. When taken beyond well supported effective pilot efforts, most comprehensive community nutrition strategies models prove difficult to scale up in broader settings.
- New experiences in operational linking and community nutrition activities with poverty alleviation programs, social safety nets, and cross-sector district and community level planning processes are expanding but lack ongoing documentation or active sharing of lessons learned.

Intervention challenges occur, and they should be expected (see Box 3). Many of the needed and potentially effective nutrition interventions programs aim toward the most disadvantaged populations and often seek change in deeply embedded social norms and behavioral practices. Some require significant levels of community or individual involvement and/or time or cash expenditures. Others interventions compete with major private sector interests and may involve substantial commodity costs borne by consumers, product manufacturers, governments, and/or donors.

Many nutrition interventions are also affected by relationships between household food security and income. Nutrition and the nutrition security of young children and women may differ significantly among households, within communities, and among different regional and cultural groups. All of these factors add to the problems of advocacy. They also increase the complexity of improving and expanding interventions known to improve maternal and child nutrition. In many cases, introduction of nutrition interventions that are well accepted in one region is stymied for long periods or progresses slowly in other regions.

Despite these constraints and challenges, "Scaling Up Nutrition: A Framework for Action," holds great promise and offers a new level of support for advocacy toward greater political commitment and larger investment in the interventions known to be effective in protecting and improving nutrition during pregnancy and early childhood. If these commitments and investments are coupled and linked to guidelines, obtain adequate technical support, and include the capacity building needed, there is reason to predict that the prevalence of undernutrition in young children in poorer countries will be greatly reduced in the decade ahead.

References

1. Black RE, Allen, LH, Bhutta ZA, et al. Maternal and child undernutrition: global and regional exposures and health consequences. *Lancet.* 2008;371(80):243–260. www.who.int/nutrition/topics/Lancetseries_Undernutritionl.pdf.
2. Policy brief: scaling up nutrition: a framework for action *Food Nutr Bull.* 2010;31(1):178–186.
3. Shekar M, Heaver R, Lee YK. *Repositioning Nutrition as Central to Development.* Washington, DC: International Bank for Reconstruction and Development/The World Bank; 2006. http://siteresources.worldbank.org/NUTRITION/Resources/281846-1131636806329/NutritionStrategy.pdf. Accessed January 14, 2010.
4. Behrman JR, Alderman H, Hoddinott J. *Challenges and Opportunities: Hunger and Malnutrition.* Copenhagen, Denmark: Copenhagen Consensus Center; 2004.
5. Bhutta ZA, Ahmed T, Black RE, et al. What works? Interventions for maternal and child undernutrition and survival, www.thelancet.com/journals/lancet/article/PIIS0140-6736(07)61693-6/fulltext. Accessed January 14, 2010.
6. Horton R. Maternal and child undernutrition. *Lancet.* 2008;371(special):9608. www.who.int/nutrition/topics/lancetseries_maternal_and_childundernutrition/en/index.html. Accessed January 14, 2010.
7. Morris SS, Cogill B, Uauy R. Effective international action against undernutrition: why has it proven so difficult and what can be done to accelerate progress. *Lancet.* 2008; 371(special):9612.
8. Horton S, Shekar M, McDonald C, Mahal A, Brooks JK. *Scaling Up Nutrition: What Will It Cost.* Washington, DC: World Bank; 2009. Report of International Conference at the World Bank, November 2009, Washington, DC. http://siteresources.worldbank.org/HEALTHNUTRITIONANDPOPULATION/Resources/ScalingUpNutritionMeetingReport.pdf. Accessed January 14, 2010.

Critical Thinking

1. Discuss the challenges of strengthening global nutrition policy and food assistance programs.
2. Identify the most cost-effective global nutrition interventions.
3. Define "human development window" and "scaling up to national standards"
4. Identify the barriers to international food assistance and education programs.

GARY R. GLEASON, PhD, is working primarily on "Fork to Fuel," a large-scale exhibition on human food and nutrition, international technical assistance on nutrition policies against child undernutrition, micronutrient deficiencies, improved management of nutrition research and communication, and social change strategies for prevention and control of HIV/AIDS. He is communication director for the International Nutrition Foundation and an adjunct associate professor at the Friedman School of Nutrition Science and Policy at Tufts University, Boston, Massachusetts.

Food Stamps for Good Food

Should the program target hunger *and* obesity by promoting consumption of fruits and veggies?

MELANIE MASON

Coretta Dudley's monthly grocery shopping strategy is as finely calibrated as a combat plan. Armed with $868 in Supplemental Nutrition Assistance Program (SNAP) benefits (the fancy new name for food stamps), she stops first at FoodMaxx, a discount supermarket in East Oakland, where she stocks up on four weeks' worth of nonperishables: cases of noodles, cans of vegetables and boxes of the sugary cereals her kids like. She also buys fresh fruit—apples and pears and bananas and grapes—but those will be gone in a week. Then she swings by Wal-Mart for bread, eggs and milk. Later, she'll hit the family-owned meat market, where she chooses hamburger and cube steaks. Other than $100 she sets aside to replenish the milk, eggs and cheese later in the month, that first multipronged attack will last her and her six children, ages 4 to 16, the whole month. That's the idea, anyway.

"At the end of the month, we'll still need something," she says. "It never fails."

Almost 500 miles away, in the City Heights neighborhood of San Diego, Tsehay Gebere has developed her own shopping plan at the Saturday farmers' market. The lines are long, and the ten-pound sacks of oranges, plentiful at 9 AM, will have disappeared by noon. But Gebere, a weekly fixture at the market, has the inside track. She persuades farmer Bernardino Loera to sock away four bags in his van. Forty-five minutes later, she gets back to Loera's stall and collects her hoarded prize.

Like Dudley, Gebere receives food stamp benefits, for herself and her four children. Like Dudley, Gebere shops at discount supermarkets like Food 4 Less for most of her groceries. But while Dudley buys four bags of fruit every month, Gebere buys at least four bags every week—made possible by the free money she gets at the farmers' market.

Yes, free money—though the technical name is "double voucher." The market matches a certain amount of money from a customer's federal food assistance benefits, essentially doubling the customer's purchasing power. City Heights was one of the first double voucher markets in the country; there are now more than 160 participating farmers' markets in twenty states. They reach just a tiny fraction of the more than 43 million Americans receiving food stamps. But their very existence raises questions about SNAP's identity: is it a welfare program or, as its recent name change suggests, a nutrition program?

These questions are the subject of lively debate in USDA offices and advocacy circles, where the idea of giving extra money for fruits and veggies, innocuous as it may seem, is exposing fault lines between traditional advocates for the poor and a new coalition of healthy-food activists.

The underlying premise of the modern food stamp program, shaped in the Kennedy/Johnson years, was that the American poor were starving and in need of calories, any calories at all. But there is now a well-documented overlap between the country's staggering rate of "food insecurity" (the term used by the USDA in lieu of "hunger") and its escalating obesity rates. In 2009, 43 percent of households below the federal poverty line experienced food insecurity. And if you're poor, you're more likely to be obese. Nine of the ten states with the highest poverty levels also rank in the top ten of obesity rates.

That one can be simultaneously food insecure and obese seems like a paradox. But consider that many low-income neighborhoods have few full-service supermarkets. Grocery shopping in the neighborhood likely means buying at corner stores with limited options for healthy choices. Even if those options do exist, they are not necessarily the rational economic choice for someone on a tight budget. The cost per calorie for foods containing fats and oils, sugars and refined grains are extremely low, but these are precisely the foods linked to high obesity rates. Healthy choices like fruits and vegetables are as much as several thousand times more expensive per calorie.

In a California Department of Public Health survey of eating habits, low-income people said they knew the importance of healthy eating. But they still eat fewer fruits and vegetables than the government recommends, less than the American population as a whole. "People said they couldn't afford it," says George Manalo-LeClair, legislation director with the California Food Policy Advocates. "It's cost."

At the heart of this whole mess—poverty, hunger and declining health—is the food stamp program. Nationwide, the average SNAP beneficiary received $125.31 per month in fiscal year 2009. If food stamps constitute a person's entire food budget—as often happens, even though the program is intended to supplement recipients' own money—that translates to just under $1.40 per meal. If you're looking to buy something that will satiate you for $1.40, you probably won't be buying broccoli.

Researchers have long studied whether food stamps contribute to obesity. Previously the conclusion was, probably not. But in an Ohio State University study released in the summer of 2009 the finding was, quite possibly yes. The study found that the body mass index (BMI) of program participants is more than one point higher than nonparticipants at the same income level. The longer one is on food stamps, the higher the BMI rises.

If the link exists—and it is exceedingly difficult to prove a causal relationship between food stamps and any one physical condition—it exposes a weakness in the program. The food stamp program has certainly evolved since the "war on poverty," but fundamentally it is still operating as though the only health threat facing the poor is insufficient calories.

The roots of the City Heights farmers' market date back thirty years, to an incident in 1980 Gus Schumacher calls "the case of the broken pear box." Schumacher was helping his brother, a farmer outside Boston, load a truck after the Dorchester farmers' market closed when he dropped a box of Bosc pears in the gutter. A woman passing by bent down and retrieved the damaged fruit, explaining that she was on food stamps but still couldn't afford fresh fruits and vegetables for her children. Schumacher ended up giving her an additional ten pounds of apples and pears. "People should not be picking fruit out of a gutter," he says.

A former under secretary in the USDA, Schumacher is now vice president of policy at Wholesome Wave, a Connecticut-based nonprofit that helped City Heights and similar programs get off the ground. For him, the broken pear box was a revelation: people on food assistance desperately want the products that small farmers like his brother were selling. If those pricey pears could be made affordable for these new shoppers, it could be a win-win for buyer and seller.

City Heights was an ideal community to put Schumacher's theory to the test. The average income in the neighborhood is around $26,000, as opposed to $63,000 in the county as a whole. The types of fruits and vegetables on offer are tailored to fit the cultural preferences of shoppers, mostly Latino, Vietnamese and Somali. The market's operators say more than 1,800 customers, 250 of whom are regulars, participate in their double voucher program, dubbed "Fresh Fund." In a survey of marketgoers, 90 percent said that they include more fresh fruits and vegetables in their daily diet, thanks to Fresh Fund. The market's small farmers have reaped benefits too. Bernardino Loera, Gebere's orange vendor, says Fresh Fund dollars account for three-quarters of his sales.

City Heights customers say they love the quality of the market's produce—"the food is so fresh," "it's natural," "it's organic." But it is also surprisingly economical, given the reputation farmers' markets have for designer produce. Lemons run six for $1 here; at the Albertson's down the street, lemons were selling two for $1. Other items, like kale and onions, were pretty much equal to Albertson's offerings. Loera says he adjusts his prices to match what customers can afford. The wares are made even cheaper by the Fresh Fund. Each time shoppers visit the market, their SNAP electronic benefits transfer (EBT) card is swiped, and they receive wooden tokens in $1 denominations they can use at individual stalls. The Fresh Fund is a true match program. Customers can deduct up to $20 per month from their benefit accounts; they then receive an equal amount in Fresh Fund dollars.

In three years, Wholesome Wave and its affiliated programs have secured funds from major philanthropies, including Newman's Own Foundation and the Kresge Foundation. The group had a $1.4 million operating budget last year, and Schumacher expects $1 million more in 2011. But the real money is federal money—almost $70 billion spent in fiscal year 2010 on SNAP. If just 3 percent went to fruit and vegetable incentives, that would be more than $2 billion to make healthy food affordable at farmers' markets and grocery stores.

Incentives are already on the radar at the USDA. Later this year, a fifteen-month pilot program in Massachusetts will attempt to apply the double-voucher theory—extra money for healthy foods—to the supermarket, where most food stamp purchases are made. Taking advantage of SNAP's EBT card, which functions like a debit card, the program will add 30 cents to select recipients' SNAP balance for every dollar spent on fruits and vegetables—fresh, frozen, canned or dried. The experiment cuts to the heart of nutrition incentives: would a little extra money back change people's shopping behavior—and how much money would it take to make an impact?

Food stamps have long had a vigorous network of advocates in Washington; the healthy-food advocates are the new kids in town, with backgrounds in public health with emphasis on nutrition. The convergence of the two groups has not been particularly graceful. "I have to say we got off to kind of a rocky start," says Manalo-LeClair, whose organization has worked with both types of groups. "People were pleased that the food stamp program has the ability to fight hunger, and we haven't solved that problem. So then they were saying, 'Are we asking too much to have it do more in terms of preventing obesity as well?'"

To some in the anti-hunger lobby, the emphasis on nutrition is a political Trojan horse, a pretext for cuts or restrictions to the program. "Nine times out of ten, the people in these debates who use the term 'reform' use it as a sugarcoated way of just slashing benefits," says Joel Berg, director of the New York City Coalition Against Hunger. Indeed, the link to obesity has been raised in Congress as a reason not to increase funding for the program. Also, critics worry that it's a short road from incentives to disincentives: New York City Mayor Michael Bloomberg recently suggested banning the use of SNAP benefits for sugary soda, and Schumacher once proposed a surcharge for Coke and Twinkies (he has since dropped the idea). To some, this approach smacks of paternalism, implying that low-income people cannot be trusted to make their own decisions. "The right and left said we were being nannies," says Schumacher.

The people who run City Heights argue that their initiative would actually expand choices for low-income people who want to include fruits and vegetables in their everyday diet. Imagine if everyone on food stamps enjoyed the same choice. What if there was a place like City Heights in East Oakland, where Dudley could get $20 more each month to spend on fresh produce? Is that something she'd be interested in?

"If they'd match me? Yeah. . . ." She trails off, imagining how that would work. "Yes!" she says, getting louder now. "Oh, my God—I would love that!"

Maybe she could buy fruit all month long. Maybe fresh vegetables wouldn't just be for holidays. For a moment, Dudley adjusts her battle plan to indulge in this new fantasy.

"Twenty dollars a month," she says. "That would change a lot."

Critical Thinking

1. Explain how double vouchers could be used to increase the fruit and vegetable intake of SNAP participants.

2. What is the average amount of food "vouchers" a SNAP participant will receive per month? How does that break down to cost per meal?

3. Describe the food assistance project that occurred in City Heights, CT.

MELANIE MASON, a journalist in Washington, DC, has been published in the *New York Times, Politico,* the *Dallas Morning News* and *The New Republic.* This article was written with the support of a Kaiser Permanente Institute for Health Policy fellowship.

Address Health Disparities in American Indians

Cultivating traditions and promoting nutrition can make a difference.

ELAINE KOVACS MA, AND MELISSA IP, MA, RD

As children, we may learn about the Three Sisters—squash, corn, and beans—during elementary school explorations into American Indian life. The cultivation of the Three Sisters represented ingenuity in sustainable agricultural practices. For the Iroquois, the Three Sisters were the spiritual sustainers of life, providing complete vegetarian protein.

Yet, despite a tradition of physically active lifestyles and a diet of whole, unprocessed foods, American Indian and Alaska Native communities today are experiencing some of the worst nutrition disparities in the United States. In 2009, 67 percent of American Indians and Alaska Natives were overweight or obese.[1] (Not easily simplified, the term "American Indian and Alaska Native" describes more than 560 federally recognized tribes spread across the United States, making up 1.6 percent of the U.S. population today.[2])

With an understanding of the challenges facing this population and an awareness of the programs that are making a difference by emphasizing traditional foods and physical activity, nutrition professionals can help address the health disparities affecting American Indians.

Contextualizing American Indian Health

In addressing health disparities such as obesity, diabetes, and food insecurity, context always matters. Traditionally speaking, American Indians regard food as more than just sustenance; it is a way of life. But as American Indians face limited resources, geographic isolation, and a failing government food aid system, particularly for those living on rural reservations, they are more likely to experience malnutrition and food insecurity than the general U.S. population.[3] Food aid provided to the tribes continues to be insufficient and often of low quality, ignoring the addition of traditional American Indian foods in federal nutrition assistance programs.[4]

The spiritual value of food, as well as its use as positive reinforcement, has both positive and negative impacts on many American Indian communities. Food is respected as nourishment, but it may also be used for "rewarding children with foods such as candy, bakery sweets, pop, and ice cream that were restricted when the parents themselves were young children in extreme poverty and didn't have access to such foods and beverages," notes Karen Strauss, MS, a retired dietitian with 20 years of experience in the Indian Health Service.

These issues of poor diet and lack of resources did not happen overnight. As the 2004 U.S. Commission on Civil Rights Report "Broken Promises: Evaluating the Native American Health Care System" notes, "The nation's lengthy history of failing to keep its promises to Native Americans, including the failure of Congress to provide the resources necessary to create and maintain an effective health care system for Native Americans," has been deeply detrimental to the long-term health of many American Indian and Alaska Native populations. Current funding appropriated for the Indian Health Service provides only 55 percent of what is needed to ensure standard mainstream personal healthcare services for American Indians.[5] In addition, more than one-quarter of American Indians are living in poverty, a rate that is more than double that of the general U.S. population.[6]

Given this reality of severely underfunded healthcare services, the need to focus on preventive healthcare measures (eg, healthful eating, exercise, routine care) becomes all the more vital in American Indian communities. Strauss recommends that public health strategies "involve the community via coalitions or similar organizations in developing and implementing interventions" rather than imposing a vision of public health from an outsider's perspective. Local culture and traditions should be integrated into any public health policy by accounting for the diversity of beliefs and traditions among American Indians.

Nutrition Transitions in American Indian Communities

Like many communities in the United States, many American Indian tribes have undergone nutrition transitions whereby chronic diseases are becoming more prevalent. According to one study in the August 2006 issue of *Diabetes Care*, when comparing two groups of Pima Indians with similar genetic makeup—one in traditional environments in Mexico and the other in Western environments in the United States—the prevalence of type 2 diabetes was overwhelmingly higher among Pima Indians in the United States. With many American Indians adopting a sedentary lifestyle typical of rural America, the lack of physical activity and oversupply of fatty, sugary foods has become a recipe for disaster.

With American Indian families ill equipped with financial resources, parenting support, and access to healthful foods, current generations of American Indians are struggling with obesity and prediabetes. Despite categorizing American Indians as part of the same racial or ethnic group, American Indian tribes are not all the same—not in culture or even in diabetes rates (with some at 5 percent and others at 33 percent).[7] Therefore, interventions must be uniquely planned and implemented with the individual situations in mind. The focus should be on prevention with cultural competency at the heart of these programs.

Promoting Health and Heritage

Many efforts have focused on preventing diabetes and obesity in American Indian communities by promoting the consumption of local and traditional foods. In her book *Recovering Our Ancestors' Gardens: Indigenous Recipes and Guide to Diet and Fitness*, Devon Abbott Mihesuah, PhD, a historian and member of the Choctaw Nation of Oklahoma, asserts that fry bread and Indian tacos are not traditional fare. While many American Indians have grown up eating these foods, Mihesuah points out that traditional American Indian diets did not include wheat or dairy products. Fry bread, like other foods made from wheat, came from the federal commodity food program, which provided surplus white flour, cheese, sugar, lard, and canned foods to American Indian reservations.

By contrast, traditional American Indian diets featured a wide range of meats, vegetables, fruits, and herbs. Some traditional foods popularly appeared in Thanksgiving dinners—for example, turkey, corn, green beans, potatoes, squash, cranberries, pumpkin, and beans—and the variety of foods did not end there. Walnuts, avocados, red and yellow bell peppers, strawberries, cactus, guava, papaya, and artichokes are all indigenous to the Americas. American Indian tribes also included wild plants such as dandelion, elderberry, mint, purslane, and watercress in their diet.

Community-based organizations such as Tohono O'odham Community Action in Sells, Ariz., are taking steps to promote healthful lifestyles among American Indians. In 2000, Tohono O'odham Community Action helped organize the Desert Walk for Health and Heritage, a march that lasted more than a week and took participants more than 200 miles from El Desemboque, a Mexican village on the Sea of Cortez, across the Sonoran Desert to Tucson, Ariz. The aim was to raise awareness of healthful, traditional foods, particularly as a solution to the diabetes epidemic that has affected one-half of Tohono O'odham adults,[8] through the revival of a heritage walk traditionally undertaken by young Tohono O'odham men. During the event, walkers ate stewed nopalitos (cactus pads), mesquite and amaranth pancakes with prickly pear syrup, and punch made with ocotillo flowers.

Tohono O'odham Community Action is currently working with the Indian Oasis-Boboquivari School District to improve the nutritional quality of meals by serving students healthful, local, and traditional foods. Teachers are also trained to use lesson plans that promote traditional foods and healthful eating through garden-based activities.

Urban health centers are also addressing nutrition disparities among American Indians. (Contrary to popular belief, almost two-thirds of American Indians and Alaska Natives reside off reservation in metropolitan areas.[9]) One urban effort to improve American Indian health is the Running Is My High event hosted by the Native American Health Center in Oakland, Calif. The annual event celebrates sobriety and wellness by bringing back the tradition of running among American Indians. In addition, the American Indian Health Service of Chicago offers The Healing Circle, a community diabetes program for urban American Indians. The program provides outreach screenings, educational sessions, and home visits to promote the prevention and management of diabetes while linking community members to medical care at the clinic.

Nutrition Professionals' Role

Dietitians can also do their part to make a difference in improving the health of American Indians.

Strauss recalls an overweight patient in his late 20s who had recently been diagnosed with diabetes. "As a clinical dietitian, I always looked for one, maybe two often-eaten foods that could quickly make a difference to blood sugar levels," she says. Following a now-common practice in American Indian communities, this man consumed a large amount (1 liter) of soda per day. "My only recommendation that day was for him to switch to water or diet soda." On his return visit, his blood sugar had dropped to normal levels.

The young man continued to meet with Strauss weekly, and she became his friend and partner in nutrition care. On subsequent visits, he seemed thrilled to show Strauss his progressively smaller waistline.

Strauss offers some advice: Dietitians considering offering consultant nutrition services to American Indian communities should become involved in the community and get to know its people. "Clients may be reluctant to keep appointments with a dietitian they consider an outsider," she says. RDs should also learn about the history and the challenges in the community in which they are working. While serving as the nutrition authority, they should take a collaborative rather than an authoritarian approach, serving as an advisor and friend, not the all-knowing professional. Dietitians can best work with the American Indian community by advising or loosely leading community coalitions and advisory groups. They should also withhold judgment when the social and cultural characteristics of a community or family are not consistent with their own personal experiences and ideals.

Diversifying Dietetics Practice

In trying to explain the disproportionate burden of obesity and diabetes in American Indian communities, Mihesuah asserts in Recovering Our Ancestors' Gardens that there are "not enough native nutritionists. If more people were nutritionists, then Native people would be more inclined to listen to health advice." Indeed, in 2005, less than 1 percent of American Dietetic Association members and dietetics students were American Indian, Alaska Native, or Hawaiian Native.[10]

In attempts to bridge this gap, the Southwestern Dietetic Internship Consortium prepares dietetics professionals to work in both urban and rural American Indian communities. Its goals are to improve American Indians' access to nutrition care with a qualified dietetics professional and increase the number of American Indian dietitians. In addition, the Multicultural Scholars in Dietetics Program at the University of North Dakota offers financial assistance to undergraduate students majoring in dietetics or community nutrition.

Coming Full Circle

Addressing health disparities takes a socioecological approach. Culturally appropriate food services, nutrition education and medical nutrition therapy, school gardens, and farm-to-school initiatives all have important roles to play in tackling the epidemic of obesity and chronic disease among American Indians, as they do in all communities across the United States.

While many see a return to tradition as the best way to combat diabetes and obesity, Mihesuah and others advocate for combining the best of the old and new, such as choosing traditional American Indian ingredients and adding healthful foods and flavors from other continents. Someone could put a twist on the Three Sisters stew by combining the traditional lima beans, yellow squash, and hominy corn and adding a bit of olive oil, thyme, and fresh homegrown cilantro. Such a tasty meal both preserves long-held traditions and allows new ingredients to make a healthful impact.

References

1. Henry J. Kaiser Family Foundation. Overweight and obesity rates for adults by race/ethnicity, 2009. Available at: www.statehealthfacts.org/comparetable.jsp?ind=91& cat=2&sort=137. Accessed April 10, 2011.
2. Centers for Disease Control and Prevention. American Indian & Alaska Native populations. Updated November 30, 2010. Available at: www.cdc.gov/omhd/populations/aian/aian.htm. Accessed March 1, 2011.
3. Gundersen C. Measuring the extent, depth, and severity of food insecurity: An application to American Indians in the USA. *J Popul Econ.* 2008;21:191–215.
4. Edwards K, Patchell B. State of the science: A cultural view of Native Americans and diabetes prevention. *J Cult Divers.* 2009;16(1):32–35.
5. Indian Health Service. Facts on Indian health disparities. January 2006. Available at: http://info.ihs.gov/Files/ DisparitiesFacts-Jan2006.pdf. Accessed March 1, 2011.
6. Sarche M, Spicer P. Poverty and health disparities for American Indian and Alaska Native children: Current knowledge and future prospects. *Ann N Y Acad Sci.* 2008;1136:126–136.
7. Centers for Disease Control and Prevention. National diabetes fact sheet: National estimates and general information on diabetes and prediabetes in the United States, 2011. Available at: www.cdc.gov/diabetes/pubs/pdf/ndfs_2011.pdf.
8. *Unnatural Causes: Is Inequality Making Us Sick* [DVD/VHS]. San Francisco: California Newsreel; 2008.
9. Urban Indian Health Commission. Invisible tribes: Urban Indians and their health in a changing world. 2007. Available at: www.rwjf.org/files/research/uihc2007report.pdf.
10. University of North Dakota College of Nursing. Multicultural scholars into dietetics program (MSDP). Available at: www.nursing.und.edu/nutrition-dietetics/msdp.cfm. Accessed April 10, 2011.

Critical Thinking

1. What percentage of American Indians and Alaska Natives are overweight or obese?
2. Evaluate the causes of the nutrition and health disparities among native people.
3. Summarize the findings of the Commission on Civil Rights Report Broken Promises: Evaluating the Native American Health Care System.

ELAINE KOVACS, MA, is currently pursuing her master's degree in social work while working in Austin, Tex. **MELISSA IP, MA, RD,** is a health educator in New York City.

From *Today's Dietitian*, June 2011, pp. 36–38. Copyright © 2011 by *Today's Dietitian*. Reprinted by permission.

Fixing the Global Nitrogen Problem

Humanity depends on nitrogen to fertilize croplands, but growing global use is damaging the environment and threatening human health. How can we chart a more sustainable path?

ALAN R. TOWNSEND AND ROBERT W. HOWARTH

Billions of people today owe their lives to a single discovery now a century old. In 1909 German chemist Fritz Haber of the University of Karlsruhe figured out a way to transform nitrogen gas—which is abundant in the atmosphere but nonreactive and thus unavailable to most living organisms—into ammonia, the active ingredient in synthetic fertilizer. The world's ability to grow food exploded 20 years later, when fellow German scientist Carl Bosch developed a scheme for implementing Haber's idea on an industrial scale.

Over the ensuing decades new factories transformed ton after ton of industrial ammonia into fertilizer, and today the Haber-Bosch invention commands wide respect as one of the most significant boons to public health in human history. As a pillar of the green revolution, synthetic fertilizer enabled farmers to transform infertile lands into fertile fields and to grow crop after crop in the same soil without waiting for nutrients to regenerate naturally. As a result, global population skyrocketed from 1.6 billion to six billion in the 20th century.

But this good news for humanity has come at a high price. Most of the reactive nitrogen we make—on purpose for fertilizer and, to a lesser extent, as a by-product of the fossil-fuel combustion that powers our cars and industries—does not end up in the food we eat. Rather it migrates into the atmosphere, rivers and oceans, where it makes a Jekyll and Hyde style transformation from do-gooder to rampant polluter. Scientists have long cited reactive nitrogen for creating harmful algal blooms, coastal dead zones and ozone pollution. But recent research adds biodiversity loss and global warming to nitrogen's rap sheet, as well as indications that it may elevate the incidence of several nasty human diseases.

Today humans are generating reactive nitrogen and injecting it into the environment at an accelerating pace, in part because more nations are vigorously pursuing such fertilizer-intensive endeavors as biofuel synthesis and meat production (meat-intensive diets depend on massive growth of grain for animal feed). Heavy fertilizer use for food crops and unregulated burning of fossil fuels are also becoming more prevalent in regions such as South America and Asia. Not surprisingly then, dead zones and other nitrogen-related problems that were once confined to North America and Europe are now popping up elsewhere.

At the same time, fertilizer is, and should be, a leading tool for developing a reliable food supply in sub-Saharan Africa and other malnourished regions. But the international community must come together to find ways to better manage its use and mitigate its consequences worldwide. The solutions are not always simple, but nor are they beyond our reach.

The world is capable of growing MORE FOOD with LESS FERTILIZER.

Too Much of a Good Thing

Resolving the nitrogen problem requires an understanding of the chemistry involved and a sense of exactly how nitrogen fosters environmental trouble. The element's ills—and benefits—arise when molecules

Nitrogen's Dark Side

Doubled up as N_2 gas, the most abundant component of the earth's atmosphere, nitrogen is harmless. But in its reactive forms, which emanate from farms and fossil-fuel-burning factories and vehicles, nitrogen can have a hand in a wide range of problems for the environment and human health.

1. The nitrogen produced during fossil-fuel combustion can cause severe air pollution . . .
2. Before it then combines with water to create nitric acid in rain . . .
3. And joins with nitrogen leaking from fertilized fields, farm animal excrement, human sewage and leguminous crops.
4. When too much nitrogen enters terrestrial ecosystems, it can contribute to biodiversity decline and perhaps to increased risk for several human illnesses.
5. A single nitrogen atom from a factory, vehicle or farm can acidify soil and contaminate drinking water before entering rivers . . .
6. Where it can travel to the oceans and help fuel toxic algal blooms and coastal dead zones.
7. At any point along this chain, bacteria may transform the rogue atom into nitrous oxide, a potent greenhouse gas that also speeds the loss of protective stratospheric ozone. Only bacteria that convert the atom back to innocuous N_2 gas can halt its ill effects.

of N_2 gas break apart. All life needs nitrogen, but for the vast majority of organisms, the biggest reservoir—the atmosphere—is out of reach. Although 78 percent of the atmosphere consists of N_2, that gas is inert. Nature's way of making nitrogen available for life relies on the action of a small group of bacteria that can break the triple bond between those two nitrogen atoms, a process known as nitrogen fixation. These specialized bacteria exist in free-living states on land and in both freshwater and saltwater and in symbiotic relationships with the roots of legumes, which constitute some the world's most important crops. Another small amount of nitrogen gas is fixed when lightning strikes and volcanic eruptions toast it.

Before humanity began exploiting Haber-Bosch and other nitrogen-fixation techniques, the amount of reactive nitrogen produced in the world was balanced by the activity of another small bacterial group that converts reactive nitrogen back to N_2 gas in a process called denitrification. In only one human generation, though, that delicate balance has been transformed completely. By 2005 humans were creating more than 400 billion pounds of reactive nitrogen each year, an amount at least double that of all natural processes on land combined.

At times labeled nature's most promiscuous element, nitrogen that is liberated from its nonreactive state can cause an array of environmental problems because it can combine with a multitude of chemicals and can spread far and wide. Whether a new atom of reactive nitrogen enters the atmosphere or a river, it may be deposited tens to hundreds of miles from its source, and even some of the most remote corners of our planet now experience elevated nitrogen levels because of human activity. Perhaps most insidious of all: a single new atom of reactive nitrogen can bounce its way around these widespread environments, like a felon on a crime spree.

Reaping the Consequences

When nitrogen is added to a cornfield or to a lawn, the response is simple and predictable: plants grow more. In natural ecosystems, however, the responses are far more intricate and frequently worrisome. As fertilizer-laden river waters enter the ocean, for example, they trigger blooms of microscopic plants that consume oxygen as they decompose, leading later to so-called dead zones. Even on land, not all plants in a complex ecosystem respond equally to nitrogen subsidies, and many are not equipped for a sudden embarrassment of riches. Thus, they lose out to new species that are more competitive in a nutrient-rich world. Often the net effect is a loss of biodiversity. For example, grasslands across much of Europe have lost a quarter or more of their plant species after decades of human-created nitrogen deposition from the atmosphere. This problem is so widespread that a recent scientific assessment ranked nitrogen pollution as one of the top three threats to biodiversity around the globe, and the United Nations Environment Program's Convention on Biological Diversity considers reductions of nitrogen deposition to be a key indicator of conservation success.

The loss of a rare plant typically excites little concern in the general public or among those who forge policy. But excess nitrogen does not just harm other species—it can threaten our own. A National Institutes of Health review suggests that elevated nitrate concentrations in drinking water—often a product of water pollution from the high nitrate levels in common fertilizers—may contribute to multiple health problems, including several cancers. Nitrogen-related air pollution, both particulates and ground-level ozone, affects hundreds of millions of people, elevating the incidence of cardiopulmonary ailments and driving up overall mortality rates.

Ecological feedbacks stemming from excess nitrogen (and another ubiquitous fertilizer chemical, phosphorus) may be poised to hit us with a slew of other health threats as well. How big or varied such

Fast Facts

More than half the synthetic nitrogen fertilizer ever produced was applied in the past 20 years.

The production of synthetic nitrogen has skyrocketed 80 percent since 1960, dwarfing the 25 percent increase in atmospheric carbon dioxide over that same period.

If Americans were to switch to a typical Mediterranean diet, the country's fertilizer use would be cut in half.

responses will become remains to be seen, but scientists do know that enriching ecosystems with nitrogen changes their ecology in myriad ways. Recent evidence suggests that excess nitrogen may increase risk for Alzheimer's disease and diabetes if ingested in drinking water. It may also elevate the release of airborne allergens and promote the spread of certain infectious diseases. Fertilization of ragweed elevates pollen production from that notorious source, for instance. Malaria, cholera, schistosomiasis and West Nile virus show the potential to infect more people when nitrogen is abundant.

These and many other illnesses are controlled by the actions of other species in the environment, particularly those that carry the infective agent—for example, mosquitoes spread the malaria parasite, and snails release schistosomes into water. Snails offer an example of how nitrogen can unleash a chain reaction: more nitrogen or phosphorus run-off fuels greater plant growth in water bodies, in turn creating more food for the snails and a larger, faster-growing population of these disease-bearing agents. The extra nutrients also fuel an exponentially increasing effect of having each snail produce more parasites. It is too soon to tell if, in general, nutrient pollution will up the risk of disease—in some cases, the resulting ecological changes might lower our health risks. But the potential for change, and thus the need to understand how it will play out, is rising rapidly as greater use of fertilizers spreads to disease-rich tropical latitudes in the coming decades.

Mounting evidence also blames reactive nitrogen for an increasingly important role in climate change. In the atmosphere, reactive nitrogen leads to one of its major unwanted by-products—ground-level ozone—when it occurs as nitric oxide (NO) or as nitrogen dioxide (NO_2), collectively known as NO_X. Such ozone formation is troubling not only because of its threat to human health but also because at ground level, ozone is a significant greenhouse gas. Moreover, it damages plant tissues, resulting in billions of dollars in lost crop production every year. And by inhibiting growth, ozone curtails plants' ability to absorb carbon dioxide (CO_2) and offset global warming.

Reactive nitrogen is an especially worrisome threat to climate change when it occurs as nitrous oxide (N_2O)—among the most powerful of greenhouse gases. One molecule of N_2O has approximately 300 times the greenhouse warming potential of one molecule of CO_2. Although N_2O is far less abundant in the atmosphere than CO_2 is, its current atmospheric concentration is responsible for warming equivalent to 10 percent of CO_2's contribution. It is worth noting that excess nitrogen can at times counteract warming—by combining with other airborne compounds to form aerosols that reflect incoming radiation, for example, and by stimulating plants in nitrogen-limited forests to grow faster and thus scrub more CO_2 out of the atmosphere. But despite uncertainties regarding the balance between nitrogen's heating and cooling effects, most signs indicate that continued human creation of excess nitrogen will speed climate warming.

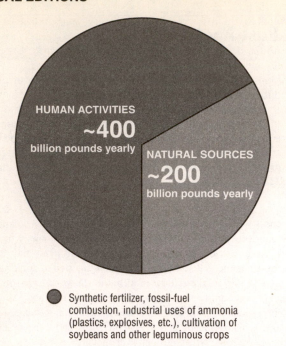

HUMAN ACTIVITIES
~400
billion pounds yearly

NATURAL SOURCES
~200
billion pounds yearly

● Synthetic fertilizer, fossil-fuel combustion, industrial uses of ammonia (plastics, explosives, etc.), cultivation of soybeans and other leguminous crops

● Nitrogen-fixing bacteria on land, lightning, volcanoes

HUMAN ACTIVITIES have tripled the amount of reactive nitrogen released into terrestrial environments and coastal oceans every year.

Global Perspectives
Shifting Hotspots

Regions of greatest nitrogen use were once limited mainly to Europe and North America. But as new economies develop and agricultural trends shift, patterns in the distribution of nitrogen are changing rapidly. Recent growth rates in nitrogen use are now much higher in Asia and in Latin America, whereas other regions—including much of Africa—suffer from fertilizer shortages.

- **Southern Brazil:** Rapid population growth and industrialization around Sao Paulo, poor civic sewage treatment and vibrant sugar cane production all contribute to this new South American nitrogen hotspot.
- **North China Plain:** More vigorous application of fertilizer has produced stunning increases in maize and wheat production, but China now has the highest fertilizer inputs in the world.

What to Do

Although fertilizer production accounts for much of the nitrogen now harming the planet—roughly two thirds of that fixed by humans—abandoning it certainly is not an option. Fertilizer is too important for feeding the world. But an emphasis on efficient use has to be a part of the solution, in both the wealthy and the developing nations.

It's up to You

Making certain personal choices will reduce your carbon and nitrogen footprints simultaneously:

- Support wind power, hybrid cars and other policies designed to reduce fossil-fuel consumption.
- Choose grass-fed beef and eat less meat overall.
- Buy locally grown produce.

Wealthy countries have blazed a path to an agricultural system that is often exceptionally nitrogen-intensive and inefficient in the use of this key resource. Too often their use of nitrogen has resembled a spending spree with poor returns on the investment and little regard for its true costs. Elsewhere, a billion or more people stand trapped in cycles of malnutrition and poverty. Perhaps best exemplified by sub-Saharan Africa, these are regions where agricultural production often fails to meet even basic caloric needs, let alone to provide a source of income. Here an infusion of nitrogen fertilizers would clearly improve the human condition. Recent adoption of policies to supply affordable fertilizer and better seed varieties to poor farmers in Malawi, for example, led to substantial increases in yield and reductions in famine.

But this fertilizer does not need to be slathered on injudiciously. The proof is out there: studies from the corn belt of the U.S. Midwest to the wheat fields of Mexico show that overfertilization has been common practice in the breadbaskets of the world—and that less fertilizer often does not mean fewer crops. The simple fact is that as a whole, the world is capable of growing more food with less fertilizer by changing the farming practices that have become common in an era of cheap, abundant fertilizer and little regard for the long-term consequences of its use. Simply reducing total application to many crops is an excellent starting point; in many cases, fertilizer doses are well above the level needed to ensure maximum yield in most years, resulting in disproportionately large losses to the environment. In the U.S., people consume only a little more than 10 percent of what farmers apply to their fields every year. Sooner or later, the rest ends up in the environment. Estimates vary, but for many of our most common crops, a quarter to half immediately runs off the field with rainwater or works its way into the atmosphere.

Precision farming techniques can also help. Applying fertilizer near plant roots only at times of maximum demand is one example of methods that are already in play in some of the wealthier agricultural regions of the planet. By taking advantage of Global Positioning System technology to map their fields, coupled with remotely sensed estimates of plant nutrient levels, farmers can refine calculations of how much fertilizer a crop needs and when. But the high-tech equipment is costly, prohibitively so for many independent farmers, and so such precision farming is not a panacea.

The solutions are not all high tech. Cheaper but still effective strategies can include planting winter cover crops that retain nitrogen in a field instead of allowing a field to lie bare for months, as well as maintaining some form of plant cover in between the rows of high-value crops such as corn. Simply applying fertilizer just before spring planting, rather than in the fall, can also make a big difference.

The world can also take advantages of changes in meat production. Of the nitrogen that ends up in crop plants, most goes into the mouths of pigs, cows and chickens—and much of that is then expelled as belches, urine and feces. Although a reduction in global meat consumption would be a valuable step, meat protein will remain an important part of most human diets, so efficiencies in its production must also improve. Changing animal diets—say, feeding cows more grass and less corn—can help on a small scale, as can better treatment of animal waste, which, like sewage treatment facilities for human waste, converts more of the reactive nitrogen back into inert gas before releasing it into the environment [see "The Greenhouse Hamburgerr" by Nathan Fiala; *Scientific American,* February 2009].

On the energy side, which represents about 20 percent of the world's excess nitrogen, much reactive nitrogen could be removed from current fossil-fuel emissions by better deployment of NO_x-scrubbing technologies in smokestacks and other sources of industrial pollution. Beyond that, a sustained global effort to improve energy efficiency and move toward cleaner, renewable sources will drop nitrogen emissions right alongside those for carbon. Removing the oldest and least-efficient power plants from production, increasing vehicle emission standards and, where possible, switching power generation from traditional combustion to fuel cells would all make a meaningful difference.

Of course, one source of renewable energy—biofuel made from corn—is generating a new demand for fertilizer. The incredible increase in the production of ethanol from corn in the U.S.—a nearly fourfold rise since 2000—has already had a demonstrable effect on increased nitrogen flows down the Mississippi River, which carries excess fertilizer to the Gulf of Mexico, where it fuels algal blooms and creates dead zones. According to a report last April by the Scientific Committee on Problems of the Environment (then part of the International Council for Science), a business-as-usual approach to biofuel production could exacerbate global warming, food security threats and human respiratory ailments in addition to these familiar ecological problems.

How to Get It Done

Society already has a variety of technical tools to manage nitrogen far more effectively, retaining many of its benefits while greatly reducing the risk. As for our energy challenges, a switch to more sustainable nitrogen use will not come easily, nor is there a silver bullet. Furthermore, technological know-how is not enough: without economic incentives and other policy shifts, none of these solutions will likely solve the problem.

The speed at which nitrogen pollution is rising throughout the world suggests the need for some regulatory control. Implementing or strengthening environmental standards, such as setting total maximum daily loads that can enter surface waters and determining the reactive nitrogen concentrations allowable in fossil-fuel emissions, is probably

essential. In the U.S. and other nations, regulatory policies are being pursued at both national and regional scales, with some success [see "Reviving Dead Zones," by Laurence Mee; *Scientific American,* November 2006]. And as much needed policy changes bring fertilizer to those parts of the world largely bypassed by the green revolution, those areas should employ sustainable solutions from the outset—to avoid repeating mistakes made in the U.S. and elsewhere.

Promising improvements could occur even without the regulatory threat of monetary fines for exceeding emissions standards. Market-based instruments, such as tradable permits, may also be useful. This approach proved remarkably successful for factory emissions of sulfur dioxide. Adoption of similar approaches to NO_x pollution are already under way, including the U.S. Environmental Protection Agency's NO_x Budget Trading Program, which began in 2003. Such policies could be extended to fertilizer runoff and livestock emissions as well—although the latter are more difficult to monitor than the smokestacks of a coal-burning power plant.

Other approaches to the problem are also beginning to take hold, including better use of landscape design in agricultural areas, especially ensuring that crop fields near bodies of water are fringed by intervening wetlands that can markedly reduce nitrogen inputs to surface waters and the coastal ocean. Protected riparian areas, such those promoted by the U.S. Conservation Reserve Program, can do double duty: not only will they reduce nitrogen pollution, but they also provide critical habitat for migratory birds and a host of other species.

Substantial progress may also require a rethinking of agricultural subsidies. In particular, subsidies that reward environmental stewardship can bring about rapid changes in standard practice. A recent not-for-profit experiment run by the American Farmland Trust shows promise. Farmers agreed to reduce their fertilizer use and directed a portion of their cost savings from lowered fertilizer purchases to a common fund. They then fertilized the bulk of the crop at reduced rates, while heavily fertilizing small test plots. If such plots exceeded the average yield of the entire field, the fund paid out the difference.

As one of us (Howarth) reported in a Millennium Ecosystem Assessment in 2005, such pay-outs would rarely be required, given the current tendency to overfertilize many crops. The average farmer in the breadbasket of the upper U.S. Midwest (the source of the great majority of nitrogen pollution fueling the Gulf of Mexico dead zones) typically uses 20 to 30 percent more nitrogen fertilizer than agricultural extension agents recommend. As predicted, farmers who participated in this and similar experiments have applied less fertilizer with virtually no decrease in crop yield and have saved money as a result, because what they paid into the fund is less than the amount they saved by buying less fertilizer. As a result, such funds grow with no taxpayer subsidy.

Finally, better public education and personal choice can play critical roles. In much the way that many individuals have begun reducing their own energy consumption, so, too, can people from all walks of life learn how to select a less nitrogen-intensive lifestyle.

One big improvement would be for Americans to eat less meat. If Americans were to switch to a typical Mediterranean diet, in which average meat consumption is one sixth of today's U.S. rates, not only would Americans' health improve, the country's fertilizer use would be cut in half. Such shifts in dietary and agricultural practices could simultaneously lower environmental nitrogen pollution and improve public health: nitrogen-intensive agricultural practices in wealthier nations contribute to overly protein-rich, often unbalanced diets that link to health concerns from heart disease and diabetes to childhood obesity.

Making personal choices designed to reduce an individual's carbon footprint can help—not just on the industrial side, as in supporting wind power and hybrid cars, but on the agricultural side as well. Eating less meat, eating locally grown food and eating grass-fed rather

Solutions Are within Reach

- Industry can install more NO_x-scrubbing technologies in smokestacks and other sources of pollution.
- Farmers can use less fertilizer. For many crops, applying less fertilizer would not sacrifice yield.
- Community officials can ensure that crop fields are fringed by wetlands that can absorb nitrogen-laden runoff before it enters streams or lakes.
- Nations can institute farm subsidies that reward environmental stewardship.

Where Fertilizer *Shortage* Is the Problem

Synthetic fertilizer has been, and will continue to be, critical to meeting world food demands, particularly in malnourished regions, such as sub-Saharan Africa, where increased fertilizer use is one of the leading strategies for developing a reliable food supply.

Humans already produce more than enough fertilizer to feed the world, but inequitable and inefficient distribution means that excessive use is causing problems in some places while poverty-stricken regions are mired in a cycle of malnutrition. Making synthetic fertilizer available to those who typically cannot afford it has clearly played a role in bettering food security and the human condition in parts of rural sub-Saharan Africa, where wide-spread malnutrition stems directly from nutrient depletion and soil erosion.

Fertilizer subsidies are one pillar of the African Millennium Villages Project, an ambitious proof-of-concept project in which coordinated efforts to improve health, education and agricultural productivity are now under way in a series of rural villages across Africa. Launched in 2004, the project was implemented on a national scale in Malawi. After a decade of repeated food shortages and famine, Malawi created subsidies that provided poor farmers with synthetic fertilizer and improved seed varieties. Although better climate conditions played a role, the approach clearly worked: Malawi went from a 43 percent food deficit in 2005 to a 53 percent surplus in 2007.

—A.R.T. and R.W.H.

More to Explore

Nutrient Management. R. W. Howarth et al. in *Ecosystems and Human Well-Being: Policy Responses.* Millennium Ecosystem Assessment. Island Press, 2005.
Transformation of the Nitrogen Cycle: Recent Trends, Questions, and Potential Solutions. James N. Galloway et al. in *Science,* Vol. 320, pages 889–892; May 16, 2008.
Biofuels: Environmental Consequences and Interactions with Changing Land Use. Edited by R. W. Howarth and S. Bringezu. *Proceedings of the SCOPE International Biofuels Project Rapid Assessment,* Cornell University, April 2009. http://cip.cornell.edu/biofuels.
Nutrient Imbalances in Agricultural Development. P. M. Vitousek et al. in *Science,* Vol. 324, pages 1519–1520; June 19, 2009.

nitrogen production continuing to rise, we will face a future in which the enormous benefits of Fritz Haber's discovery become ever more shrouded by its drawbacks.

Still, as we have argued here, nitrogen cycle problems could be significantly reduced with current technology at relatively affordable costs. We can and must do better. It will take immediate and ongoing effort, but a sustainable nitrogen future is entirely achievable.

Critical Thinking

1. How did the creation of nitrogen-based synthetic fertilizers change agricultural production?
2. How do synthetic fertilizers affect the atmosphere, rivers, and oceans?
3. Why does raising animals for consumption require more fertilizer than raising vegetable, fruit, legumes, and grain crops for consumption?

than corn-fed beef all tackle the carbon and nitrogen problems simultaneously. Individual choices alone are unlikely to solve the problems, but history shows they can spur societies to move down new paths. The well-known trade-offs between climate and energy production that were long ignored as hypothetical now appear everywhere from presidential speeches to roadside billboards to budding regulatory schemes.

Unfortunately, the nitrogen problem is in one critical way tougher than the carbon problem. In solving the latter, it is reasonable to work toward a future of one day producing energy without CO_2-emitting fossil fuels. But it is not possible to envision a world free of the need to produce substantial amounts of reactive nitrogen. Synthetic fertilizer has been, and will continue to be, critical to meeting world food demands. Yet if we stay on a business-as-usual trajectory, with

ALAN R. TOWNSEND is incoming director of the Environmental Studies Program at the University of Colorado at Boulder and is a professor in the university's Institute of Arctic and Alpine Research and department of ecology and evolutionary biology. He studies how changes in climate, land use and global nutrient cycles affect the basic functioning of terrestrial ecosystems. **ROBERT W. HOWARTH,** who is David R. Atkinson Professor of Ecology and Environmental Biology at Cornell University, studies how human activities alter ecosystems, with an emphasis on fresh water and marine locales.

Perennial Grains
Food Security for the Future

Developing perennial versions of our major grain crops would address many of the environmental limitations annuals while helping to feed an increasingly hungry planet.

JERRY D. GLOVER AND JOHN P. REGANOLD

Colorful fruits and vegetables piled to overflowing at a farmer's market or in the produce aisle readily come to mind when we think about farming and food production. Such images run counter to those of environmental destruction and chronic hunger and seem disconnected from the challenges of climate change, energy use, and bio-diversity loss. Agriculture, though, has been identified as the greatest threat to biodiversity and ecosystem function of any human activity. And because of factors including climate change, rising energy costs, and land degradation, the number of "urgently hungry" people, now estimated at roughly 1 billion, is at its highest level ever. More troubling, agriculture-related problems will probably worsen as the human population expands—that is, unless we reshape agriculture.

The disconnect between popular images of farming and its less rosy reality stems from the fact that fruits and vegetables represent only a sliver of farm production. Cereal, oilseed, and legume crops dominate farming, occupying 75% of U.S. and 69% of global croplands. These grains include crops such as wheat, rice, and maize and together provide more than 70% of human food calories. Currently, all are annuals, which means they must be replanted each year from seed, require large amounts of expensive fertilizers and pesticides, poorly protect soil and water, and provide little habitat for wildlife. Their production emits significant greenhouse gases, contributing to climate change that can in turn have adverse effects on agricultural productivity.

These are not the inevitable consequences of farming. Plant breeders can now, for perhaps the first time in history, develop perennial versions of major grain crops. Perennial crops have substantial ecological and economic benefits. Their longer growing seasons and more extensive root systems make them more competitive against weeds and more effective at capturing nutrients and water. Farmers don't have to replant the crop each year, don't have to add as much fertilizer and pesticide, and don't burn as much diesel in their tractors. In addition,

soils are built and conserved, water is filtered, and more area is available for wildlife. Although perennial crops such as alfalfa exist, there are no commercial perennial versions of the grains on which humans rely. An expanding group of plant breeders around the world is working to change that.

Although annual grain crops have been with us for thousands of years and have benefited from many generations of breeding, modern plant breeding techniques provide unprecedented opportunities to develop new crops much more quickly. During the past decade, plant breeders in the United States have been working to develop perennial versions of wheat, sorghum, sunflowers, and legumes. Preliminary work has also been done to develop a perennial maize, and Swedish researchers see potential in domesticating a wild mustard species as a perennial oilseed crop. Relatively new breeding programs in China and Australia include work to develop perennial rice and wheat. These programs could make it possible to develop radically new and sustainable farming systems within the next 10 to 20 years.

Currently, these efforts receive little public funding in marked contrast to the extensive public support for cellulosic ethanol technologies capable of converting perennial biomass crops into liquid fuels. Yet perennial grain crops promise much larger payoffs for the environment and food security and have similar timelines for widespread application. Public research funds distributed through the U.S. Department of Agriculture (USDA) and the National Science Foundation (NSF) could greatly expand and accelerate perennial grain breeding programs. Additionally, the farm bill could include support for the development of perennial breeding programs.

The Rise of Annuals

Since the initial domestication of crops more than 10,000 years ago, annual grains have dominated food production. The agricultural revolution was launched when our Neolithic ancestors began harvesting and sowing wild seed-bearing plants. The earliest cultivators had long collected seed from both annual and perennial plants; however, they found the annuals to be better adapted to the soil disturbance and annual sowing they had adopted in order to maintain a convenient and steady supply of grains harvested from the annual plants.

Although some of the wild annuals first to be domesticated, such as wheat and barley, were favored because they had large seeds, others had seeds comparable in size to those of their wild perennial counterparts. With each year's sowing of the annuals, desirable traits were selected for and carried on to the next generation. Thus, selection pressure was applied, albeit unintentionally, to annual plants but not to perennials. Evidence indicates that selection pressures on wild annuals quickly resulted in domesticated plants with more desirable traits than their wild relatives. The unchanged wild perennials probably would have been ignored in favor of the increasingly large, easily harvested seeds of the modified annual plants.

The conversion of native perennial landscapes to the monocultures of annual crops characteristic of today's agriculture has allowed us to meet our increasing food needs. But it has also resulted in dramatic changes. Fields of maize and wheat require frequent, expensive care to remain productive. Compared to perennials, annuals typically grow for shorter lengths of time each year and have shallower rooting depths and lower root densities, with most of their roots restricted to the surface foot of soil or less. Even with crop management advances such as no-tillage practices, these traits limit their access to nutrients and water, increase their need for nutrients, leave croplands more vulnerable to degradation, and reduce soil carbon inputs and provisions for wildlife. These traits also make annual plants less resilient to the increased environmental stress expected from climate change.

Even in regions best suited for annual crops, such as the Corn Belt, soil carbon and nitrogen levels decreased by 40 to 50% or more after conversion from native plants to annuals. Global data for maize, rice, and wheat indicate that they take up only 20 to 50% of the nitrogen applied in fertilizer; the rest is lost to surrounding environments. Runoff of nitrogen and other chemicals from farm fields into rivers and then coastal waters has triggered the development of more than 400 "dead zones" that are depleted of fish and other sea dwellers.

Annual crops do, however, have some advantages over perennial crops in terms of management flexibility. Because they are short-lived, they offer farmers opportunities to quickly change crops in response to changing market demands as well as environmental factors such as disease outbreaks. Thus, annual grain production will undoubtedly be important far into the future. Still, the expanded use of perennial grain crops on farms would provide greater biological and economic diversity and yield additional environmental benefits.

Perennial Advantages

Developing new crop species capable of significantly replacing annuals will require a major effort. During the past four decades, breeders have had tremendous success in doubling,

tripling, and even quadrupling the yields of important annual grains, success that would seem to challenge the notion that a fundamental change in agriculture is needed. Today, however these high yields are being weighed against the negative environmental effects of agriculture that are increasingly seen around the world. And with global grain demand expected to double by 2050, these effects will increase.

The development of perennial crops through breeding would help deal with the multiple issues involving environmental conservation and food security in a world of shrinking resources. We know that perennials such as alfalfa and switchgrass are much more effective than annuals in maintaining topsoil. Soil carbon may also increase 50 to 100% when annual fields are converted to perennials. With their longer growing seasons and deeper roots, perennials can dramatically reduce water and nitrate losses. They require less field attention by the farmer and less pesticide and fertilizer inputs, resulting in lower costs. Wildlife benefit from reduced chemical inputs and from the greater shelter provided by perennial cover.

There are other benefits as well. Greater soil carbon storage and reduced input requirements mean that perennials have the potential to mitigate global warming, whereas annual crops tend to exacerbate the problem. With more of their reserves protected belowground and their greater access to more soil moisture, perennials are also more resilient to temperature increases of the magnitude predicted by some climate change models. Although perennials may not offer farmers the flexibility of changing crops each year, they can be planted on more-marginal lands and can be used to increase the economic and biological diversity of a farm, thereby increasing the flexibility of the farming system. Perhaps most important in a crowded world with limited resources, perennials are more resilient to social, political, health, and environmental disruptions because they don't rely on annual seedbed preparation and planting. A farmer suffering from illness might be unable to harvest her crop one season, but a new crop would be ready the next season when she recovers. Meanwhile, the soil is protected and water has been captured.

The increased use of perennials could also slow, reverse, or prevent the increased planting of annuals on marginal lands, which now support more than half the world's population. Because marginal lands are by their nature fragile and subject to rapid degradation, large areas of these lands now being planted with annuals are already experiencing declining productivity. This will mean that additional marginal lands will be cultivated. This troubling reality makes the development of crops that can be more sustainably produced a matter of necessity. Developing perennial versions of our major grain crops would address many of the environmental limitations of annuals while helping to feed an increasingly hungry planet.

Perennial Possibilities

Recent advances in plant breeding, such as the use of marker-assisted selection, genomic in situ hybridization, transgenic technologies, and embryo rescue, coupled with traditional breeding techniques, make the development of perennial grain crops possible in the next 10 to 20 years. Two traditional approaches to developing these crops are direct domestication and wide hybridization, which have led to the wide variety of crops on which humans now rely. To directly domesticate a wild perennial, breeders select desirable plants from large populations of wild plants with a range of characteristics. Seeds are collected for replanting in order to increase the frequency of genes for desirable traits, such as large seed size, palatability, strong stems, and high seed yield. In wide hybridization, breeders cross an annual grain such as wheat with one of its wild perennial relatives, such as intermediate wheatgrass. They manage gene flow by making a large number of crosses between the annual and perennial plants, selecting offspring with desirable traits and repeating this cycle of crossing and selection multiple times. Ten of the 13 most widely grown grain and oilseed crops are capable of hybridization with perennial relatives.

The idea that plants can build and maintain perennial root systems and produce sufficient yields of edible grains seems counterintuitive. After all, plant resources, such as carbon captured through photosynthesis, must be allocated to different plant parts, and more resource allocation to roots would seem to mean that less can be allocated to seeds. Fortunately for the breeder, plants are relatively flexible organisms that are responsive to selection pressures, able to change the size of their resource "pies" depending on environmental conditions, and able to change the size of the slices of the resource pie. For example, when plant breeders take the wild plant out of its resource-strapped natural environment and place it into a managed environment with greater resources, the plant's resource pie can suddenly grow bigger, typically resulting in a larger plant.

Many perennial plants, with their larger overall size, offer greater potential for breeders to reallocate vegetative growth to seed production. Additionally, for a perennial grain crop to be successful in meeting our needs, it may need to live for only 5 to 10 years, far less than the lifespan of many wild perennials. In other words, the wild perennial is unnecessarily overbuilt for a managed agricultural setting. Some of the resources allocated to the plant's survival mechanisms, such as those allowing it to survive infrequent droughts or pest attacks, could be reallocated to seed production, and the crop would still persist in normal years.

Breeders see several other opportunities for perennials to achieve high seed yield. Perennials have greater access to resources over a longer growing season. They also have greater ability to maintain, over longer periods of time, the health and fertility of the soils in which they grow. Finally, the unprecedented success of plant breeders in recent decades in selecting for the simultaneous improvement of two or more characteristics that are typically negatively correlated with one another (meaning that as one characteristic increases, the other decreases, as is typical of seed yield and protein content) can be applied to perennial crop development.

Although current breeding efforts focused on developing perennial grain crops have been under way for less than a decade, the idea isn't new. Soviet researchers abandoned their attempts to develop perennial wheat through wide hybridization in the 1960s, in part because of the inherent difficulties of developing new crops at the time. California plant scientists in the 1960s also developed perennial wheat lines with yields similar to the then-lower-yielding annual wheat cultivars. At the time, large yield increases achieved in annuals overshadowed the modest success of these perennial programs, and the widespread environmental problems of annual crop production were not generally acknowledged.

In the late 1970s, Wes Jackson at the Land Institute revisited the possibility of developing perennial grain crops in his book *New Roots for Agriculture*. In the 1990s, plant breeders at the Land Institute initiated breeding programs for perennial wheat, sunflowers, sorghum, and some legumes. Some preliminary genetics work and hybridization research have also focused on perennial maize. Washington State University scientists have initiated a perennial wheat breeding program to address the high rates of erosion resulting from annual wheat production in eastern Washington. In 2001, some of those perennial wheat lines yielded 64% of the of the yield produced by the annual wheat cultivars grown in the region. Scientists at Kansas State University, the Kellogg Biological Station at Michigan State, the University of Manitoba, Texas A&M, and the University of Minnesota are carrying out additional plant breeding, genetics, or agronomic research on perennial grain crops.

The potential for perennial crops to tolerate or prevent adverse environmental conditions such as drought or soil salinity has attracted interest in other parts of the world. The conversion of native forests for annual wheat production in southwest Australia resulted in the rise of subsurface salts to the surface. This salinization threatens large areas of this non-irrigated, semi-arid agricultural region, and scientists there believe perennial crops would use more subsurface water, which would keep salts from rising to the surface and produce high-value crops. During the past decade, Australian scientists have been working to develop perennial wheat through wide hybridization and to domesticate a wild perennial grass for the region. More recently, plant breeders at the Food Crops Research Institute in Kunming, China, initiated programs to develop perennial rice to address the erosion problems associated with upland rice production. It is believed that perennial rice would also be more tolerant of the frequent drought conditions of some lowland areas. Scientists at the institute have also been evaluating perennial sorghum, sunflower, and intermediate wheatgrass for their potential as perennial grain crops.

Vision of a New Agriculture

The successful development of perennial grain crops would have different effects on the environment, on life at the dinner table, and on the farm. Producing grains from perennials rather than from annuals will have large environmental implications, but the consumer will see little if any difference at the dinner table. On the farm, whether mechanically harvested from large fields or hand-harvested in the parts of the world where equipment is prohibitively expensive, perennial grains 20 to 50 years from now will also look much the same to the farmer. The addition, however, of new high-value perennial crops to the farm would increase farmers' flexibility.

Farmers could use currently available management practices, such as no-till or organic approaches, but with a new array of high-value perennial grain crops. These would give farmers more options to have long rotations of perennial crops or rotations in which annuals are grown for several years followed by several years of perennials. Crop rotation aids in managing pests, diseases, and weeds but is often limited by the number of profitable crops from which farmers can choose. There are also opportunities to simultaneously grow annual and perennial grain crops or to grow multiple species of perennials together because of differences in rooting characteristics and growth habits. And because perennial grains regrow after seed harvest, livestock can be integrated into the system, allowing for greater use of the crops and therefore greater profit.

Although the environmental and food-security benefits of growing perennial grain crops are attractive, much work remains to be completed. For the great potential of perennial grain crops to be realized, more resources are needed to accelerate plant breeding programs with more personnel, land, and technological capacity; expand ecological and agronomic research on improved perennial germplasm; coordinate global activities through germplasm and scientist exchanges and conferences; identify global priority crop-lands; and develop training programs for young scientists in ecology, perennial plant breeding, and crop management.

Where, then, should the resources come from to support these objectives? The timeline for widespread production of perennials, given the need for extensive plant breeding work first, discourages private-sector investment at this point. As has occurred with biofuel production R&D, large-scale funding by governments or philanthropic foundations could greatly accelerate perennial grain crop development. As timelines for the release and production of perennial grain crops shorten, public and philanthropic support could increasingly be supplanted by support from companies providing agricultural goods and services. Although perennial grain crops might not initially interest large agribusinesses focused on annual grain crop production, the prospect of developing a suite of new goods and services, including equipment management consulting, and seeds, would be attractive to many entrepreneurial enterprises.

Although public support for additional federal programs is problematic given the current economic conditions, global conditions are changing rapidly. Much of the success of modern intensive agricultural production relies on cheap energy, a relatively stable climate, and the public's willingness to overlook widespread environmental problems. As energy prices increase and the costs of environmental degradation are increasingly appreciated, budgeting public money for long-term projects that will reduce resource consumption and depletion will probably become more politically popular. Rising food and fuel prices, climatic instability that threatens food production, and increased concern about the degradation of global ecological systems should place agriculture at the center of attention for multiple federal agencies and programs.

The USDA has the greatest capability to accelerate perennial grain crop development. Most important would be the use of research funds for the rapid expansion of plant breeding programs. Funds for breeding could be directed through the Agricultural Research Service and the competitive grant programs. Such investments directly support the objectives of the National Institute of Food and Agriculture (NIFA), created by the Food, Conservation and Energy Act of 2008, which will be responsible for awarding peer-reviewed grants for agricultural research. Modeled on the National Institutes of Health, NIFA objectives include enhancing agricultural and environmental sustainability and strengthening national security by improving food security in developing countries.

As varieties of perennial grain crops become available for more extensive testing, additional funds will be needed for agronomic and ecological research at multiple sites in the United States and elsewhere. This would include support for the training of students and scientists in managing perennial farming systems. Currently, less than $1.5 million directly supports perennial grain R&D projects around the world. USDA funds will provide less than $300,000 annually over the next few years through competitive grant awards, primarily for the study and development of perennial wheat and wheatgrass. Much of the rest is provided by the Land Institute.

Once the suitability of a perennial grain crop is well established, support from federal programs for farmers might be needed to encourage the initial adoption of new crops and practices. Farm subsidies, distributed through the USDA and which now primarily support annual cropping systems, could be used to encourage fundamental changes in farming practices, such as those offered by perennial grain crop development. Public funds supporting the Conservation Reserve Program (CRP) could be redirected toward transitioning CRP lands, once the federal contracts have expired, to perennial grain production. The CRR initially established in the 1985 farm bill, pays farmers to remove highly erodible croplands from production and to plant them for 10 years with grasses, trees, and other long-term cover to stabilize the soil. Some 36 million acres are enrolled in the program, and most are unsuitable or marginal for annual grain crop production but would be suitable for the production of perennials.

One obstacle to supporting programs necessary to achieve such long-term goals is the short timeframes of current policy agencies. The farm bill is revisited every five years and focuses primarily on farm exports, commodities, subsidies, food programs, and some soil conservation measures. Thus, it is poorly suited to deal with long-term agendas and larger objectives. The short-term objectives can change with changes in the political fortunes of those in charge of approving the bill. The Land Institute's Jackson has proposed a 50-year farm bill to serve as compass for the five-year bills. This longer-term agenda would focus on the larger environmental issues and on rebuilding and preserving farm communities. In the near term, Jackson proposes that, during an initial buildup phase, the federal government should fund 80 plant breeders and geneticists who would develop perennial grain, legume, and oilseed crops, and 30 agricultural and ecological scientists to develop the necessary agronomic systems. They would work on six to eight major crop species at diverse locations. Budgeting $400,000 per scientist-year for salaries and research costs would add less than $50 million annually to the farm bill, a blip in a bill that will cost taxpayers $288 billion between 2008 and 2012.

Some limited federal money has already been awarded for research related to perennial grain through the USDAs, competitive grants programs. Most recently, researchers at Michigan State University received funding to study the ecosystem services and performance of perennial wheat lines obtained from Washington State University and the Land Institute. The Green Lands Blue Waters Initiative, a multistate network of universities, individual scientists, and nonprofit research organizations, is also advocating the development of perennial grain crops, along with other perennial forage, biofuel, and tree crops.

Although agriculture has traditionally been primarily the concern of the USDA, it now plays an increasingly important role in how we meet challenges—international food security, environmental protection, climate change, energy supply, economic sustainability, and human health—beyond the primary concerns of that agency. Public programs intended to address these challenges should consider the development of perennial grain crops a priority. For example, programs at the NSF, Department of Energy (DOE), Environmental Protection Agency, and the National Oceanic and Atmospheric Administration and U.S. international assistance and development programs could provide additional incentives through research programs or subsidies.

Currently, no government funding agencies, including the USDA, specifically target the development of perennial crops as they do for biofuels. In the 2009 federal economic stimulus package alone, the DOE was appropriated $786.5 million in funds to accelerate biofuels research and commercialization. The displacement of food crops by biofuel crops recently played a significant role in the rise of global food prices and resulted in increased hunger and social unrest in many parts of the world. Although some argue that biofuel crops should be grown only on marginal lands unsuited for annual food crops, perennial crops have the potential to be grown on those same lands and be used for food, feed, and fuel.

Substantial public funding of perennial grain crops need not be permanent. As economically viable crops become widely produced, farmers and businesses will have opportunities to market their own seeds and management inputs just as they do with currently available crops. Although private-sector companies may not profit as much from selling fertilizers and pesticides to farmers producing perennial grains, they will probably adapt to these new crops with new products and services. The ability of farmers to spread the initial planting costs over several seasons rather than meet these costs each year opens up opportunities for more expensive seed with improved characteristics.

Although the timelines for development and widespread production of perennial grain crops may seem long, the potential payoffs stretch far into the future, and the financial costs are low relative to other publicly funded agricultural expenditures. Adding perennial grains to our agricultural arsenal will give farmers more choices in what they can grow and where, while sustainably producing food for the growing population.

Adding perennial grains to our agricultural arsenal will give farmers more choices in what they can grow and where, while sustainably producing food for the growing population.

Recommended Reading

T. S. Cox, J. D. Glover, D. L. Van Tassel, C. M. Cox, and L. R. DeHaan, "Prospects for Developing Perennial Grain Crops," *BioScience* 56 (2006): 649–659.

J. D. Glover, C. M. Cox, and J. P. Reganold, "Future Farming: A Return to Roots?" *Scientific American* 297 (2007): 66–73.

Green Lands, Blue Waters, *A Vision and Roadmap for the Next Generation of Agricultural Systems* (www.greenlandsbluewaters.org).

W. Jackson, *New Roots for Agriculture* (Lincoln, NE: University of Nebraska, 1980).

W. Jackson, *A 50-year Farm Bill* (www.landinstitute.org/pages/50yrfb-booklet_7-29-09.pdf).

N. Jordan, G. Boody, W. Broussard, J. D. Glover, D. Keeney, B. H. McCown, G. McIsaac, M. Muller, H. Murray, J. Neal, C. Pansing, R. E. Turner, K. Warner, and D. Wyse, "Sustainable Development of the Agricultural Bio-Economy," *Science* 316 (2007): 1570–1571.

Critical Thinking

1. Are the current grains that feed the world annual crops or perennial crops?

2. How do perennial grain crops differ from annual grain crops?

3. What are the advantages and disadvantages of creating perennial grain crops?

4. Identify the three grain crops that provide 70 percent of calories for human consumption worldwide.

JERRY D. GLOVER is an agroecologist with the Land Institute in Salina, Kansas. **JOHN P. REGANOLD** (reganold@wsu.edu) is a Regents professor in the Department of Crop and Soil Sciences at Washington State University in Pullman, Washington.

Test-Your-Knowledge Form

We encourage you to photocopy and use this page as a tool to assess how the articles in *Annual Editions* expand on the information in your textbook. By reflecting on the articles you will gain enhanced text information. You can also access this useful form on a product's book support website at www.mhhe.com/cls.

NAME: DATE:

_____

TITLE AND NUMBER OF ARTICLE:

_____

BRIEFLY STATE THE MAIN IDEA OF THIS ARTICLE:

_____

LIST THREE IMPORTANT FACTS THAT THE AUTHOR USES TO SUPPORT THE MAIN IDEA:

_____

WHAT INFORMATION OR IDEAS DISCUSSED IN THIS ARTICLE ARE ALSO DISCUSSED IN YOUR TEXTBOOK OR OTHER READINGS THAT YOU HAVE DONE? LIST THE TEXTBOOK CHAPTERS AND PAGE NUMBERS:

_____

LIST ANY EXAMPLES OF BIAS OR FAULTY REASONING THAT YOU FOUND IN THE ARTICLE:

_____

LIST ANY NEW TERMS/CONCEPTS THAT WERE DISCUSSED IN THE ARTICLE, AND WRITE A SHORT DEFINITION:

NOTES

NOTES

NOTES

NOTES